Knee Osteoarthritis: Advances in Diagnosis and Treatment

Knee Osteoarthritis: Advances in Diagnosis and Treatment

Editor: Connor Santiago

AMERICAN
MEDICAL PUBLISHERS
www.americanmedicalpublishers.com

AMERICAN
MEDICAL PUBLISHERS
www.americanmedicalpublishers.com

Cataloging-in-Publication Data

Knee osteoarthritis : advances in diagnosis and treatment / edited by Connor Santiago.
p. cm.
Includes bibliographical references and index.
ISBN 978-1-63927-397-3
1. Osteoarthritis. 2. Knee. 3. Knee--Diseases. I. Santiago, Connor.
RC931.O67 O88 2021
616.722 3--dc23

American Medical Publishers,
41 Flatbush Avenue,
1st Floor, New York,
NY 11217, USA

ISBN 978-1-63927-397-3 (Hardback)

Contents

Preface

I am honored to present to you this unique book which encompasses the most up-to-date data in the field. I was extremely pleased to get this opportunity of editing the work of experts from across the globe. I have also written papers in this field and researched the various aspects revolving around the progress of the discipline. I have tried to unify my knowledge along with that of stalwarts from every corner of the world, to produce a text which not only benefits the readers but also facilitates the growth of the field.

Osteoarthritis is a degenerative condition in which the cartilage between joints wears away and bones rub against each other without the natural cushioning. It is characterized by pain, stiffness, swelling and restricted ability to move. Osteoarthritis of the knee is a form of arthritis affecting the knee joint which usually occurs in people above the age of 45. However, it can also affect younger individuals. This may be due to genetic mutations that lend a susceptibility to the disease, obesity, inherited abnormalities around the knee joint, repetitive stress injuries and other clinical conditions such as excess growth hormone or iron overload disorders. Knee osteoarthritis can take several years to develop. It progresses in stages with symptoms ranging from minor to severe. An examination of the joints, evaluation of their range of motion, blood tests, fluid scan tests and MRI scans can help establish a diagnosis. The treatment of knee osteoarthritis depends on the stage of progression of the disease. Exercises that build strength and mobility, and acetaminophens can address early osteoarthritis. Physical therapy and the practice of wearing braces are recommended for managing mild symptoms. This book aims to shed light on some of the unexplored aspects of osteoarthritis of the knee joint and the recent researches in this condition. The objective of this book is to give a general view of the different symptoms and effects of this condition, and their management strategies. This book is a vital tool for all researching or studying knee osteoarthritis as it gives incredible insights into emerging trends and concepts.

Finally, I would like to thank all the contributing authors for their valuable time and contributions. This book would not have been possible without their efforts. I would also like to thank my friends and family for their constant support.

Editor

1

Meta-analysis of serum C-reactive protein and cartilage oligomeric matrix protein levels as biomarkers for clinical knee osteoarthritis

Junfeng Zhang

Abstract

Background: The roles of C-reactive protein (CRP) and cartilage oligomeric matrix protein (COMP) in knee osteoarthritis (KOA) remain controversial, thus the present study is aimed to explore the relationships between CRP, COMP, and the incidence/progression of KOA.

Methods: A systematic search was conducted on PubMed and Embase until September, 2016 for all the relevant studies. The pooled mean difference (MD) with its 95% confidence interval (95% CI) based on fixed effects model or random effects model was calculated to assess the potential role of CRP and COMP in the incidence or progression of KOA. Heterogeneity was evaluated by Cochran's Q and I^2 tests. When $P < 0.05$ or $I^2 > 50\%$, a random effects model was chosen, otherwise, a fixed effects model was used. Moreover, the role of CRP in different degrees of pain was also analyzed. Sensitivity analysis was performed to evaluate the strength of the meta-analysis.

Results: Fourteen studies were enrolled in the meta-analysis. No difference was found between baseline CRP and CRP levels in the last follow-up period of KOA (MD = – 0.09, 95% CI: -0.30, 0.13). Pooled data showed higher CRP concentration in patients with incident KOA when compared with controls (MD = 0.33, 95% CI: 0.04, 0.63). Moreover, higher serum COMP levels were found in patients with incident KOA (MD = 1.69, 95% CI: 0.61, 2.76) Additionally, significant higher CRP concentration was observed in KOA patients with highest degree of pain (MD = 1.60, 95% CI: 0.52, 2.67).

Conclusion: CRP and COMP serum levels were both associated with the incidence of KOA. Patients with a higher CRP and COMP concentration might have an increased probability of developing KOA. However, higher CRP serum levels was not related with KOA progression. Furthermore, KOA patients with more pain had higher CRP concentrations.

Keywords: C-reactive protein, Knee osteoarthritis, Pain, Meta-analysis

Background

Osteoarthritis (OA), the most common type of arthritis, is characterized by joint space deterioration, pain, and loss of motion. Epidemiology studies have observed high prevalence of OA both in developed countries and developing countries. For example, the overall prevalence of knee OA was found to be 28.7% in India [1], the prevalence was highest (13.7%) in subjects living in the South-West region in China [2], and OA affected nearly 27 million Americans [3]. Additionally, the prevalence and incidence of the disease continue to increase. OA can become both a financial and health burden to patients and can affect their quality of life. Therefore, it is urgent to find an effective way to diagnosis and prevent the incidence or progression of OA in the early stage of disease.

Inflammation plays an important role in the pathogenesis of OA, although the specific correlations between biomarkers of inflammation and knee osteoarthritis (KOA) remain controversial. C-reactive protein(CRP) is a pentameric protein found in blood plasma associated with

Correspondence: sxzhangjf163@163.com
Department of Health Statistics / the Publishing house, Public Health of Shanxi Medical University / Chinese Journal of Rheumatology, Taiyuan, Shanxi 030001, China

inflammation, infection, and injury. Studies demonstrated that CRP was correlated with complications, such as hypertension, cardiovascular disease, and diabetes [4, 5]. Studies have suggested that KOA was significantly related with CRP concentration [6, 7]. Other studies suggested that there were significant association between CRP concentration and KOA incidence [8–10]. Cartilage oligomeric matrix protein (COMP) is a 535-kDa non-collagen protein which has strong relation with the incidence of KOA. Some evidence has demonstrated that COMP serum levels in OA was different from healthy controls.

Because of these conflicting reports, the purpose of this study was to evaluate the association between CRP concentration, COMP serum levels and the incidence/progression of KOA. The relationship between CRP concentration and pain in KOA patients was also assessed.

Methods

Search strategy and study selection

A systematic search was performed on PubMed and Embase from database inception through September 2016. The following search terms were used: "osteoarthritis", "knee osteoarthritis", "C-reactive protein", "CRP", "cartilage oligomeric matrix protein", "COMP". Search terms were combined with OR and AND. All the reference list of retrieved studies and any additional publication were also searched and screened. The study was conducted based on the PRISMA guidelines [11].

Inclusion criteria

The included studies were in line with the following criteria: 1) subjects had clinical KOA; 2) investigated the association between KOA incidence and progression and the concentration of CRP or COMP serum levels; 3) parameter of CRP or COMP could be extracted or calculated; 4) published in English.

We excluded studies in which KOA patients were formerly treated by medication. In addition, repeated studies, reviews, comments, and letters were also excluded.

Data extraction and quality assessment

Data were extracted by two independent researchers following pre-designed form. The quality assessment was performed independently by two reviewers, and disagreement would be solved by the third reviewer.

Baseline characteristics of the eligible studies included first author, publication year, patients' demographic, study design, research area, the concentration of CRP and COMP serum levels, and the number of the number of KOA and control patients. The quality of the studies was assessed by Newcastle-Ottawa Scale (NOS) [12]. In brief, NOS contains 8 items, categorizes into three groups, and with a total score of 9 stars. Each eligible study was graded according to this tool. In the current study, a cohort study with a follow-up rate > 75% was assigned one star. If NOS score of the study reached more than 5, it was considered as high quality literature, and was suitable for the meta-analysis.

Statistical analysis

We extracted mean difference(MD) and standard deviation(SD) of CRP and COMP levels at baseline and at the end of the follow-up period of study subjects and controls. Heterogeneity among the included studies was calculated by Cochran's Q-test and I^2 test [13]. $P < 0.05$ or $I^2 > 50\%$ was defined as significant heterogeneity between individual studies. Then, the random effects model was selected for pooling MD and SD of CRP and COMP levels to assess the association between CRP and COMP concentration and KOA incidence and progression. When $P > 0.05$ or $I^2 < 50\%$, a fixed effect model was chosen to pool MD and SD of CRP and COMP levels. Sensitivity analyses were performed by changing one study at a time, to see what effect this produces on the outcome. All statistical analysis was performed by Cochrane Collaboration Review Manager (version 5.3). We considered $P < 0.05$ as statistically significant.

Results

Search results and study selection

As shown in Fig. 1, the initial search yielded a total of 982 articles. 537 remained after removing the duplicated articles. 392 studies were further excluded because they did not investigate the relationship between CRP or COMP concentration and the incidence/progression of KOA. A total of 145 articles were under full-text review, of which 131 studies were excluded. Among the 131 articles, 91 articles were reviews, comments or case reports, 25 studies did not provide sufficient data, 14 studies were not about KOA incidence or progression, and 1 duplicate population [9, 14]. Eventually, 14 articles were included in the meta-analysis [6, 7, 14–25].

All relevant baseline characteristics of the enrolled studies were summarized in Table 1. In general, nine studies were designed as case control, and five were designed as cohort

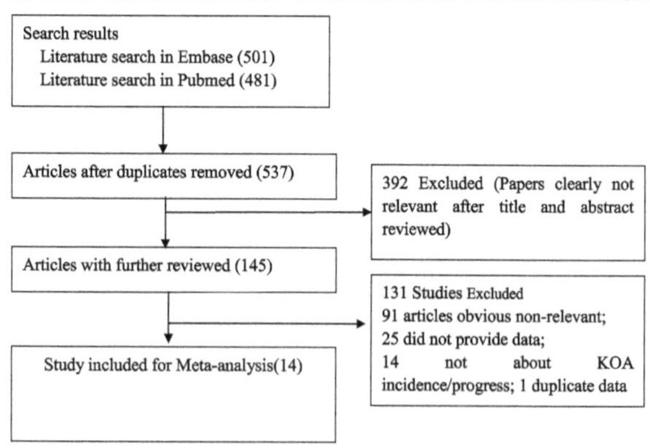

Fig. 1 Flowchart of study selection for inclusion in the systematic review

Table 1 Baseline chacteristics of enrolled studies

Study	Design	Number	Age (years)	Follow-up	area
Fernandes, 2007	Case control	KOA:75 Control: 40	KOA:56.6 ± 7.6; Control: 53.8 ± 8.5	NA	Brazil
Senolt, 2005	Case control	KOA:38 Control: 38	KOA:64.1 ± 10.1; Control: 58.3 ± 9.1	NA	USA
Wakitani, 2007	Case control	KOA:31 Control: 24	KOA:20–80; Control: 23–52	NA	Japan
Li, 2012	Case control	KOA:115 Control: 35	KOA:55 ± 13.2; Control:53 ± 12.53	2–3 years	China
Engstrom, 2009	population-based cohort	5171	57.5 + 5.9	12.4 years	Sweden
Zhang, 2015	Case control	Control: 20 KOA: 20	Control:56.3 ± 7.9; KOA: 59.2 ± 8.3	NA	China
Sowers, 2002	cohort	1025	42.9 ± 0.1	2.5 years	USA
Kerkhof,2010	Case control	KOA: 210; Control: 1360	≥55 years	NA	Netherlands
Haghighian,2014	Case control	23	58.27 ± 7.84	2 months	Iran
Ramirez, 2014	cohort	186	61 ± 7.3	2 years	Netherlands
Nielsen, 2014	Case control	281	40–80	NA	Denmark
Scorei, 2011	Case control	15	67.6 (5.5)	2 weeks	Romania
Stannus, 2012	cohort study	KOA:35; Control:114	KOA:63.2 ± 6.9 Control: 61.5 ± 6.7	5 years	Australia
Hosnijeh, 2016	population-based prospective cohort	1335	65.2 (8.43)	5-year	Netherlands

KOA knee osteoarthritis

studies. Four studies were conducted in Asia, seven were performed in Europe, one was in Australia, and two were in USA. Study sizes ranged from 15 to 5171 patients, and the follow-up period ranged from 2 weeks to 12.4 years. Furthermore, all the included studies were scored more than 5 stars based on the NOS criteria, suggesting all enrolled studies were suitable for meta-analysis.

Meta-analysis of the association between KOA progression and CRP levels

As shown in Fig. 2a, 5 studies including 836 KOA patients at baseline and 748 patients at the end of the follow-up period evaluated the association between KOA progression and CRP levels [6, 16–18, 21]. Significant heterogeneity was observed among the five studies ($P < 0.00001$, $I^2 = 93\%$). Therefore, a random effects model was used to pool data. No difference was found between baseline CRP and CRP levels at the last follow-up period in KOA patients (MD = 0.09, 95%CI: -0.30, 0.13). Because there was significant heterogeneity among the studies, sensitivity analysis was performed, and no discrepancy results were observed when we omitted one study at a time (Table 2).

Meta-analysis of the association between KOA incidence and CRP levels

Four studies including 557 KOA patients and 7417 controls were enrolled in the meta-analysis to assess the

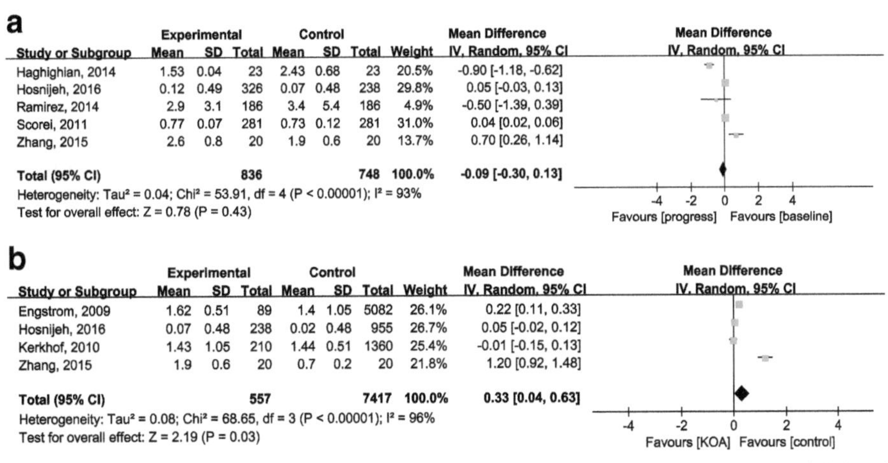

Fig. 2 Pooled effect size of the relationship between C-reactive protein (CRP) concentration and knee osteoarthritis (KOA). **a** the association between CRP concentration and KOA progression; **b** the association between CRP concentration and KOA incidence

Table 2 Sensitivity analysis for the meta-analysis

	Outcomes	No. of studies	MD(95% CI)	Heterogeneity test	
				P	I^2 (%)
KOA progress with CRP	All studies	5	0.09 [−0.30, 0.13]	< 0.00001	93.0
	Haghighian, 2014	4	0.07 [− 0.04, 0.18]	0.02	70.0
	Hosnijeh, 2016	4	−0.15 [− 0.77, 0.47]	< 0.00001	94.0
	Ramirez, 2014	4	−0.07 [− 0.29, 0.16]	< 0.00001	94.0
	Scorei, 2011	4	−0.15 [− 0.78, 0.49]	< 0.00001	94.0
	Zhang, 2015	4	−0.20 [− 0.42, 0.02]	< 0.00001	93.0
KOA incidence with CRP	All studies	4	0.33 [0.04, 0.63]	< 0.00001	96.0
	Engstrom, 2009	3	0.39 [−0.08, 0.86]	< 0.00001	97.0
	Hosnijeh, 2016	3	0.45 [−0.05, 0.95]	< 0.00001	97.0
	Kerkhof, 2010	3	0.46 [0.06, 0.86]	< 0.00001	97.0
	Zhang, 2015	3	0.09 [−0.03, 0.21]	0.01	76.0
KOA pain with CRP	All studies	3	1.60 [0.52, 2.67]	0.001	85.0
	Nielsen, 2014	2	1.69 [−0.02, 3.40]	0.03	78.0
	Sowers, 2002	2	1.13 [0.44, 1.82]	0.49	0.0
	Stannus, 2012	2	1.88 [0.76, 3.00]	0.003	89.0

KOA knee osteoarthritis, *CRP* C-reactive protein

relation between KOA incidence and CRP levels (Fig. 2b) [7, 14, 17, 21]. A random effects model was selected due to significant heterogeneity among studies ($P < 0.00001$, $I^2 = 96\%$). The pooled MD with its 95% CI suggested that CRP concentration was somewhat higher in KOA patients when compared with healthy controls (MD = 0.33, 95% CI: 0.04, 0.63). High heterogeneity also existed in this subgroup. Therefore, sensitivity analysis was conducted by deducting one study at a time. When we removed the study by Engstrom et al., Hosnijeh et al., and Zhang et al., pooled data suggested no significant difference in CRP concentration between KOA patients and healthy controls (Table 2).

Meta-analysis of the association between COMP serum levels and KOA incidence

Figure 3 shows the association between KOA incidence and COMP serum levels from 5 studies containing 259 KOA patients and 137 healthy controls. Pooled data indicated that patients with clinical KOA had a higher serum COMP levels than controls (MD = 1.69, 95% CI: 0.61, 2.76). Sensitivity analysis was performed to evaluate the strength of this conclusion, and no inconsistent results were found when we omitted each study (Table 2).

Meta-analysis of the association between CRP levels and pain in KOA patients

As shown in Fig. 4, three studies estimated the correlation between CRP levels and pain in KOA patients [15, 19, 20]. A total of 2291 patients were included, among them 1112 patients reported knee pain at baseline assessment, and 1179 patients without knee pain were set as controls. Higher mean concentrations of CRP were found in patients who self-reported the highest level of knee pain (MD = 1.60, 95% CI: 0.52, 2.67). When we removed the study by Nielsen et al. in the sensitivity analysis, the significant difference between groups disappeared.

Discussion

For inflammatory diseases, C-reactive protein (CRP) concentration is recognized as the most common laboratory marker, several clinical studies put forward that CRP

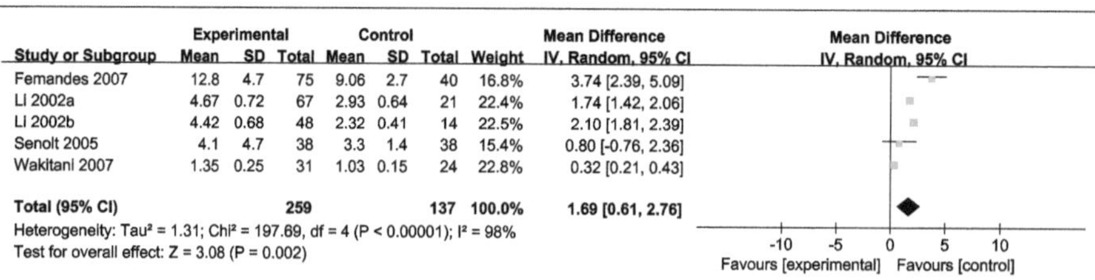

Fig. 3 Pooled effect size of the relationship between cartilage oligomeric matrix protein (COMP) serum levels and knee osteoarthritis (KOA)

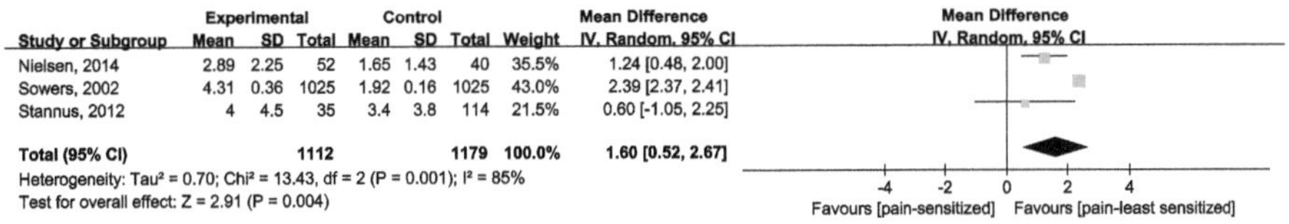

Fig. 4 Pooled effect size of the relationship between C-reactive protein (CRP) concentration and pain in knee osteoarthritis (KOA)

concentration was elevated in patients with KOA [26]. Additionally, COMP serum levels are also considered as a potential biomarker for the diagnosis of KOA. The present meta-analysis demonstrated that higher CRP concentration was associated with higher KOA incidence, however, CRP levels were not related to the progression of KOA. Moreover, CRP concentration was higher in KOA patients with higher degrees of knee pain. Higher serum COMP levels in patients with incident KOA were also observed. Thus, both CRP and COMP could serve as useful biomarkers of KOA.

The outcome of our study suggests that CRP as a biomarker plays a positive role in the diagnosis and prognosis of KOA. This finding is consistent with a previous study [27]. However, in sensitivity analysis, when removing the study by Engstrom et al. [6], Hosnijeh et al. [17], and Zhang et al. [21], the significant difference of CRP levels between KOA patients and control group diminished. Thus, further study enrolling larger sample size and balancing confounding factors such as patient's backgrounds is needed. Although significantly higher COMP serum levels was observed in incident KOA, no stratified analysis based on severity of KOA was performed due to limited enrolled studies. Further investigation is required to determine if this marker can be utilized to assess the incidence OA. Given that both CRP and COMP levels were higher in patients with KOA, the two factors could be used in combination for the prognosis of KOA.

Significant heterogeneity existed in our study. Although we conducted sensitivity analysis to assess the strength of the meta-analysis using one-at-a-time method, heterogeneity did not reduce. In patients with early KOA, many factors could affect the concentration of CRP, such as life habit and the background of KOA. For example, a previous study indicated that cigarette smoking was positively associated with serum CRP levels [28]. In addition, experimental data suggested both dietary and serum Mg were inversely related with serum CRP in early radiographic KOA patients [29]. Moreover, serum CRP was associated with knee bone marrow lesions scores [30]. Thus, future study stratified by living habit and background of patients should be performed to verify the present conclusion.

There are some limitations should be noted in the meta-analysis. First, the number of enrolled subjects was small, which limited the subgroup analysis stratified by smoking status, and other confounding factors such as hyperlipidemia. Second, we did not restrict the timing of biomarker assessment, and exercise status of the patients, also the follow-up period ranged from 2 weeks to 12.4 years, which might be one of the reasons causing significant heterogeneity among individual studies. Third, a number of studies did not provide calculated data. Moreover, other chronic diseases might influence the CRP levels in patients, and we did not eliminate the effect of those factors. Our study was designed to evaluate the relationship between biamarkers and KOA. The association between CRP and other OA types, such as hand, hip, and spine OA was not considered.

Conclusion

The present meta-analysis indicated that both CRP and COMP could serve as biomarkers for KOA. Higher CRP and COMP serum levels might be associated with a higher incidence of KOA. However, higher CRP concentration was not associated with the progression of KOA. Further study is required verify the actual relationship between CRP and KOA incidence.

Abbreviations

CI: Confidence interval; COMP: Cartilage oligomeric matrix protein; CRP: C-reactive protein; KOA: Knee osteoarthritis; MD: Mean difference; OA: Osteoarthritis

Acknowledgements

I would like to thank Dr. Liu Shaolong for his valuable guidance in every stage of the writing of this thesis.

Also, I shall extend my thanks to Haiyuan Dong from General Office of Shanxi Medical Journal and Qianqian He from Shanxi Medical University for their kind help in the data extraction and quality assessment processes.

Funding

This study was sponsored by the National Natural Science Foundation of China (No. 81573245); Shanxi provincial health and Family Planning Commission projects (No. 2014169).

Authors' contributions

Only ZJF conceived this study, participated in the experiments and finally wrote the paper. ZJF approved the final manuscript.

Consent for publication

Not applicable

Competing interests

The author declares that he/she has no competing interests.

References

1. Pal CP, Singh P, Chaturvedi S, Pruthi KK, Vij A. Epidemiology of knee osteoarthritis in India and related factors. Indian J Orthop. 2016;50:518–22.
2. Tang X, Wang S, Zhan S, Niu J, Tao K, Zhang Y, Lin J. The prevalence of symptomatic knee osteoarthritis in China: results from the China health and retirement longitudinal study. Arthritis Rheumatol. 2016;68:648–53.
3. Issa SN, Sharma L. Epidemiology of osteoarthritis: an update. Curr Rheumatol Rep. 2006;8:7–15.
4. Ablij H, Meinders A. C-reactive protein: history and revival. Eur J Intern Med. 2002;13:412.
5. Dalton RR, Hoffman WH, Passmore GG, Martin SL. Plasma C-Reactive protein levels in severe diabetic ketoacidosis. Ann Clin Lab Sci. 2003;33:435–42.
6. Engstrom G, Gerhardsson de Verdier M, Rollof J, Nilsson PM, Lohmander LS. C-reactive protein, metabolic syndrome and incidence of severe hip and knee osteoarthritis. A population-based cohort study. Osteoarthr Cartil. 2009;17:168–73.
7. Kerkhof HJ, Bierma-Zeinstra SM, Castano-Betancourt MC, de Maat MP, Hofman A, Pols HA, Rivadeneira F, Witteman JC, Uitterlinden AG, van Meurs JB. Serum C reactive protein levels and genetic variation in the CRP gene are not associated with the prevalence, incidence or progression of osteoarthritis independent of body mass index. Ann Rheum Dis. 2010;69:1976–82.
8. Garnero P, Piperno M, Gineyts E, Christgau S, Delmas PD, Vignon E. Cross sectional evaluation of biochemical markers of bone, cartilage, and synovial tissue metabolism in patients with knee osteoarthritis: relations with disease activity and joint damage. Ann Rheum Dis. 2001;60:619–26.
9. Sanchez-Ramirez DC, van der Leeden M, van der Esch M, Roorda LD, Verschueren S, van Dieen J, Lems WF, Dekker J. Increased knee muscle strength is associated with decreased activity limitations in established knee osteoarthritis: two-year follow-up study in the Amsterdam osteoarthritis cohort. J Rehabil Med. 2015;47:647–54.
10. Conrozier T, Chappuis-Cellier C, Richard M, Mathieu P, Richard S, Vignon E. Increased serum C-reactive protein levels by immunonephelometry in patients with rapidly destructive hip osteoarthritis. Rev Rhum Engl Ed. 1998;65:759–65.
11. Moher D, Liberati A, Tetzlaff J, Altman DG. Preferred reporting items for systematic reviews and meta-analyses: the PRISMA statement. Int J Surg. 2010;8:336–41.
12. Lo CK, Mertz D, Loeb M. Newcastle-Ottawa scale: comparing reviewers' to authors' assessments. BMC Med Res Methodol. 2014;14:45.
13. Lau J, Ioannidis JP, Schmid CH. Quantitative synthesis in systematic reviews. Ann Intern Med. 1997;127:820–6.
14. Sanchez-Ramirez DC, van der Leeden M, van der Esch M, Roorda LD, Verschueren S, van Dieen JH, Dekker J, Lems WF. Elevated C-reactive protein is associated with lower increase in knee muscle strength in patients with knee osteoarthritis: a 2-year follow-up study in the Amsterdam osteoarthritis (AMS-OA) cohort. Arthritis Res Ther. 2014;16:R123.
15. Arendt-Nielsen L, Eskehave TN, Egsgaard LL, Petersen KK, Graven-Nielsen T, Hoeck HC, Simonsen O, Siebuhr AS, Karsdal M, Bay-Jensen AC. Association between experimental pain biomarkers and serologic markers in patients with different degrees of painful knee osteoarthritis. Arthritis Rheumatol. 2014;66:3317–26.
16. Khadem Haghighian M, Alipoor B, Malek Mahdavi A, Eftekhar Sadat B, Asghari Jafarabadi M, Moghaddam A. Effects of sesame seed supplementation on inflammatory factors and oxidative stress biomarkers in patients with knee osteoarthritis. Acta Med Iran. 2015;53:207–13.
17. Saberi Hosnijeh F, Siebuhr AS, Uitterlinden AG, Oei EH, Hofman A, Karsdal MA, Bierma-Zeinstra SM, Bay-Jensen AC, van Meurs JB. Association between biomarkers of tissue inflammation and progression of osteoarthritis: evidence from the Rotterdam study cohort. Arthritis Res Ther. 2016;18:81.
18. Scorei R, Mitrut P, Petrisor I, Scorei I. A double-blind, placebo-controlled pilot study to evaluate the effect of calcium fructoborate on systemic inflammation and dyslipidemia markers for middle-aged people with primary osteoarthritis. Biol Trace Elem Res. 2011;144:253–63.
19. Sowers M, Jannausch M, Stein E, Jamadar D, Hochberg M, Lachance L. C-reactive protein as a biomarker of emergent osteoarthritis. Osteoarthr Cartil. 2002;10:595–601.
20. Stannus OP, Jones G, Blizzard L, Cicuttini FM, Ding C. Associations between serum levels of inflammatory markers and change in knee pain over 5 years in older adults: a prospective cohort study. Ann Rheum Dis. 2013;72:535–40.
21. Zhang Q, Li H, Zhang Z, Yang F, Chen J. Serum metabolites as potential biomarkers for diagnosis of knee osteoarthritis. Dis Markers. 2015;2015: 684794.
22. Fernandes FA, Pucinelli ML, da Silva NP, Feldman D. Serum cartilage oligomeric matrix protein (COMP) levels in knee osteoarthritis in a Brazilian population: clinical and radiological correlation. Scand J Rheumatol. 2007;36:211–5.
23. Li H, Wang D, Wu ZQ, Zhong JM, Yuan YJ. Serum levels of cartilage oligomeric matrix protein in the diagnosis of knee osteoarthritis. Zhongguo Gu Shang. 2012;25:380–3.
24. Senolt L, Braun M, Olejarova M, Forejtova S, Gatterova J, Pavelka K. Increased pentosidine, an advanced glycation end product, in serum and synovial fluid from patients with knee osteoarthritis and its relation with cartilage oligomeric matrix protein. Ann Rheum Dis. 2005;64:886–90.
25. Wakitani S, Nawata M, Kawaguchi A, Okabe T, Takaoka K, Tsuchiya T, Nakaoka R, Masuda H, Miyazaki K. Serum keratan sulfate is a promising marker of early articular cartilage breakdown. Rheumatology (Oxford). 2007; 46:1652–6.
26. Takahashi M, Naito K, Abe M, Sawada T, Nagano A. Relationship between radiographic grading of osteoarthritis and the biochemical markers for arthritis in knee osteoarthritis. Arthritis Res Ther. 2004;6:R208–12.
27. Hurter K, Spreng D, Rytz U, Schawalder P, Ott-Knusel F, Schmokel H. Measurements of C-reactive protein in serum and lactate dehydrogenase in serum and synovial fluid of patients with osteoarthritis. Vet J. 2005;169:281–5.
28. Zhang Y, Zeng C, Wei J, Li H, Yang T, Yang Y, Deng ZH, Ding X, Lei G. Associations of cigarette smoking, betel quid chewing and alcohol consumption with high-sensitivity C-reactive protein in early radiographic knee osteoarthritis: a cross-sectional study. BMJ Open. 2016;6:e010763.
29. Li H, Zeng C, Wei J, Yang T, Gao SG, Luo W, Li YS, Xiong YL, Xiao WF, Lei GH. Associations of dietary and serum magnesium with serum high-sensitivity C-reactive protein in early radiographic knee osteoarthritis patients. Mod Rheumatol. 2016:1–6.
30. Zhu Z, Jin X, Wang B, Wluka A, Antony B, Laslett LL, Winzenberg T, Cicuttini F, Jones G, Ding C. Cross-sectional and longitudinal associations between serum levels of high-sensitivity C-reactive protein, knee bone marrow lesions, and knee pain in patients with knee osteoarthritis. Arthritis Care Res (Hoboken). 2016;68:1471–7.

2

Significant pain variability in persons with, or at high risk of, knee osteoarthritis: preliminary investigation based on secondary analysis of cohort data

Emma Parry[1*], Reuben Ogollah[2] and George Peat[3]

Abstract

Background: While knee osteoarthritis (OA) is characterised as a slowly progressive disease, acute flares, episodes of severe pain, and substantial fluctuations in pain intensity appear to be part of the natural history for some patients. We sought to estimate what proportion of symptomatic community-dwelling adults might be affected, and to identify patient and problem characteristics associated with higher risk of such variability in pain.

Methods: We analysed data collected at baseline, 18, 36, 54, and 72 month follow-up of a prospective cohort of symptomatic adults aged over 50 years with current/recent knee pain. At each time point we estimated the proportion of participants reporting 'significant pain variability' (defined as worst pain intensity in the past 6 months ≥5/10 and ≥2 points higher than average pain intensity during the same 6-month period). The associations between significant pain variability and demographic, socioeconomic, lifestyle, clinical, radiographic, and healthcare utilisation factors measured at baseline were estimated by adjusted odds ratios and 95% confidence intervals (aOR; 95%CI) from multivariable discrete-time survival analysis.

Results: Seven hundred and nineteen participants were included in the final analysis. At each time point, 23–32% of participants were classed as reporting significant pain variability. Associated factors included: younger age (aOR (per year): 0.96; 95% CI 0.94, 0.97), higher BMI (per kg/m^2:1.03; 1.01, 1.06), higher WOMAC Pain score (per unit: 1.06; 1.03, 1.10), longer time since onset (e.g. 1–5 years vs < 1 year: 1.79; 1.16, 2.75) and morning stiffness (≤30 min vs none: 1.43; 1.10, 1.85). The models accounting for multiple periods of significant symptom variability found similar associations.

Conclusions: Our findings are consistent with studies showing that, for some patients OA symptoms are significantly variable over time. Future prospective studies on the nature and frequency of flare ups are needed to help determine triggers and their underlying pathophysiology in order to suggest new avenues for effective episode management of OA to complement long-term behaviour change.

Keywords: Knee, Osteoarthritis, Flare, Frequency, Association, Symptom, Variability

* Correspondence: e.clarke@keele.ac.uk
[1]NIHR In-Practice Fellow, Arthritis Research UK Primary Care Centre, Research Institute for Primary Care & Health Sciences, Keele University, Keele, Staffordshire ST5 5BG, UK
Full list of author information is available at the end of the article

Background

Longitudinal studies of knee osteoarthritis (OA) with repeated measurements over 5-6 years have suggested that symptoms typically follow relatively stable long-term trajectories [1–5]. However, these can mask considerable within-person variability [6–8]. Of particular interest are acute flares and episodes of uncharacteristically severe pain that have been suggested to occur in both the early and advanced stages of OA and which are associated with distress and loss of function, particularly when unpredictable [9].

Flare design trials, in which usual medication is withdrawn with the intention of inducing an acute increase in pain within a specified time period are well established. For example, a recent systematic review identified 33 definite or possible flare design trials evaluating non-steroidal anti-inflammatory drugs (NSAID) [10]. The 'natural occurrence' of such flares has received less attention although there is a growing body of observational research on these phenomena under a variety of labels ("flares", "acute events", "episodes", "exacerbations"). These include studies that have attempted to define an osteoarthritis flare [11, 12], to understand the role of inflammation in these acute events [13, 14], to identify triggers [15] and to describe their impact on productivity [16].

Despite this growing body of research there is an outstanding gap of epidemiological evidence on how common these flare ups may be and the type of patients that are experiencing them. The largest quantitative study by Marty et al. [11] produced a scoring tool to determine those experiencing potential knee OA flare ups but this has not yet been widely adopted clinically or in research. Factors that have been critically important in defining flare ups in other diseases may be important in osteoarthritis. These include worsening of symptoms beyond normal day-to-day variation requiring additional medication [17–19], that is progressive [20] and is clinically significant [21]. Looking at significant symptom variability in osteoarthritis is a starting point.

The aim of our study was to generate a preliminary initial estimate of the frequency of significant symptom variability in a primary care population and assess if there were any risk factors associated with them.

Methods

Design

This was a secondary analysis of prospective observational cohort data from a sample of community-dwelling symptomatic adults – the Clinical Assessment Study of the Knee (CAS(K)).

Study population

Participants were recruited from a two-stage cross-sectional postal survey of all adults ages ≥50 years registered with three general practices in North Staffordshire (irrespective of actual consulting patterns). Respondents reporting pain of any duration in or around the knee within the previous 12 months were invited to attend a research clinic at a local National Health Service Hospital Trust. The study protocol was approved by North Staffordshire Local Research Ethics Committee (project number 1430) and details have been published elsewhere [22, 23]. All participants provided written informed consent to undergo clinical and radiographic assessment. In addition, they were asked for consent to medical record review to assist in excluding pre-existing inflammatory disease. The inclusion criteria for the current analysis were as follows: age ≥50 years, registered with one of the participating general practices at the time of study, responded to both postal questionnaires, consented to further contact, and attended the research clinic. Participants were excluded if they had incomplete baseline radiographs, had not experienced knee pain within the six months prior to clinic attendance, had a pre-existing diagnosis of inflammatory arthropathy in their medical records, or had had a total knee replacement in their most affected knee. Participants who reported total knee replacement (TKR) after baseline and up to 3 years were also excluded. Patients reporting TKR after 3 years were censored at the 3 year time point.

Baseline data collection

All data were planned and gathered prospectively. At baseline, participants underwent a standardized clinical interview and physical examination conducted by one of six research therapists blinded to the findings from radiography, postal questionnaires and medical records.

Participants filled in a brief self-complete questionnaire about their knee symptoms on the day of their clinic attendance.

Plain knee radiographs were obtained on the day of clinic attendance. Three views were taken of each knee: a weight-bearing semi-flexed posteroanterior (PA) view, according to the protocol developed by Buckland-Wright et al. [24], and lateral and skyline views, both in a supine position with the knee flexed to 45°. The tibiofemoral joint was assessed using the PA view and the posterior compartment of the lateral view. The patellofemoral joint was assessed using the skyline and lateral views.

Scoring of plain radiographs

A single reader (a consultant rheumatologist with extensive training in assessing knee radiographs for knee OA), blinded to all other information on participants, scored all films. Films were scored for individual radiographic features, including osteophytes, joint space width, sclerosis, subluxation and chondrocalcinosis. PA and skyline views were assigned a Kellgren and Lawrence (K&L) grade based on these authors' original written descriptions [25]. The atlas developed by Burnett et al. [26] was used for the lateral view.

For PA, K&L score, skyline K&L score and lateral osteophytes, intra- and inter-reader reliability were assessed in a subsample of 50 participants (100 knees) and found to be very good (κ = 0.81–0.98 and 0.49–0.76, respectively) [27].

Follow-up data collection

Follow up surveys, which included 11-point numerical rating scales (NRS) on current, average and worst knee pain intensity over the past 6 months [28], were mailed to Phase 2 participants at 18 months, 36 months, 54 months and 72 months.

Outcome measure

At baseline and at each follow-up point we classed participants as reporting 'significant pain variability' if their recalled worst pain intensity in the past 6 months was ≥5 out of 10 and at least 2 points higher than recalled average pain intensity in the same 6 month period. To be included in the denominator, individuals had to be 'at risk' during that interval (i.e. average pain intensity <9 out of 10).

This definition was chosen after referring to previous studies of osteoarthritis flares which were described as worsening usual pain [11, 13], within defined limits using equivocal pain scales from flare design trials which set a minimum threshold of 50 mm on a 100 mm visual analogue scale (VAS) [29] and a pain increase of at least 20 mm on a 100 mm VAS or an increase of at least two points on a 10 point scale, from baseline [30, 31]. Definitions used in other musculoskeletal disorders such as lower back pain [32] and non-musculoskeletal conditions such as Chronic Obstructive Pulmonary Disease (COPD) were used [33, 34] where worsening of symptoms is used in addition to requiring different or extra medication. The definitions are all reliant on change and difference in pain.

Putative predictors

Predictors available in the CAS(K) dataset were selected for analysis on the basis of being shown in previous studies to be associated with incidence and progression of knee osteoarthritis [15, 35–39], pain outcomes [15] or acute flare-ups [11] (Table 1).

Statistical analysis

The proportion of participants classed as experiencing significant symptom variability was reported for each time point. For each follow-up time point those experiencing symptom variability at baseline were compared between those followed up and not followed up to identify any differences.

To estimate the association between the putative predictor variables and significant pain variability, we used discrete-time survival analysis. For clinical history/examination and radiographic severity predictors we used information from only one knee per individual, the "index knee": the single painful knee in participants with unilateral knee pain or the most painful knee in

Table 1 Summary of putative predictors and their source

Domain	Indicator
Demographic	Age; gender
Socioeconomic	Employment Status(employed, other); Occupational class[a] (managerial and professional, intermediate, routine and manual)
	Attended further education; Married/cohabiting
Clinical history/Examination	Time since onset of problem (<1 year, 1 to <5 years, 5 to <10 years, 10+ years); Problem started following injury; Bilateral knee pain; Duration of morning stiffness; Knee given way during previous month; Visited a hospital doctor about knee problem; Presence and severity of palpable knee effusion (none, mild, moderate/gross); Nodal symptomatic hand OA
Radiographic Severity	Overall severity of radiographic OA: index knee (none, mild, moderate/severe)[b]
	Compartmental distribution of radiographic OA: index knee (none, isolated TFJ, isolated PFJ, combined PFJ-TFJ)
Lifestyle factors	Body mass index (kg/m^2); Current smoker (Yes/No); Physical activity level[c] : sedentary (Yes/No); moderate (Yes/No); high (Yes/No)
Mental Health	HADS Anxiety and Depression subscale scores scale
Physical function	SF-36 (PF-10 subscale)
Knee-specific pain and functional limitation	WOMAC Pain and Function subscale scores

Hospital Anxiety and Depression scale [54]; OA Osteoarthritis; PF-10 Medical Outcomes Study SF-36 Physical Functioning subscale [55]; SD Standard deviation; WOMAC Western Ontario & McMaster Universities Osteoarthritis Index [56]

[a] Derived from National Socio-economic Classification [57]

[b] Mild = KL2 (PA or skyline view) or grade 1 osteophytes (lateral view); Moderate/severe = KL ≥ 3 (PA or skyline view) or grade 3 osteophytes (lateral view) [58]

[c] Twenty-three physical activity items were originally included. Those that were difficult to quantify were excluded from this analysis for example; 'go out for a walk' and 'go out to work'. We chose 6 items which were then categorised into sedentary ('spend most or all of day in bed or chair'), moderate ('walks of a least a quarter of a mile' and 'walks of two miles') and vigorous physical activity ('play a sport', 'heavy gardening' and 'heavy DIY work at home'). These measures were included if it was reported that they were done on 'all, most or some days'

individuals with bilateral knee pain. Discrete-time hazard survival models become models for dichotomous response when the data have been expanded to person-period data with one observation for each year the person is at risk. For each follow-up time point, we constructed an indicator variable on whether the patient had experienced significant pain variability in the 6 month period or not and estimated the hazard of significant pain variability using logistic discrete-time hazards model. The outcome was right censored at 72 months, which was the last follow-up time. Individuals who were lost to follow-up or withdrew from the study before the period of significant symptom variability was recorded, were also censored. To adjust for changes in proportion reporting significant pain variability over time, we included dummy variables for each follow-up time in all models. Two sets of analyses were conducted. We first modelled the time to first period of significant pain variability, ignoring additional subsequent periods of significant pain variability reported by the participant. We then used multilevel discrete-time survival (frailty) models to take into account recurrent periods of significant pain variability within participants. In the frailty model method, the association between periods of significant pain variability is explicitly modelled as a random-effect term. The frailty model was estimated using logistic discrete-time hazards model with random effects.

The association between each predictor and outcome was estimated and those with *P*-value <0.20 were selected for inclusion in the multivariable models. Tests of multicollinearity were performed first by pairwise correlations (one variable excluded if correlation coefficient >0.7) and then by variance inflation factor (VIF >5 considered as evidence of collinearity). We used a manual backward elimination procedure to remove variables from the multivariable model until only factors with a *P*-value <0.05 were retained in the final model. An a priori decision was made to include age and gender in the final models. All analyses were performed using Stata 13 [40].

Results

Eight hundred and nineteen people attended the research clinic, of whom 719 participants were eligible for inclusion for the baseline analysis (54% female; mean age 67.3 (SD 8.5) years; mean BMI 29.3 (SD 5.0) kg/m^2). There was no strong evidence of selective loss to follow-up related to presence of significant pain variability at baseline (Additional file 1 Table S1).

Participants classed as having at least one period of 'significant pain variability'

Between 23 and 32% of participants were estimated to have experienced significant pain variability at each of the five time points (Table 2). Across the entire cohort follow up period 363 (47%) participants reported no periods, 202 (27%) reported one period, 90 (12%) reported two periods, 63 (8%) reported three periods, 30 (4%) reported four periods and 13 (2%) reported five periods of significant pain variability. Table 3 presents the descriptive statistics for participants reporting at least one period of significant pain variability.

Factors associated with time to first period of significant pain variability

Based on the outcome of time to first period of significant symptom variability, baseline measures associated with a higher risk of symptom variability in the adjusted analysis were: younger age (OR (per year): 0.96; 95% CI 0.94, 0.97), higher BMI (per kg/m^2: 1.03; 1.01, 1.06), higher WOMAC knee pain scores (per unit: 1.05; 1.03, 1.10), longer time since onset (e.g. 1–5 years vs < 1 year:

Table 2 Proportion of patients reporting significant pain variability at each time point

	Measurement point				
	Baseline (*n* = 761)	18 months (*n* = 679)	36 months (*n* = 610)	54 months (*n* = 503)	72 months (*n* = 410)
Eligible respondents reporting significant pain variability[a]: n (%)	227 (32)	163 (26)	126 (23)	129 (27)	114 (30)
Average pain intensity in past 6 months (0-10NRS)	4.7 (1.7)	4.6 (1.8)	4.5 (1.6)	4.4 (1.5)	4.9 (1.9)
Worst pain intensity in past 6 months (0-10NRS)	7.6 (1.6)	7.5 (1.5)	7.3 (1.5)	7.1 (1.5)	7.6 (1.6)
Eligible respondents reporting no significant pain variability: n (%)	493 (68)	462 (74)	433 (77)	336 (72)	260 (70)
Average pain intensity in past 6 months (0-10NRS)	3.9 (2.3)	3.5 (2.5)	3.9 (2.6)	3.5 (2.7)	3.8 (2.5)
Worst pain intensity in past 6 months (0-10NRS)	4.1 (2.3)	3.7 (2.4)	4.1 (2.6)	3.8 (2.7)	4.1 (2.5)
Ineligible respondents[b]: n (%)	41 (5)	42 (6)	40 (7)	31 (6)	30 (7)
Missing: n (%)	0 (0)	12 (2)	11 (2)	10 (2)	6 (1)

Figures are mean (standard deviation) unless otherwise stated. NRS Numerical Rating Scale
[a]worst pain intensity in past 6 months ≥5 and ≥2 points higher than average pain intensity in past 6 months
[b]average pain intensity in past 6 months ≥ 9/10

Table 3 Comparison of patient baseline characteristics of participants reporting at least one period of significant pain variability potential flare

	Periods of significant pain variability	
	≥1	None
	n = 398	*n* = 363
Female gender	53	56
Age (years): mean (SD)	63.6 (8.2)	67.4 (8.7)
Employed	27	17
Attended full time education after school	17	13
Married/cohabiting	76	68
Current smoker	11	10
Body Mass Index (kg/m^2): mean (SD)	30.0 (5.3)	28.7 (4.8)
Routine/manual occupational class[a]	48	56
PF-10 physical function subscale (0–100): mean (SD)	56.1 (27.9)	58.7 (30.1)
WOMAC knee pain (0–20): mean (SD)	6.5 (4.2)	5.6 (4.3)
WOMAC knee function (0–68): mean (SD)	21.1 (14.3)	18.5 (14.7)
HADS Anxiety (0–21): mean (SD)	6.8 (4.1)	6.3 (4.0)
HADS Depression (0–21): mean (SD)	4.8 (3.4)	4.2 (3.1)
Compartmental distribution of radiographic OA – index knee		
Normal	33	31
Isolated tibiofemoral	5	3
Isolated patellofemoral	23	25
Combined tibiofemoral and patellofemoral	40	41
Overall severity of radiographic OA - index knee		
Normal	33	31
Mild	28	30
Moderate/severe	39	39
Severity of knee effusion – index knee		
None	67	66
Mild	23	23
Moderate/gross	10	11
Nodal symptomatic hand OA	15	18
Previous knee injury		
None	65	71
Unilateral	26	23
Bilateral	9	5
Time since onset of knee problem		
< 12 months	8	16
1 year to < 5 years	36	35
5 years to < 10 years	21	19
≥ 10 years	35	30
Duration of morning stiffness		
None	35	46
≤30 min	60	50
>30 min	6	4

Table 3 Comparison of patient baseline characteristics of participants reporting at least one period of significant pain variability potential flare *(Continued)*

Knee given way during past month	32	27
Seen hospital doctor about knee	27	20
Frequent sedentary activity	11	8
Frequent moderate activity	54	55
Frequent vigorous activity	28	28

Figures are column percentages unless otherwise stated. Hospital Anxiety and Depression scale [54]; OA Osteoarthritis; PF-10 Medical Outcomes Study SF-36 Physical Functioning subscale [55]; SD Standard deviation; WOMAC Western Ontario & McMaster Universities Osteoarthritis Index [56]
[a] Derived from National Socio-economic Classification [57]

1.79; 1.16, 2.75) and morning stiffness (≤30 min vs none: 1.43; 1.10, 1.85) (Table 4).

Factors associated with recurrent periods of significant pain variability

Based on the outcome of recurrent periods of significant symptom variability, i.e. allowing for those experiencing more than one episode, baseline measures associated with a higher risk of potential symptom variability in the adjusted analysis were: younger age (0.94; 0.91, 0.98), higher BMI (1.04; 1.00,1.08), higher WOMAC knee pain scores (1.10; 1.03,1.17), longer time since onset (e.g. 1–5 years vs < 1 year: (2.23; 1.11, 4.46) and morning stiffness (≤30 min vs none: 1.67; 1.07, 2.61) (Table 5).

Discussion

From our study we estimate that between a quarter and a third of adults aged over 50 years with knee pain report significant symptom variability. Such variability was associated with younger age, longer history of knee problem, higher BMI and more severe knee symptoms. Variability was also more common in people reporting previous bilateral knee injury, greater functional limitation, frequent sedentary behaviour and higher anxiety and depression scores at baseline although these associations were not statistically significant after adjusting for covariates.

In the context of previous studies it appears that significant variability in pain affects a large minority of persons with, or at risk, of knee OA but that estimates are sensitive to the definition and period of time and frequency of measurement. Of previous studies employing latent class growth analysis or growth mixture modelling to cohort data with repeated measures of pain only the study by Leffondre et al [41] identified a group of patients characterised by pain variability. Their group of patients with 'highly unstable WOMAC total scores, with abrupt changes or short-term fluctuations' accounted for 18% of the community-dwelling sample of adults aged over 55 years with hip or knee pain. The failure of other studies to extract such a 'fluctuating pain' latent class using similar methodology [2–5], may well reflect the long intervals between re-measurements (typically a year). In studies of low back pain, those with weekly or fortnightly pain measurements classed twice as many patients into a 'fluctuating' trajectory than studies using monthly measurement [42]. It must also be stressed that within trajectory groups that have an average 'stable' trajectory, members of these groups can still experience significant variability in their pain at an individual level. A further source of comparison is Ricci et al.'s [16] estimate from NHANES I data that 38% of US workers aged 40–65 years with arthritis (predominantly hip or knee pain) report 'pain exacerbations'. Like our study, they adopted the same magnitude of increase in pain intensity to define these events (2 or more points on 0-10NRS) although the Ricci study was based on a 2-week recall period.

The extent to which our own, and any of these previous studies, provides insights into the frequency of pain exacerbations or flares is limited by the data available. As noted by Marty [11] and in consensus work for flare definition in other rheumatic diseases [43, 44], flares are probably best thought of as multidimensional constructs. With the data available to us we could not verify the speed of onset, duration, or other features (e.g. swelling, limping) that may be important in distinguishing acute flares from other forms of variability within the natural history of osteoarthritis pain. An important limitation of our study is the potential misclassification bias as a result of recall error. We hypothesise that patients with increased pain closer to the measurement time points may have overestimated their average and worst pain scores whereas those with fewer pain fluctuations or no increase in pain close to the measurement time points are likely to have underestimated their pain scores over the previous 6 months. The overall impact of this on our results is uncertain. In addition, the long period of recall may be particularly prone to 'forward telescoping' where an event is reported more recently than it actually happened [45, 46]. In our analysis we have used the 'average' and 'worst' pain scores taken from the Von Korff pain grade. These were chosen as they were similar but unfortunately not comparable to outcomes used in flare design trials. Flare-ups are identified in drug withdrawal trials by comparing baseline pain scores to worst pain scores. These limitations are only likely to be resolved by prospective studies with frequent repeated measures over clinically relevant time periods incorporating the concept of pain variability

Table 4 Patient baseline characteristics associated with significant pain variability based on discrete-time logit model (first outcome)

		Unadjusted		Adjusted[a]	
	Reference	OR	(95% CI)	aOR	(95% CI)
Male gender	Female	1.15	(0.92, 1.45)	1.22	(0.96, 1.55)
Age (years)	per year	0.96	(0.95, 0.98)	0.96	(0.94, 0.97)
Body mass index (kg/m^2)	per kg/m^2	1.05	(1.03, 1.08)	1.03	(1.01, 1.06)
Occupational class	Managerial/professional				
Intermediate		0.90	(0.56, 1.45)		
Routine and manual		0.76	(0.51, 1.12)		
PF-10 physical function (0–100)	per unit	0.99	(0.99, 0.99)	ns	ns
WOMAC knee pain (0–20)	per unit	1.08	(1.05, 1.11)	1.06	(1.03, 1.10)
WOMAC knee function (0–68)	per unit	1.02	(1.01, 1.03)	mc	mc
Compartmental distribution of radiographic OA[b]	Normal				
Isolated tibiofemoral		1.03	(0.58, 1.81)		
Isolated patellofemoral		0.94	(0.70, 1.28)		
Combined tibiofemoral and patellofemoral		1.06	(0.81, 1.38)		
Overall severity of radiographic OA[b]	Normal				
Mild		0.94	(0.70, 1.25)		
Mod/severe		1.08	(0.82, 1.41)		
HADS anxiety (0–21)	per unit	1.04	(1.01, 1.07)	mc	mc
HADS depression (0–21)	per unit	1.07	(1.03, 1.10)	ns	ns
Previous knee injury	None			ns	ns
Unilateral		1.25	(0.95, 1.64)		
Bilateral		1.82	(1.17, 2.85)		
Time since onset of knee problem[b]	<1 year				
1 year to < 5 years		1.97	(1.29, 3.01)	1.79	(1.16, 2.75)
5 years to < 10 years		1.94	(1.23, 3.05)	1.82	(1.15, 2.89)
≥10 years		2.02	(1.32, 3.08)	1.82	(1.18, 2.82)
Duration of morning stiffness[b]	None				
≤30 min		1.63	(1.28, 2.07)	1.43	(1.10, 1.85)
>30 min		2.26	(1.34, 3.81)	1.44	(0.83, 2.50)
Knee given way during past month[b]	No	1.38	(1.08, 1.77)	ns	ns
Seen hospital doctor about knee[b]	No	1.61	(1.23, 2.10)	ns	ns
Severity of effusion[b]	None				
Mild		0.99	(0.77, 1.30)		
Moderate/gross		1.15	(0.79, 1.67)		
Nodal symptomatic hand OA	No	0.90	(0.66, 1.24)		
Frequent sedentary activity	No	1.59	(1.07, 2.35)		
Frequent moderate activity	No	0.85	(0.68, 1.07)		
Frequent vigorous activity	No	0.88	(0.68, 1.13)		

[a] Adjusted for all other variables; - indicates variables entered but not retained in multivariable model
[b] For index (most problematic) knee
Hospital Anxiety and Depression scale [54]; OA Osteoarthritis; OR Odds ratio; PF-10 Medical Outcomes Study SF-36 Physical Functioning subscale [55]; WOMAC Western Ontario & McMaster Universities Osteoarthritis Index [56]; 95%CI 95% confidence interval
ns Non-significant in multivariable model
mc Variables omitted in the multivariable model due to multi-collinearity

Table 5 Patient baseline characteristics associated with significant pain variability based on discrete-time frailty model (recurrent outcome)

		Unadjusted		Adjusted[a]	
	Reference	OR	(95% CI)	aOR	(95% CI)
Male gender	Female	1.30	(0.86, 1.97)	1.40	(0.93, 2.09)
Age (years)	per year	0.95	(0.92, 0.98)	0.94	(0.91, 0.98)
Body mass index (kg/m^2)	per kg/m^2	1.07	(1.02, 1.12)	1.04	(1.00, 1.08)
Occupational class	Managerial/professional				
Intermediate		0.95	(0.53, 1.70)		
Routine and manual		0.77	(0.49, 1.22)		
PF-10 physical function (0–100)	per unit	0.99	(0.99, 0.99)	ns	ns
WOMAC knee pain (0–20)	per unit	1.12	(1.04, 1.21)	1.10	(1.03, 1.17)
WOMAC knee function (0–68)	per unit	1.03	(1.01, 1.05)	mc	mc
Compartmental distribution of radiographic OA[b]	Normal				
Isolated tibiofemoral		1.05	(0.49, 2.24)		
Isolated patellofemoral		0.93	(0.62, 1.40)		
Combined tibiofemoral and patellofemoral		1.07	(0.75, 1.53)		
Overall severity of radiographic OA[b]	Normal				
Mild		0.93	(0.63, 1.36)		
Mod/severe		1.10	(0.77, 1.57)		
HADS anxiety (0–21)	per unit	1.05	(1.00, 1.10)	mc	mc
HADS depression (0–21)	per unit	1.11	(1.02, 1.21)	ns	ns
Previous knee injury	No			ns	ns
Unilateral		1.27	(0.92, 1.76)		
Bilateral		1.96	(1.02, 3.79)		
Time since onset of knee problem[b]	<1 year				
1 year to < 5 years		2.38	(1.14, 4.97)	2.23	(1.11, 4.46)
5 years to < 10 years		2.32	(1.10, 4.89)	2.20	(1.08, 4.48)
≥10 years		2.40	(1.18, 4.92)	2.11	(1.12, 4.05)
Duration of morning stiffness[b]	None				
≤30 min		2.23	(1.17, 4.23)	1.67	(1.07, 2.61)
>30 min		3.75	(1.16, 12.16)	1.71	(0.73, 3.98)
Knee given way during past month	No	1.42	(1.06, 1.90)	ns	ns
Seen hospital doctor about knee	No	1.89	(1.41, 3.13)	ns	ns
Severity of effusion	None				
Mild		0.99	(0.69, 1.42)		
Moderate/gross		1.18	(0.72, 1.92)		
Nodal symptomatic hand OA	No	0.80	(0.48, 1.35)		
Frequent sedentary activity	No	2.00	(0.96, 4.19)		
Frequent moderate activity	No	0.79	(0.56, 1.13)		
Frequent vigorous activity	No	0.79	(0.51, 1.23)		

[a] Adjusted for all other variables; - indicates variables entered but not retained in multivariable model

[b]relates to index (most problematic) knee

Hospital Anxiety and Depression scale [54]; OA Osteoarthritis; OR Odds ratio; PF-10 Medical Outcomes Study SF-36 Physical Functioning subscale [55]; WOMAC Western Ontario & McMaster Universities Osteoarthritis Index [56]; 95%CI 95% confidence interval

ns Non-significant in final model

mc Variables omitted in the multivariable model due to multi-collinearity

The pattern of associations found in our study is consistent with previous findings for some risk factors but not others. Higher BMI, pain intensity, stiffness, and functional limitation have been found to be associated with flares in previous studies [11, 16]. By contrast, our finding of an increased risk of potential flare with younger age was found by neither Marty nor Ricci which may reflect the duration of data collection. Bouts of heavy physical activity [47], buckling and knee injury [48] and worsening mental health [37] have previously been shown in case-crossover designs to be associated with pain flares. The fact that our study found no association between these factors measured at baseline and episodes of worsened pain occurring months and years later may simply affirm the need to regard these factors as time-varying, proximal triggers. From influential qualitative studies by Gooberman-Hill et al [49] and Hawker et al [9], pain variability is thought to be a particular feature in the early and the advanced stages of osteoarthritis. In our study we found no strong relationship between significant variability in pain and severity of radiographic knee OA suggesting that this may happen across the spectrum of the disease. As noted above, our data do not permit us to explore further the quality or predictability of episodes of severe pain: dimensions identified by patients as critical to their ability to cope [12, 50]. If correct, our finding that younger age, male gender, and BMI are associated with higher risk of significant symptom variability, might imply an important role for joint loading in provoking episodes of severe pain and acute flares.

Conclusion

Up to a third of community-dwelling symptomatic adults recall significant variability in knee pain that includes periods of severe pain. Such variability occurs across the spectrum of radiographic severity of knee osteoarthritis. A larger body of work, as has been done for other diseases such as COPD (Chronic Obstructive Pulmonary Disease), is needed to reliably determine the characteristics of those who experience significant symptom variability, including acute flares [51], to assess burden [52], and to guide prevention [53].

Abbreviations

BMI: Body mass index; CAS(K): The knee clinical assessment study; COPD: Chronic obstructive pulmonary disease; OA: Osteoarthritis; PA: Postero-anteriorly; PFJ: Patellofemoral joint; SD: Standard deviation; SF-36: 36 item short form health survey; TFJ: Tibiofemoral joint; WOMAC: Western Ontario & McMaster Universities Osteoarthritis index

Acknowledgements

The authors thank Professor Peter Croft, Professor Elaine Hay, Dr Elaine Thomas, Dr Laurence Wood, Dr Michelle Marshall, June Handy, Professor Krysia Dziedzic, Dr Helen Myers, Dr Ross Wilkie, Dr Rachel Duncan, Dr Jonathan Hill, Charlotte Clements, Professor Chris Buckland-Wright and Professor Iain McCall for their contributions to the design and acquisition of data for the CAS(K) study. We also thank the administrative and health informatics staff at the Arthritis Research UK Primary Care Centre, staff of the participating general practices and Haywood Hospital, especially Dr Jackie Sakhlatvala, Carole Jackson, Julia Myatt and the Radiographers at the Department of Radiography.

Funding

The CAS(K) cohort was supported by the Medical Research Council (Grant G9900220), Arthritis Research UK (Grant 18174), and by Support for Science funding secured by North Staffordshire Primary Care Research Consortium for National Health Service support costs. EP is currently funded by a NIHR In-Practice Fellowship and was previously funded by a NIHR Academic Clinical Fellowship. The views expressed are those of the author(s) and not necessarily those of the NHS, the NIHR or the Department of Health.

Authors' contributions

The authors contributed to the manuscript as follows: conception and design - GP, EP,RO; analysis and interpretation of data - EP, RO, GP; drafting of the article - EP, GP, RO; final approval - EP, GP, RO. All authors read and approved the final manuscript.

Competing interests

GP has received consultancy fees from InFirst Healthcare Ltd. The authors have no other competing interests to declare.

Consent for publication

Not applicable.

Author details

[1]NIHR In-Practice Fellow, Arthritis Research UK Primary Care Centre, Research Institute for Primary Care & Health Sciences, Keele University, Keele, Staffordshire ST5 5BG, UK. [2]Research Fellow in Biostatistics, Arthritis Research UK Primary Care Centre, Research Institute for Primary Care & Health Sciences, Keele University, Keele ST5 5BG, Staffordshire, UK. [3]Professor of Clinical Epidemiology, Arthritis Research UK Primary Care Centre, Research Institute for Primary Care & Health Sciences, Keele University, Keele ST5 5BG, Staffordshire, UK.

References

1. Holla JF, van der Leeden M, Heymans MW, et al. Three trajectories of activity limitations in early symptomatic knee osteoarthritis: a 5-year follow-up study. Ann Rheum Dis. 2014;73:1369–75.
2. Collins JE, Katz JN, Dervan EE, Losina E. Trajectories and risk profiles of pain in persons with radiographic, symptomatic knee osteoarthritis: data from the osteoarthritis initiative. Osteoarthr Cartil. 2014;22:622–30.
3. Nicholls E, Thomas E, van der Windt DA, Croft PR, Peat G. Pain trajectory groups in persons with, or at high risk of, knee osteoarthritis: findings from the Knee Clinical Assessment Study and the Osteoarthritis Initiative. Osteoarthr Cartil. 2014;22:2041–50.

4. Wesseling J, Bastick AN, ten Wolde S, et al. Identifying Trajectories of Pain Severity in Early Symptomatic Knee Osteoarthritis: A 5-year Followup of the Cohort Hip and Cohort Knee (CHECK) Study. J Rheumatol. 2015;42:1470–7.
5. Bastick AN, Wesseling J, Damen J, et al. Defining knee pain trajectories in early symptomatic knee osteoarthritis in primary care: 5-year results from a nationwide prospective cohort study. Br J Gen Pract. 2016;66:e32–9.
6. Soni A, Kiran A, Hart DJ, et al. Prevalence of reported knee pain over twelve years in a community-based cohort. Arthritis Rheum. 2012;64:1145–52.
7. Cedraschi C, Delézay S, Marty M, et al. Let's talk about OA pain": A Qualitative Analysis of the Perceptions of People Suffering from OA. Towards the Development of a Specific Pain OA-Related Questionnaire, the Osteoarthritis Symptom Inventory Scale (OASIS). PLoS One. 2013;8:e79988.
8. Schneider S, Junghaenel DU, Keefe FJ, et al. Individual differences in the day-to-day variability of pain, fatigue, and well-being in patients with rheumatic disease: Associations with psychological variables. Pain. 2012;153:813–22.
9. Hawker GA, Stewart L, French MR, et al. Understanding the pain experience in hip and knee osteoarthritis – an OARSI/OMERACT initiative. Osteoarthr Cartil. 2008;16:415–22.
10. Smith TO, Zou K, Abdullah N, Chen X, Kingsbury SR, Doherty M, Zhang W, Conaghan PG. Does flare trial design affect the effect size of non-steroidal anti-inflammatory drugs in symptomatic osteoarthritis? A systematic review and meta-analysis. Ann Rheum Dis. 2016; doi: 10.1136/annrheumdis-2015-208823.
11. Marty M, Hilliquin P, Rozenberg S, Valat JP, Vignon E, Coste P, Savarieau B, Allaert FA. Validation of the KOFUS (Knee Osteoarthritis Flare-Ups Score). Joint Bone Spine. 2009;76:268–72.
12. Rayahin JE, Chmiel JS, Hayes KW, et al. Factors Associated with Pain Experience Outcome in Knee Osteoarthritis. Arthritis Care Res. 2014;66:1828–35.
13. Esen S, Akarirmak U, Aydin FY, Unalan H. Clinical evaluation during the acute exacerbation of knee osteoarthritis: the impact of diagnostic ultrasonography. Rheumatol Int. 2013;33(3):711–7.
14. Conrozier T, Mathieu P, Vignon E, et al. Differences in the osteoarthritic synovial fluid composition and rheology between patients with or without flare: a pilot study. Clin Exp Rheumatol. 2010;30:729–34.
15. Wise BL, Niu J, Zhang Y, Wang N, Jordan JM, Choy E, et al. Psychological factors and their relation to osteoarthritis pain. Osteoarthr Cartil. 2010;18(7):883–7.
16. Ricci JA, Stewart WF, Chee E, Leotta C, Foley K, HochbergG MC. Pain exacerbation as a major source of lost productive time in US workers with arthritis. Arthritis Care Res. 2005;53:673–81.
17. NICE: Chronic Obstructive Pulmonary Disease in over 16 s: diagnosis and management. NICE guidelines [CG101]. https://www.nice.org.uk/Guidance/CG101 (2010). Accessed 19 July 2016.
18. Global Initiative for Chronic Obstructive Lung Disease. COPD diagnosis, management and prevention. https://www.guidelines.co.uk/gold/copd (2016). Accessed 19 July 2016.
19. Stone MA, Pomeroy E, Keat A, et al. Assessment of the impact of flares in ankylosing spondylitis disease activity using the Flare Illustration. Rheumatology. 2008;47:1213–8.
20. Global Initiative for Asthma. Global Strategy for Asthma Management and Prevention. http://ginasthma.org/wp-content/uploads/2016/01/GINA_Report_2015_Aug11-1.pdf (2015). Accessed 19 July 2016.
21. Ruperto N, Hanrahan LM, Alarcón GS, et al. International consensus for a definition of disease flare in lupus. Lupus. 2011;20:453–62.
22. Peat G, Thomas E, Handy J, Wood L, Dziedzic K, Myers H. The Knee Clinical Assessment Study – CAS(K). A prospective study of knee pain and knee osteoarthritis in the general population. BMC Musculoskelet Disord. 2004;5:4.
23. Peat G, Thomas E, Handy J, Wood L, Dziedzic K, Myers H. The Knee Clinical Assessment Study – CAS(K). A prospective study of knee pain and knee osteoarthritis in the general population: baseline recruitment and retention at 18-months. BMC Musculoskelet Disord. 2006;7:30.
24. Buckland-Wright JC, Ward RJ, Peterfy C, et al. Reproducibility of the semiflexed (metatarsophalangeal) radiographic knee position and automated measurements of medial tibiofemoral joint space width in a multicenter clinical trial of knee osteoarthritis. J Rheumatol. 2004;31:1588–97.
25. Lawrence JS. Rheumatism in Populations. London: Heinemann; 1977. p. 99–100.
26. Burnett S, Hart D, Cooper C, Spector T. A Radiographic Atlas of OA. London: Springer; 1994.
27. Duncan RC, Hay E, Saklatvala J, Croft PR. Prevalence of radiographic osteoarthritis - it all depends on your point of view. Rheumatology (Oxford). 2006;45:757–60. doi:10.1093/rheumatology/kei270.
28. Von Korff M, Ormel J, Keefe FJ, Dworkin SF. Grading the severity of chronic pain. Pain. 1992;50:133–49.
29. Kivitz A, Makarowski W, Fiechtner J, et al. A flexible daily dosage regimen of oxaprozin potassium in patients with acute knee pain associated with knee osteoarthritis- 24-h analgesic durability and safety. Clin Drug Investig. 2001;21:745–53.
30. Scott-Lennox JA, Mclaughlin-Miley C, Lennox RD, Bohlig AM, Cutler BL, Yan C, Jaffe M. Stratification of flare intensity identifies placebo responders in a treatment efficacy trial of patients with osteoarthritis. Arthritis Rheum. 2001;44:1599–607.
31. Baer PA, Thomas LM, Shainhouse Z. Treatment of osteoarthritis of the knee with a topical diclofenac solution: a randomised controlled, 6-week trial ISRCTN53366886]. BMC Musculoskelet Disord. 2005;6.
32. Suri P, Saunders KW, Von Korff M. Prevalence and characteristics of flare-ups of chronic nonspecific back pain in primary care: A telephone survey. Clin J Pain. 2012;28:573–80.
33. Burge S, Wedzicha JA. COPD exacerbations: definitions and classifications. Eur Respir J. 2003;21(41 suppl):46s–53s.
34. Wedzicha JA, Seemungal TA. COPD exacerbations: defining their cause and prevention. Lancet. 2007;9:786–96.
35. Grotle M, Hagen K, Natvig B, Dahl F, Kvien T. Obesity and osteoarthritis in knee, hip and/or hand: An epidemiological study in the general population with 10 years follow-up. BMC Musculoskelet Disord. 2008;9:132.
36. Felson DT, Naimark A, Anderson J, Kazis L, Castelli W, Meenan RF. The prevalence of knee osteoarthritis in the elderly. The Framingham Osteoarthritis Study. Arthritis Rheum. 1987;30(8):914–8.
37. Chapple CM, Nicholson H, Baxter GD, Abbott JH. Patient characteristics that predict progression of knee osteoarthritis: A systematic review of prognostic studies. Arthritis Care Res. 2011;63:1115–25.
38. Conaghan PG, D'Agostino MA, Le Bars M, Baron G, Schmidely N, Wakefield R, et al. Clinical and ultrasonographic predictors of joint replacement for knee osteoarthritis: results from a large, 3-year, prospective EULAR study. Ann Rheum Dis. 2010;69(4):644–7.
39. Cheung PP, Gossec L, Dougados M. What are the best markers for disease progression in osteoarthritis (OA)? Best Pract Res Clin Rheumatol. 2010;24:81–92.
40. StataCorp. Stata Statistical Software: Release 13. College Station, TX: StataCorp LP; 2013.
41. Leffondré K, Abrahamowicz M, Regeasse A, et al. Statistical measures were proposed for identifying longitudinal patterns of change in quantitative health indicators. J Clin Epidemiol. 2004;57:1049–62.
42. Kongsted A, Kent P, Axen I, Downie AS, Dunn KM. What have we learned from ten years of trajectory research in low back pain? BMC Musculoskelet Disord. 2016;17:220.
43. Alten R, Pohl C, Choy EH, et al. Developing a construct to evaluate flares in rheumatoid arthritis: a conceptual report of the OMERACT RA Flare Definition Working Group. J Rheumatol. 2011;38:1745–50.
44. Gossec L, Portier A, Landewé R, et al. Preliminary definitions of 'flare' in axial spondyloarthritis, based on pain, BASDAI and ASDAS-CRP: an ASAS initiative. Ann Rheum Dis. 2016;75:991–6.
45. Cohen G, Conway MA, editors. Memory in the real world. 3rd ed. New York, NY: Psychology Press; 2008.
46. Tourangeau R, Rips LJ, Rasinski K. The psychology of survey response. Cambridge, UK: Cambridge University Press; 2000.
47. Zhang Y, Wheaton D, Niu J, Wise B, Havey W, Goggins J, et al. Recent heavy physical activities trigger knee pain exacerbation in persons with symptomatic knee osteoarthritis. Arthritis Rheum. 2011;63.
48. Zobel I, Erfani T, Bennell KL, et al. Relationship of Buckling and Knee Injury to Pain Exacerbation in Knee Osteoarthritis: A Web-Based Case-Crossover Study. Int J of Med Res. 2016. doi:10.2196/ijmr.5452.
49. Gooberman-Hill R, Woolhead G, Mackichan F, Ayis S, Williams S, Dieppe P. Assessing chronic joint pain: lessons from a focus group study. Arthritis Rheum. 2007;57:666–71.
50. Hawker GA, Wright JG, Badley EM, Coyte PC. Perceptions of, and willingness to consider, total joint arthroplasty in a population-based cohort of individuals with disabling hip and knee arthritis. Arthritis Rheum. 2004;15:635–41.
51. Beeh KM, Glaab T, Stowasser S et al. Characterisation of exacerbation risk and exacerbator phenotypes in the POET-COPD trial. Respir Res. 2013; doi: 10.1186/1465-9921-14-116.
52. Barnes N, Calverley PM, Kaplan A, Rabe KF. Chronic obstructive pulmonary disease and exacerbations: patient insights from the global Hidden Depths of COPD survey. BMC Pulm Med. 2013. doi:10.1186/1471-2466-13-54.

53. Larsson K, Janson C, Lisspers K, et al. Combination of budesonide/formoterol more effective than fluticasone/salmeterol in preventing exacerbations in chronic obstructive pulmonary disease: the PATHOS study. J Internal Med. 2013;273:584–94.
54. Zigmond AS, Snaith RP. The hospital anxiety and depression scale. Acta Psychiatr Scand. 1983;67:361–70.
55. Ware Jr J, Kosinski M, Keller SD. A 12-item Short-Form Health Survey: construction of scales and preliminary tests of reliability and validity. Med Care. 1996;34:220–33.
56. Bellamy N. WOMAC Osteoarthritis Index. 1996. A Users Guide.
57. Office for National Statistics. National Statistics Socio-economic Classification (NS-SEC 2002). London: Stationery Office; 2002.
58. Peat G, Thomas E, Duncan R, Wood L, Hay E, Croft P. Clinical classification criteria for knee osteoarthritis: performance in the general population and primary care. Ann Rheum Dis. 2006;65:1363–7.

3

Detecting functional change in response to exercise in knee osteoarthritis: a comparison of two computerized adaptive tests

Feng-Hang Chang[1], Alan M. Jette[2], Mary D. Slavin[3], Kristin Baker[4], Pengsheng Ni[5] and Julie J. Keysor[6*]

Abstract

Background: The intent of this study was to examine and compare the ability to detect change of two patient reported outcome (PRO) instruments that use a computerized adaptive test (CAT) approach to measurement. The Patient Reported Outcomes Measurement Information System (PROMIS®) Physical Function scale is a generic PRO, while the Osteoarthritis Computerized Adaptive Test (OA-CAT) is an osteoarthritis-specific PRO.

Methods: This descriptive, longitudinal study was conducted in a community setting, involving individuals from the greater Boston area. Inclusion criteria: age > 50, self-reported doctor-diagnosed knee osteoarthritis (OA) and knee pain. The PROMIS® Physical Function CAT and OA-CAT Functional Difficulty scale were administered at baseline and at the conclusion of a 6-week exercise program. Effect sizes (ES) were calculated for both measures, and bootstrap methods were used to construct confidence intervals and to test for significant ES differences between the measures.

Results: The OA-CAT Functional Difficulty scale achieved an ES of 0.62 (0.43, 0.87) compared to the PROMIS® Physical Function CAT ES of 0.42 (0.24, 0.63). ES estimates for the two CAT measures were not statistically different.

Conclusions: The condition-specific OA-CAT and generic PROMIS® Physical Function CAT both demonstrated the ability to detect change in function. While the OA-CAT scale showed larger effect size, no statistically significant difference was found in the effect size estimates for the generic and condition-specific CATs. Both CATs have potential for use in arthritis research.

Trial registration: This trial is registered with ClinicalTrials.gov on 6/21/11 (Identifier NCT01394874)

Keywords: Osteoarthritis, Measurement, Patient reported outcomes, Computerized adaptive testing

Background

Function is a widely targeted area for osteoarthritis (OA) treatment, including pharmacological and non-pharmacological approaches. Patient reported outcomes (PROs) that assess quality of life such as decreased function are increasingly recognized as an important component of OA intervention outcome assessment. Numerous PRO measures are used in OA research [1–6], but a review of the psychometric properties of 32 OA outcome measures concluded that these measures are uniformly rated low in terms of their ability to detect change [1]. The ability of a measure to detect change is of utmost importance when considering which measure to use for research trials and to monitor clinical progress.

Traditional fixed-form PRO measures, such as the 36-Item Short Form Health Survey (SF-36) and the Western Ontario and McMaster Universities Osteoarthritis Index (WOMAC), are comprised of a fixed number of items that are administered to all participants. To reduce administration burden, measures are constrained to a limited number of items, often lacking coverage of the broad range of ability typically observed in patient populations [5–7]. This limitation of fixed-form PRO measures raises concerns about the loss of score precision and the reduced ability to measure clinically meaningful change [8, 9]. Furthermore, these measures require respondents to answer every question even though some may be redundant and inappropriate for an individual [10–12].

* Correspondence: JKEYSOR@MGHIHP.EDU
[6]MGH Institute of Health Professions, Department of Physical Therapy, 36 1st Avenue, Boston, MA 02129, USA
Full list of author information is available at the end of the article

Item response theory (IRT) [13] and computerized adaptive testing (CAT) [14] are advances in measurement that have great potential to overcome limitations of fixed-form PRO measures and improve the ability to assess the wide range in functional ability seen in persons with OA. IRT-based measures use calibrated banks of items that are hierarchically organized from low to high ability for the outcome of interest. These banks of items can be administered as CATs, which employ computer-based algorithms to select items that match an individual's ability based on his/her responses to previously administered items. Using this approach, a relatively small number of items (e.g., 4–10) can generate a precise estimate of the individual's ability for a specific outcome domain. In this way, IRT/CAT measures can provide adequate measurement breadth, precision and sensitivity to change without being burdensome, characteristics that are important for measures used in research and clinical practice [15].

Two IRT/CAT measures are available for use in OA, one is disease-specific and one is generic. The Osteoarthritis Computerized Adaptive Test (OA-CAT) is an IRT/CAT measure developed specifically for use in OA [16, 17]. Disease-specific measures contain items, responses, or other aspects of the measurement that are developed specifically for the disease or condition being measured. In contrast, generic measures are designed to assess outcomes with the expectation that the measurement models can be applied across populations without regard to the patient's specific condition [18]. The Patient Reported Outcomes Measurement Information System (PROMIS®), funded by the National Institutes of Health, was designed as a generic measure to promote comparability across studies and clinical diagnoses [19]. Several PROMIS® domains, including physical functioning [19], can be used to assess outcomes in persons with osteoarthritis.

Faced with measurement choices among emerging PROs for OA research, it is important to examine an instrument's psychometric properties in the population of interest. Indeed, to date there is no sensitivity to change data among persons with OA for either the OA-CAT or PROMIS® instruments. The intent of this study, therefore, was to examine the ability of two PRO CATs – the generic PROMIS® Physical Function (PF) CAT v1.0 and the osteoarthritis-specific OA-CAT Functional Difficulty (FD) scale – to detect change in physical function in a sample of adults with knee OA engaged in an exercise program designed to improve physical function.

Methods

Design and participants

This study, part of a randomized controlled trial to examine the effects of an intervention to improve long-term exercise adherence, reports on data collected at baseline and at the conclusion of a 6-week exercise program designed to improve function in persons with OA. The sample included 120 persons with knee osteoarthritis. The two CAT PRO measures were administered to all participants prior to engaging in a 6-week structured exercise program (baseline) and again after the exercise program was completed (post-exercise training). The exercise program was the same for all participants. OA-CAT FD and PROMIS® PF CAT data reported in this study were collected prior to randomization into intervention and control groups for the exercise adherence study.

Participants were recruited from the greater Boston area. Inclusion criteria were age > 50 years with self-reported, doctor-diagnosed knee OA and knee pain, which was determined by answering yes to both "Have you had pain on most days of the previous month?" and "Have you had pain for most months of the past year?" Exclusion criteria included a medical condition precluding exercise (stroke or myocardial infarction in the past 3 months, treatment for cancer, severe systemic disease), a medical condition that limits physical function more than the knee pain (including back or hip pain more severe than knee pain), inflammatory arthritis, current regular exerciser, regular resistance training (one or more times per week) in the last 6 months, plan for knee replacement during the trial, dementia or inability to follow exercise instructions and use the exercise adherence intervention.

Measures

Characteristics of study measures are summarized in Table 1. Study measures included two IRT-based PRO measures that use a CAT approach: the PROMIS® PF CAT v 1.0 scale and the OA-CAT FD scale. Development of PROMIS® measures was initiated by the National Institute of Health Roadmap for Medical Research to advance the science and application of PROs in chronic diseases [18, 20]. The PROMIS® PF CAT is linked to a U.S. general population and the scale has a mean of $T = 50$ with an SD of 10 [21]. The PROMIS® PF scale assesses one's capability to perform a variety of physical activities, including mobility (lower extremity function), dexterity (upper extremity function), axial (neck and back function), and ability to carry out instrumental activities of daily living. The PROMIS® PF v 1.0 CAT was administered using the default stopping rule (minimum of 4 items and maximum of 12 items) or reaching a standard error of 0.40. The OA-CAT [16, 17] was developed to measure conceptually distinct dimensions of functional pain, functional difficulty, and disability that are relevant for OA clinical practice and research. OA-CAT was developed based on an osteoarthritis sample with a scale range from 10 (lowest score) to 90 (highest score). The OA-CAT stopping rule

Table 1 Summary of Measures

Measure (N = items)	Item Stem	Response Options
OA-CAT Item Bank Functional difficulty (N = 125)	Because of the arthritis in your legs, how much difficulty did you have on an average day, over the past month when....?	• None • A little • A lot • Did not do the activity because of the arthritis in his/her legs • Did not do the activity for reasons other than the arthritis in his/her legs
PROMIS® CAT Item Bank v1.0 Physical Function (N = 124)	Does your health now limit you in...?	• Not at all • Very little • Somewhat • Quite a lot • Cannot do
	Are you able to...?	• Without any difficulty • With a little difficulty • With some difficulty • With much difficulty • Unable to do

is a maximum number of items (10) or reaching a standard error < 0.25. Preliminary studies show that the OA-CAT has improved breadth, precision and reliability and reduced floor and ceiling effects compared with the WOMAC, a traditional fixed-form PRO instrument [16, 17]. In this study, the OA-CAT FD scale was compared to the PROMIS® PF CAT. The OA-CAT was developed and its psychometric properties were examined using an analytic approach similar to PROMIS, but there are a few differences. Instead of using Graded Response model (GRM), we calibrated the OA-CAT item bank using Generalized Partial Credit model (GPCM). Because those two models have exact the same number of parameters and usually data fits one of the model will also fit the other model [22], so different models should have little impact on calibrating the item bank. Second, we didn't remove the local dependent items as PROMIS did, instead in the CAT program we treated those local dependent items as "enemy" items – the CAT program only allows to select one item within a set of locally dependent items. Third, we applied weighted maximum likelihood (WML) estimation method in estimating the person score not Expected A Posterioi (EAP) method. The studies have shown WML estimator had less bias than EAP estimator [23, 24].

Data analyses

Descriptive analysis: Descriptive analyses were performed on assessments completed at baseline and post-exercise training. Means and standard deviations (SD) were computed for each measure: PROMIS® PF CAT and OA-CAT FD.

OA-CAT FD and PROMIS® PF comparability: It is important to examine comparability when assessing ability of the measures to detect change. Four analyses were conducted to compare measures: 1.) Pearson correlations examined the degree to which the OA-CAT FD and PROMIS® PF CAT assess a similar construct; 2.) score reliability, calculated as [1-average (squared standard error/variance of score)]; 3.) score distributions; and 4.) the number of items administered and time to complete each instrument.

Ability to detect change: Change scores were calculated based on assessments completed at baseline and post-exercise training. The Cohen effect size (ES) was computed as a standardized indicator of the ability of each instrument to detect true change [25]. The ES expresses change scores in terms of the underlying sampling distribution using SD estimates [26], and was calculated as $(M2\text{-}M1)/S_b$ [27]. M2 is the mean post-intervention score and M1 is the mean pre-intervention score of each assessment; S_b is the baseline SD. The larger values of ES indicate greater ability to detect change. An ES of 0.2 reflects small change, an ES of 0.5 reflects moderate change, and an ES of 0.8 reflects large change [27].

The bootstrap method was used to calculate the 95% confidence intervals (CI) for ES estimates of each measure and to test for significant differences in ES estimates of the two measures [27]. Five thousand bootstrap samples of the difference in ES estimates across the measures were generated and estimates of differences in ES values were rank-ordered, and the 95% CI for the differences in ES estimates between the measures was calculated.

Results

Table 2 shows the baseline demographic characteristics of the 120 participants consented into the study; of these, 104 completed the exercise program for whom we had follow-up data. Demographic characteristics of the sample are not statistically different for those enrolled at baseline and those who completed the 6-week exercise program, except for the percent of the sample identified as obese, which was significantly lower for exercise program completers.

Table 2 Sample Demographics

Variable	Mean (SD) or Frequency (%)	
	Baseline Sample (*N* = 120)	Post-Exercise training Sample (*N* = [104), *p* value*
Age (years)	65.06 (SD = 7.39)	65.57(SD = 7.38), *P* = 0.05
Gender		
Female	95 (79.2%)	85(81.7%)
Male	25 (20.8%)	19(18.3%), *P* = 0.1
Race		
White, Non-Hispanic	70 (58.3%)	62(59.6%)
Black, Non-Hispanic	33 (27.5%)	28(26.9%)
Hispanic	4 (3.3%)	2(1.9%)
Others	13 (10.8%)	12(11.6%), *p* = 0.1494
Body Mass Index (BMI)		
Underweight (< 18.50)	1 (0.83%)	1(0.96%)
Normal range (18.50–24.99)	24 (20%)	22(21.15%)
Overweight (25.00–29.99)	36 (30.0%)	28(26.92%)
Obese (> = 30.00)	59 (49.17%)	53(50.96%), *P* = 0.1587**
Knee replacement		
Yes	12 (10.1%)	9(8.7%)
No	107 (89.2%)	94(90.4%)
Missing	1(0.8%)	1(1%), *P* = 0.2042

*: *p* value of testing the demographic variables for subjects with and without Post-Exercise training data
**: categories (underweight and normal range) were merged; categories (overweight and obese) were merged
Note: BMI is calculated by body weight divided by the square of the height

Instrument comparability

OA-CAT FD and PROMIS® PF CAT scores were strongly correlated, with similar correlation coefficients at baseline and post-exercise training (0.65 and 0.69, respectively). OA-CAT FD and PROMIS® PF CAT score reliability values were similar at baseline (0.90 and 0.85, respectively) and post-exercise training (0.89 and 0.85, respectively). OA-CAT FD and PROMIS® PF CAT score distributions at baseline and post exercise training have similar distributions. (See Fig. 1a and Fig. 1b.)

The average number of items administered by the OA-CAT FD at baseline was 10.03 (SD = 2.62) and the time to complete was 2.76 (SD = 1.48) minutes. For the PROMIS® PF, an average of 4.14 (SD = 0.54) items were administered and it took 1.8 (SD = 0.66) minutes to complete.

Sensitivity to change

The mean change of OA-CAT FD and the PROMIS® PF CAT scores from baseline to post-exercise training are presented in Table 3. Findings for both the OA-CAT FD and the PROMIS® PF CAT instruments show significant ESs, with the OA-CAT FD having a somewhat greater ES [0.62 (CI = 0.43, 0.87) compared to the PROMIS® PF CAT [(0.42 (CI = 0.24, 0.63). A statistical comparison of ES for the two measures is displayed in Fig. 2, demonstrating no significant differences in ES values between the OA-CAT FD and the PROMIS® PF CAT [95% CI = (− 0.43, 0.004)].

Discussion

This study compared the relative ability of two PROs – OA-CAT FD, an OA-specific measure, and the PROMIS® PF CAT, a generic measure – in a sample of adults at risk of knee OA who completed in an exercise program designed to improve physical function. Results demonstrated that both instruments are able to detect change in function after participation in an exercise program known to have a beneficial effect on functional outcomes. The strong correlation between the two instruments provides evidence that they measure the same construct. Both scales were similar in terms of score reliability and score distribution. The OA-CAT administered more items and took longer to administer. This is likely due to the fact that OA-CAT includes a response option 'Did not do the activity for reasons other than the arthritis in his/her legs.' If this response is selected, the item is not included in the score determination. While more items are administered and it takes an additional minute to administer, the OA-CAT score may more accurately reflect the impact of arthritis on function. While no statistically significant difference in ES values was noted between the two instruments, trends suggest that the OA-CAT scale achieved a larger ES. These findings may indicate that the exercise intervention for more effective for improving function impacted by OA than it was for improving general physical function. Thus, the OA-CAT FD may be preferred for use in clinical trials, particularly when study power is somewhat compromised by sample size. Nonetheless, our study also supports use of the PROMIS® PF CAT to measure change in function among people with OA. PROMIS CAT PF mean score and range at baseline are similar to reports using the PROMIS PF short forms to assess function in a sample with symptomatic knee OA [28]. This study used Physical Function item bank v1.0 and newer, refined PROMIS® items banks include the addition of a Mobility v1.2 item bank focused on a range of activities from getting out of a bed or chair to activities such as running. This item bank may function better in a sample of persons with osteoarthritis than the Physical Function v1.0 item bank, which includes upper extremity activities and instrumental activities of daily living [29].

Performance-based measures were collected in this study, include the five-time-sit-to stand test (FTSST) shown to detect change in persons with OA completing a strength training program [30]. We examined FTSST baseline and post-exercise training scores to

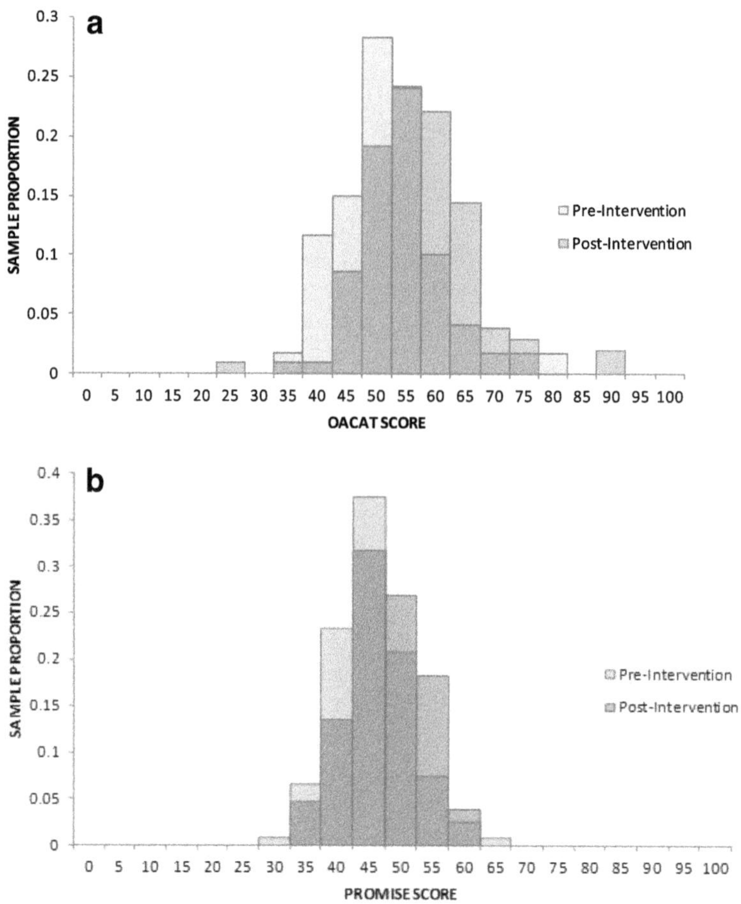

Fig. 1 **a** OA-CAT Functional Difficulty Score Distribution: Baseline and Post-Exercise Training. **b** PROMIS® Physical Function CAT Score Distribution: Baseline and Post Exercise Training

provide additional evidence that the exercise program resulted in change. The FTSST ES (0.5) is similar to the ES reported for the OA-CAT (0.62) and PROMIS (0.54), indicating that the exercise program produced similar change in a measure of performance. However, changes in strength may not translate into a similar change in function. In fact, correlations between FTSST times and OA-CAT and PROMIS scores were weak at baseline and post exercise training (− 0.21 to − 0.34), indicating that the FTSST measures a different construct.

Both the OA-CAT FD and the PROMIS® PF CATs provide the many advantages of contemporary measurement approaches compared to traditional fixed form PROs [31]. The primary difference between the two instruments is that the PROMIS® Physical Function CAT is a generic PRO measure and the OA-CAT is an osteoarthritis-specific PRO. Debates over the pros and cons of generic and disease-specific functional measures are frequently found in the literature [32, 33]. The generic instruments are universally applicable across diseases by measuring an overall condition, while the disease-specific instruments can usually tap into more and deeper disease-specific effects. Our study findings indicated that both the generic PRO measure and the osteoarthritis-specific PRO measure showed significant sensitivity to change and that both have potential usefulness.

Table 3 Descriptive statistics of PROMIS® PF CAT and OA-CAT FD

Measure/Domain	Baseline (*N* = 120)	Post-Exercise Training (*N* = 104)	Effect Size (ES)
	Mean ± SD (Range)	Mean ± SD (Range)	ES (95%CI)
OA-CAT Functional Difficulty	49.53 ± 8.29 (33.35, 75.72)	54.75 ± 9.28 (24.17, 88.17)	0.62[a] (0.43, 0.87)
PROMIS® Physical Function CAT	42.96 ± 5.72 (28.60, 60.70)	45.27 ± 5.67 (31.90, 57.20)	0.42[a] (0.24, 0.63)

Note: [a] The 95% Confidence interval of the effect size (ES) does not contain 0, indicating that the change of score is significant

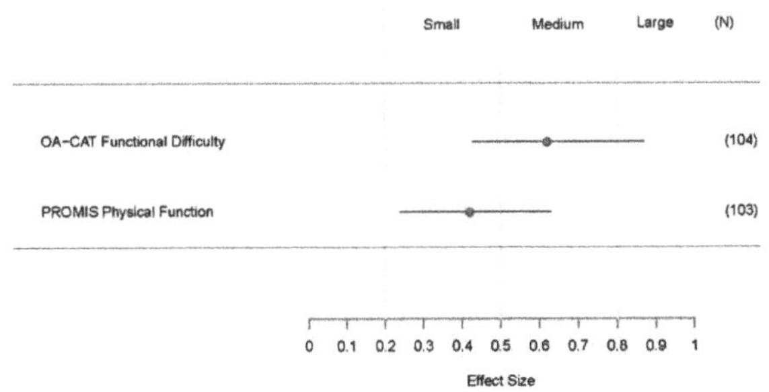

Fig. 2 OA-CAT Functional Difficulty and PROMIS Physical Function Effect Size

Study limitations include a relatively small sample size and loss to follow-up. With a larger sample size, a significant difference in ESs may have been detected. Second, we did not compare the sensitivity to change of these instruments to other standard patient reported outcomes (e.g., Western Ontario and McMaster Universities Osteoarthritis Index (WOMAC)). Third, the exercise program was relatively brief and a longer duration could have resulted in greater 'true' change, enhancing the ability of these instruments to detect change. Fourth, we only have one follow-up data point and are unable to determine the sensitivity to change over longer periods of time which is often needed for chronic conditions such as OA.

Conclusions

The investigation of the sensitivity to change for the OA-CAT FD and PROMIS® PF CAT suggests that both instruments have significant sensitivity to change in persons with OA. While no statistically significant difference was found in the sensitivity to change between the two instruments, the trends revealed that the OA-CAT achieved larger ES. Both instruments have potential usefulness in arthritis research.

Abbreviations

CAT: Computerized Adaptive Test; CI: Confidence Intervals; ES: Cohen Effect Size; IRT: Item Response Theory; OA: Osteoarthritis; OA-CAT FD: Osteoarthritis Computerized Adaptive Test Functional Difficulty; PRO: Patient Reported Outcome; PROMIS® PF CAT: Patient Reported Outcomes Measurement Information System Physical Function scale; SD: Standard Deviation; SF-36: Short Form Health Survey; WOMAC: Western Ontario and McMaster Universities Osteoarthritis Index

Acknowledgements

Not applicable

Funding

ENACT/NIDILRR Grant number: HHS90RT5009
Boston ROC/MRRIN Grant number: 5R24HD065688-05
NIDILRR ARRT Grant number: H113P120001

Authors' contributions

FC analyzed and interpreted the data for both measures and was a major contributor to the manuscript. AJ provided measurement expertise, oversaw analysis design, and edited the manuscript. MS provided measurement and study design expertise and wrote sections of the manuscript and edited the full manuscript. KB oversaw data collection, database development and contributed to the manuscript. PN developed the statistical analysis approach and interpreted the results. JK provided expertise on study design and wrote sections of the manuscript and edited the full manuscript. All authors read and approved the final manuscript.

Consent for publication

Not applicable

Competing interests

The authors declare that they have no competing interests.

Author details

[1]Graduate Institute of Injury Prevention and Control, College of Public Health, Taipei Medical University, 250 Wu-Hsing Street, Taipei City 11031, Taiwan. [2]MGH Institute of Health Professions, 36 1st Avenue, Charlestown Navy Yard, Boston, MA 02129-4557, USA. [3]Health Law, Policy and Management, Boston University School of Public Health, 715 Albany St., 5th floor West, Boston, MA 02118, USA. [4]Boston University College of Health and Rehabilitation Sciences: Sargent College, Boston, USA. [5]Health Law, Policy and Management, Boston University School of Public Health, 715 Albany St., 5th floor West, Boston, MA 02118, USA. [6]MGH Institute of Health Professions, Department of Physical Therapy, 36 1st Avenue, Boston, MA 02129, USA.

References

1. Veenhof C, Bijlsma JW, van den Ende CH, van Dijk GM, Pisters MF, Dekker J. Psychometric evaluation of osteoarthritis questionnaires: a systematic review of the literature. Arthritis Rheum. 2006;55(3):480–92.
2. Rat AC, Coste J, Pouchot J, Baumann M, Spitz E, Retel-Rude N, Le Quintrec JS, Dumont-Fischer D, Guillemin F. OAKHQOL: a new instrument to measure quality of life in knee and hip osteoarthritis. J Clin Epidemiol. 2005;58(1):47–55.
3. Bruce B, Fries JF. The Stanford health assessment Questionnaire: a review of its history, issues, progress, and documentation. J Rheumatol. 2003;30(1): 167–78.
4. Fries JF, Spitz P, Kraines RG, Holman HR. Measurement of patient outcome in arthritis. Arthritis & Rheumatism. 1980;23(2):137–45.
5. Ware JE Jr. Conceptualization and measurement of health-related quality of life: comments on an evolving field. Arch Phys Med Rehabil. 2003;84(4 Suppl 2):S43–51.
6. Wolfe F, Michaud K, Pincus T. Development and validation of the health assessment questionnaire II: a revised version of the health assessment questionnaire. Arthritis Rheum. 2004;50(10):3296–305.
7. McHorney CA. Generic health measurement: past accomplishments and a measurement paradigm for the 21st century. Ann Intern Med. 1997;127(8 Pt 2):743–50.
8. Backman CL. Outcome measures for arthritis care research: recommendations from the CARE III conference. J Rheumatol. 2006;33(9):1908–11.
9. Rubenach S, Shadbolt B, McCallum J, Nakamura T. Assessing health-related quality of life following myocardial infarction: is the SF-12 useful? J Clin Epidemiol. 2002;55(3):306–9.
10. Beaton DE, Richards RR. Measuring function of the shoulder. A cross-sectional comparison of five questionnaires. J Bone Joint SurgAm Vol. 1996; 78(6):882–90.
11. Chen AL, Broadhead WE, Doe EA, Broyles WK. Patient acceptance of two health status measures: the medical outcomes study short-form general health survey and the Duke health profile. Fam Med. 1993; 25(8):536–9.

12. CA MH, Earl Bricker D Jr. A qualitative study of patients' and physicians' views about practice-based functional health assessment. Med Care. 2002; 40(11):1113–25.
13. Hambleton RK. Emergence of item response modeling in instrument development and data analysis. Med Care. 2000;38(9 Suppl):II60–5.
14. Wainer H. Computerized adaptive testing: a primer. Mahwah: Lawrence Erlbaum Associates; 2000.
15. Jette AM, Haley SM. Contemporary measurement techniques for rehabilitation outcomes assessment. J Rehabil Med. 2005;37(6):339–45.
16. Jette AM, CM MD, Haley SM, Ni P, Olarsch S, Latham N, Hambleton RK, Felson D, Kim YJ, Hunter D. A computer-adaptive disability instrument for lower extremity osteoarthritis research demonstrated promising breadth, precision, and reliability. J Clin Epidemiol. 2009;62(8):807–15.
17. Jette AM, McDonough CM, Ni P, Haley SM, Hambleton RK, Olarsch S, Hunter DJ, Kim YJ, Felson DT. A functional difficulty and functional pain instrument for hip and knee osteoarthritis. Arthritis Res Therapy. 2009;11(4):R107.
18. Fries JF, Bruce B, Bjorner J, Rose M: More relevant, precise, and efficient items for assessment of physical function and disability: moving beyond the classic instruments. Ann Rheum Dis 2006, 65 Suppl 3(Journal Article):iii16–21.
19. Cella D, Riley W, Stone A, Rothrock N, Reeve B, Yount S, Amtmann D, Bode R, Buysse D, Choi S, et al. The patient-reported outcomes measurement information system (PROMIS) developed and tested its first wave of adult self-reported health outcome item banks: 2005-2008. J Clin Epidemiol. 2010; 63(11):1179–94.
20. Cella D, Yount S, Rothrock N, Gershon R, Cook K, Reeve B, Ader D, Fries JF, Bruce B, Rose M, et al. The patient-reported outcomes measurement information system (PROMIS): progress of an NIH roadmap cooperative group during its first two years. Med Care. 2007;45(5 Suppl 1):S3–S11.
21. Rose M, Bjorner JB, Gandek B, Bruce B, Fries JF, Ware JE. The PROMIS physical function item bank was calibrated to a standardized metric and shown to improve measurement efficiency. J Clin Epidemiol. 2014;67(5): 516–26.
22. Bjorner JB, Chang CH, Thissen D, Reeve BB. Developing tailored instruments: item banking and computerized adaptive assessment. Qual Life Res. 2007; 16(Suppl 1):95–108.
23. Randall DP, Jennifer MB. Applying a weighted maximum Likelihood Latent Trait Estimator to the Generalized Partial Credit Model. Appl Psychol Meas. 2005;29(3):218–33.
24. Warm TA. Weighted likelihood estimation of ability in item response theory. Psychometrika. 1989;54(3):427–50.
25. Kazis LE, Anderson JJ, Meenan RF. Effect sizes for interpreting changes in health status. Med Care. 1989;27(3 Suppl):S178–89.
26. Haley SM, Fragala-Pinkham MA. Interpreting change scores of tests and measures used in physical therapy. Phys Ther. 2006;86(5):735–43.
27. Cohen J: Statistical Power Analysis. Current Directions in Psychological Sciences, 1, 98–101. In.; 1992.
28. Driban JB, Morgan N, Price LL, Cook KF, Wang C. Patient-reported outcomes measurement information system (PROMIS) instruments among individuals with symptomatic knee osteoarthritis: a cross-sectional study of floor/ceiling effects and construct validity. BMC Musculoskelet Disord. 2015;16(1):253.
29. PHYSICAL FUNCTION: A brief guide to the PROMIS Physical Function instruments. https://www.assessmentcenter.net/documents/PROMIS%20Physical%20Function%20Scoring%20Manual.pdf. Accessed 18 Jan 2018.
30. French HP Fitzpatrick M, FitzGerald O: Responsiveness of physical function outcomes following physiotherapy intervention for osteoarthritsi of the knee: an outcome comparison study. Physiotherapy 2011, 97(4):302-308.
31. Spadoni GF, Stratford PW, Solomon PE, Wishart LR. The evaluation of change in pain intensity: a comparison of the P4 and single-item numeric pain rating scales. J Orthop Sports Phys Ther. 2004;34(4):187–93.
32. Engström CP, Persson LO, Larsson S, Sullivan M. Health-related quality of life in COPD: why both disease-specific and generic measures should be used. Eur Respir J. 2001;18(1):69–76.
33. Juhl C, Lund H, Roos EM, Zhang W, Christensen R. A hierarchy of patient-reported outcomes for meta-analysis of knee osteoarthritis trials: empirical evidence from a survey of high impact journals. Arthritis. 2012;2012:136245. http://dx.doi.org/10.1155/2012/136245. Epub 2012 Jun 26.

4

Efficacy of nerve growth factor antibody in a knee osteoarthritis pain model in mice

Masayuki Miyagi[1*], Tetsuhiro Ishikawa[2], Hiroto Kamoda[2], Miyako Suzuki[2], Gen Inoue[1], Yoshihiro Sakuma[2], Yasuhiro Oikawa[2], Sumihisa Orita[2], Kentaro Uchida[1], Kazuhisa Takahashi[2], Masashi Takaso[1] and Seiji Ohtori[2]

Abstract

Background: Nerve growth factor (NGF) is not only an important factor in nerve growth but also a major contributor to the production of inflammation. It has been reported that inhibiting NGF could reduce several types of pain in several animal models. Here, we aimed to clarify the efficacy of NGF antibody in a knee osteoarthritis (OA) pain model in mice.

Method: Six-week-old male C57BR/J mice were used ($n = 30$). Ten mice comprised the control group, which received saline injection into the right knee joints; the other 20 mice comprised the experimental group, which received monoiodoacetate (MIA) injection into the right knee joints. Three weeks after surgery, the 20 experimental mice were randomly placed into treatment groups which received either sterile saline (non-treat group: 10 mg/kg, i.p.) or an anti-NGF antibody (anti-NGF group: 10 mg/kg, i.p.). Simultaneously, all mice received fluorogold (FG) retrograde neurotracer injection into their right joints. In a behavioral study, we evaluated gait using the CatWalk quantitative gait analysis system before surgery, 3 weeks after surgery (before treatment), 4 weeks after surgery (one week after surgery), and 5 weeks after surgery (2 weeks after surgery). In immunohistochemical analysis, the right dorsal root ganglia (DRGs) from the L4–L6 levels were resected 5 weeks after surgery (2 weeks after surgery). They were immunostained for calcitonin gene-related peptide (CGRP), and the number of FG-labeled or CGRP-immunoreactive (IR) DRG neurons was counted.

Results: On gait analysis using the CatWalk system, duty cycle, swing speed, and print area were decreased in non-treat group compared with those in control group and improved in the anti-NGF group compared with those in non-treat group. CGRP expression in DRGs was up-regulated in non-treat group compared with that in control group and suppressed in the anti-NGF group compared with that in non-treat group (both $p < 0.05$).

Conclusions: MIA injection into the knee joint induced gait impairment and the up-regulation of CGRP in DRG neurons in a knee OA pain model in mice. Intraperitoneal injection of anti-NGF antibody suppressed this impairment of gait and up-regulation of CGRP in DRG neurons. These finding suggest that anti-NGF therapy might be valuable in the treatment of OA pain in the knee.

Keywords: Nerve growth factor, Anti-nerve growth factor therapy, Knee osteoarthritis, Monoiodoacetate, CatWalk, Calcitonin gene-related peptide, Dorsal root ganglia

* Correspondence: masayuki008@aol.com
[1]Department of Orthopaedic Surgery, Kitasato University, School of Medicine, 1-15-1, Kitasato, Minami-ku, Sagamihara city, Kanagawa 252-0374, Japan
Full list of author information is available at the end of the article

Background

Knee osteoarthritis (OA) is a common chronic degenerative disease characterized by degeneration of articular cartilage components, synovitis, remodeling of subchondral bone and atrophy of joint muscles. Knee OA patients usually suffer from knee pain and are treated with several treatment modes, including medication, intraarticular injection of hyaluronic acid, and surgery [1]. Understanding of the mechanism of knee OA pain is incomplete, and medication for knee OA pain were sometimes insufficient.

As part of studies into new targets of knee OA pain, we have focused on pain-related molecules, including nerve growth factor (NGF) [2]. NGF not only plays an important role in the maintenance and development of the sensory nervous system [3] but is also a major contributor to inflammation and nociception [4]. Lewin et al. reported that the systemic injection of NGF induced thermal and mechanical hyperalgesia [5]. In addition, systemic injection of anti-NGF antibody reduced allodynia and hyperalgesia in animal models of neuropathic pain, including nerve trunk or spinal nerve ligation [6–8].

Basic research into knee OA has been aided by the development of several animal models, including the anterior cruciate ligament transection model [9], destabilization of the medial meniscus model [10], the rat medical meniscal tear model [11], GDF5 deficiency mice [12], and monoiodoacetate (MIA) injection model [13–16]. The MIA injection model has been reported to result in progressive joint damage, with some features that may be considered similar to OA [14–16] and significant pain-related behavior [13, 16]. The MIA injection model is superior for evaluating knee pain; although it seems animal models including the medical meniscus model better approximate the anatomic pathology found in OA in humans. Some of these previous reports evaluated pain-related behavior using the von Frey test, which is for evaluation of mechanical allodynia. Clinically, however, knee OA patients suffer from knee pain that includes gait impairment but not mechanical allodynia. Several authors have evaluated knee pain behavior using weight bearing assays [17–20]. For instance, the CatWalk gait analysis system can provide quantitative assessment of gait and motor function in rats and mice. This system has recently been used to assay impaired gait function in knee OA pain models [17–19]. Regarding the pathological mechanism of knee OA pain, our previous immunohistochemical analysis showed that the expression of pain-related molecules in the sensory nervous system was increased in a knee OA pain model [16]. Thus, this finding demonstrated the upregulation of pain-related molecules in the sensory nervous system in the pain state.

We therefore hypothesized that anti-NGF therapy was effective for knee pain in a mouse model of knee OA. The aim of the current study is to evaluate the efficacy of NGF antibody in a knee OA pain model using the CatWalk gait analysis system and immunohistochemical analysis of the sensory nervous system in mice.

Method

Knee osteoarthritis pain model

Thirty 8-week-old male C57 BL/6 mice were used. (Control group: n = 10, Monoiodeacete (MIA) without treatment (non-treat) group: n = 10, and MIA + anti-NGF therapy (anti-NGF) group: n = 10) Animals were anesthetized with sodium pentobarbital (40 mg/kg, intraperitoneal) and treated aseptically throughout the experiments. In the non-treatment group and anti-NGF group, the right knees were treated with a single intraarticular injection of 0.2 mg of MIA (Sigma-Aldrich, St. Louis, MO) in 10 μl of sterile saline. The solution was injected through the patellar ligament by using a 27G needle with the leg flexed at a 90 degrees angle at the knee as described previously [16]. Three weeks after surgery, mice were randomly assigned to treatment groups receiving either sterile saline (10 mg/kg, i.p.) (non-treat group) or an anti-NGF antibody (L148 M; Exalpha Biological Inc., Shirley, MA) (10 mg/kg, i.p.) (anti-NGF group). We have previously confirmed this medication's efficacy for treating neuropathic pain [2]. Simultaneously, to detect dorsal root ganglia (DRG) neurons innervating the right knee joint, the right knees of all 20 animals were treated with intraarticular injection of 2% retrograde neurotracer FG (Fluorochrome, Denver, CO) as we have previously described [16]. The control group was treated with a single intraarticular injection of 10 μl of sterile saline to the right knee, followed three weeks later by intraarticular injection of 2% retrograde neurotracer FG.

Behavioral evaluation (gait analysis)

Gait was analysed in detail using the CatWalk system (Noldus Information Technology, Wageningen, The Netherlands). This system has been described in detail elsewhere [19]. Briefly, mice are placed on a glass plate located in a darkened room and allowed to walk freely. A light beam from a fluorescent lamp is aimed through the glass plate. The light beams are completely reflected internally. However, when a paw touches the glass plate, the light beams are reflected downwards. This results in a sharp bright image of the paw print. The entire run is recorded with a video camera. The data are acquired, compressed, and analyzed using CatWalk software as described previously [21].

Before surgery and 3 (before treatment; pre-treat) 4, or 5 weeks (1 or 2 weeks after treatment, respectively; treat-1w or treat-2w) after surgery, all mice were walked on the glass plate three times. The gait of all mice was recorded three times and analyzed using the CatWalk system. We compared the ratio of movement of the ipsi and contralateral hind paws with regard to three variables, namely duty cycle (standing as a percentage of the step cycle: stand/(stand time + swing time) × 100%); swing speed (speed of the paw during swing: stride length/swing time); and print area (surface area of the complete print) among the three groups.

Immunohistochemical analysis

All procedure, including anesthetization, perfusion, sectioning, immunostaining and the observation and evaluation of immunoreactive neurons, were used the same manner as discribed previously [21, 22].

In all three groups, four (n = 5, each) or five (n = 5, each) weeks after surgery (one or two weeks after treatment), mice were anesthetized with sodium pentobarbital (40 mg/kg, intraperitoneal) and perfused transcardially with 0.9% saline, followed by 30 mL of 4% paraformaldehyde in phosphate buffer (0.1 M, pH 7.4). Next, the right DRGs from the L3 to L5 levels were resected and the specimens were immersed in the same fixative solution overnight at 4 °C, and then stored in 0.01 M phosphate-buffered saline (PBS) containing 20% sucrose for 20 h at 4 °C.

For DRGs, each ganglion was sectioned at a 10 μm thickness on a cryostat and mounted on POLY-L-LYSINE-coated slides. Endogenous tissue peroxidase activity was quenched by soaking sections in 0.3% hydrogen peroxide solution in 0.01 M PBS for 30 min. Specimens were then treated for 90 min at room temperature in blocking solution consisting of 0.01 M PBS containing 0.3% Triton X-100 and 3% skim milk. To evaluate the expression of neuropeptides in DRGs, the sections were processed for CGRP immunohistochemistry using a rabbit antibody to CGRP (1:1000; Chemicon, Temecula, CA) diluted in blocking solution, and incubated for 20 h at 4 °C. To detect CGRP in the DRGs, sections were incubated for 3 h with goat antirabbit Alexa 488 fluorescent antibody conjugate (1:400; Molecular Probes, Eugene, OR).

Thirty sections in each group (two sections per each DRG (L3, L4, L5) in 5 animals) were examined using a fluorescence microscope. For each DRG section, we counted the number of all Fluoro-Gold-labeled neurons and the number of Fluoro-Gold-labeled and CGRP-immunoreactive (IR) neurons per 0.45 mm^2 in 10 randomly-selected fields among 30 sections in each group at ×400 magnification using a counting grid, as we have previously reported [16]. The proportion of FG-labeled and CGRP-IR DRG neurons among all FG-labeled neurons was then calculated. All FG-labeled neurons indicated neurons innervating the right knee joint, while FG-labeled and CGRP-IR neurons indicated pain-related neurons innervating the right knee joint.

Statistical analysis

Using the ratio of ipsi and contralateral hind paw values for the three CatWalk variables of duty cycle, swing speed, and print area, the proportion of FG-labeled and CGRP-IR DRG neurons among all FG-labeled DRG neurons was compared among the three groups using a non-repeated measures ANOVA with Bonferroni's correction. A p-value less than 0.05 was considered statistically significant.

Results

Behavioral analysis

In the non-treatment group, the ratio of ipsi to contralateral hind paw values for duty cycle was significantly decreased at pre-treat, treat-1w, and treat-2w compared with that in control group. ($p < 0.05$) In contrast, in the anti-NGF group, the ratio of ipsi to contralateral hind paws values for duty cycle were significantly decreased only at pre-treat ($p < 0.05$) compared with that in control group, and not at treat-1w and treat-2w ($p > 0.05$). In addition, the ratio in the anti-NGF group was significantly improved at treat-1w compared with that in the non-treat group. ($p < 0.05$) (Fig. 1).

In the non-treated group, the ratio of ipsi to contralateral hind paw values for swing speed were significantly decreased at pre-treat, treat-1w, and treat-2w compared with that in the control group. ($p < 0.05$) In contrast, in the anti-NGF group, this ratio was significantly decreased only at pre-treat ($p < 0.05$) compared with that

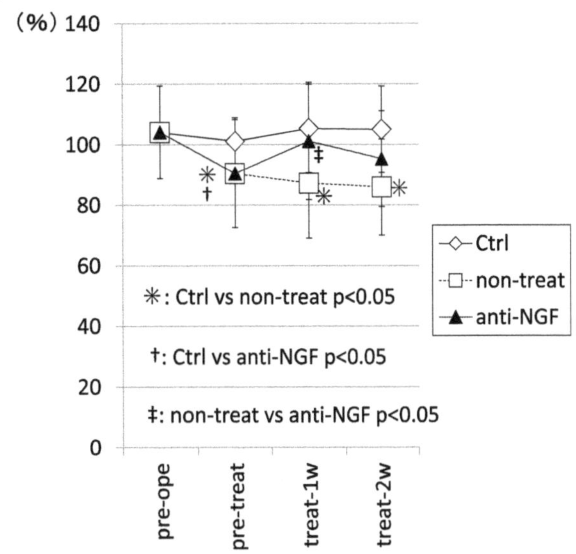

Fig. 1 Ratio of ipsi and contralateral hind paw values of the duty cycle from the CatWalk system. ($p < 0.05$, compared among 3 groups using with a non-repeated measures ANOVA with Bonferroni's *post-hoc* correction.). MIA injection of the knee joint induced a significant small duty cycle within 5 weeks after injection. In contrast, systemic injection of anti-NGF antibody induced significant improvement after only one week of treatment

in control group, and not at treat-1w and treat-2w ($p > 0.05$). In addition, this ratio in the anti-NGF group was significantly improved at treat-1w compared with that in the non-treat group. ($p < 0.05$) (Fig. 2).

In the non-treated group, the ratio of ipsi and contralateral hind paw values for print area were significantly decreased at pre-treat, treat-1w, and treat-2w compared with that in control group. ($p < 0.05$) In contrast, in the anti-NGF group, this ratio was significantly decreased only at pre-treat ($p < 0.05$) compared with that in control group, and not at treat-1w and treat-2w ($p > 0.05$). In addition, the ratio in the anti-NGF group was significantly improved at treat-1w and treat-2w compared with that in the non-treat group. ($p < 0.05$) (Fig. 3).

Immunohistochemical analysis

FG-labeled DRG neurons, which indicated where FG was transported from the right knee, were present in the right L3 to L5 DRGs in all 3 groups (Fig. 4).

The proportion of FG-labeled/CGRP-IR neurons among all FG-labeled neurons was significantly increased in the non-treated group at treat-1w and treat-2w compared with that in control group. ($p < 0.05$) Conversely, the expression of CGRP was significantly decreased in the anti-NGF group at treat-1w and treat-2w compared with the non-treated group ($p < 0.05$). (Figs. 4 and 5).

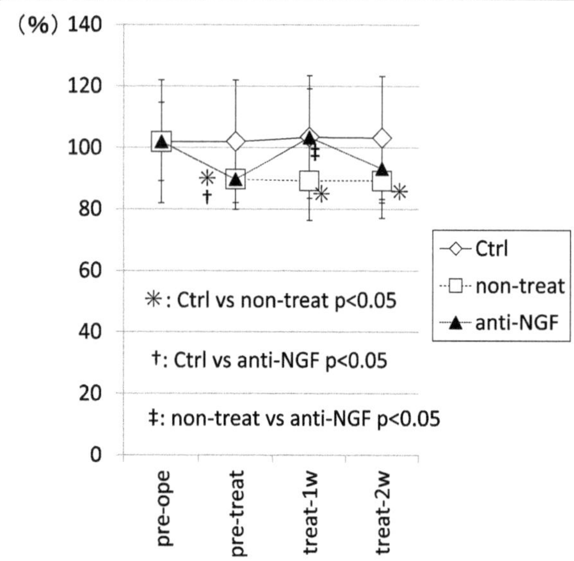

Fig. 2 The ratio of ipsi and contralateral hind paw values for swing speed from the CatWalk system. ($p < 0.05$, compared among 3 groups using with a non-repeated measures ANOVA with Bonferroni's *post-hoc* correction.). MIA injection of the knee joint induced a significant small swing speed within 5 weeks after injection. In contrast, systemic injection of anti-NGF antibody induced significant improvement after only one week of treatment

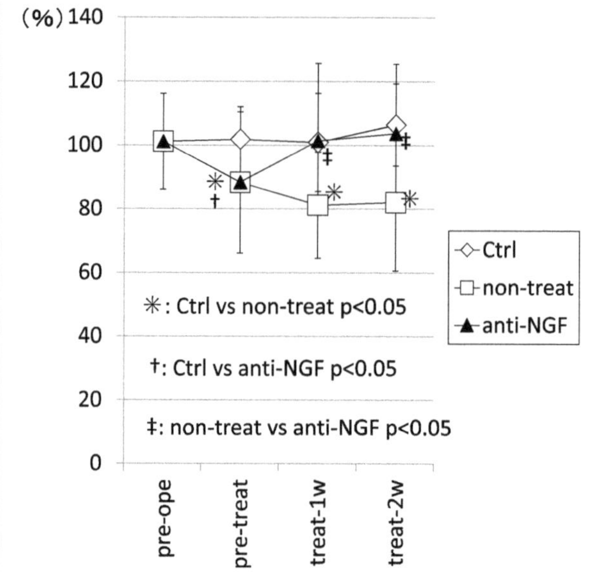

Fig. 3 The ratio of ipsi and contralateral hind paw values of print area from the CatWalk system. ($p < 0.05$, compared among 3 groups using with a non-repeated measures ANOVA with Bonferroni's *post-hoc* correction.). MIA injection of the knee joint induced a significant small print area within 5 weeks after injection. In contrast, systemic injection of anti-NGF antibody induced significant improvement after only 2 weeks of treatment

Discussion

In this study, intraarticular injection of MIA to the knee joints induced gait disturbances, including a small duty cycle, small swing speed, and small print area, and the up-regulation of neuropeptides in DRG neurons innervating the knee joints. Systemic injection of anti-NGF antibody improved these gait disturbances and the expression of neuropeptides in DRG neurons in this model.

Regarding the Knee OA model, multiple authors have reported various surgery-induced animal models. Myers et al. reported that anterior cruciate ligament transection induced changes in the articular cartilage of the unstable knee that are consistent with OA [23]. In addition, Marijnissen et al. reported the usability of the "Groove" model, in which knee articular cartilage is damaged as a knee OA model [24]. Further, Bendele AM report that medial meniscal tear in rats results in rapidly progressive degenerative changes to the cartilage with similarities to OA [11]. These surgically induced knee OA models are suitable for basic research, to the extent that they simulate clinical situations. Nevertheless, the MIA injection model which results in severe joint damage seems superior for evaluating knee pain. MIA injection to the knee joints has been reported to cause joint pathology via the inhibition of glycolysis, and thereby targets avascular cartilage and causes chondrocyte death [25]. We also previously reported that MIA-treated knees exhibited behavioral disturbances within four days and osteoarthritic histological

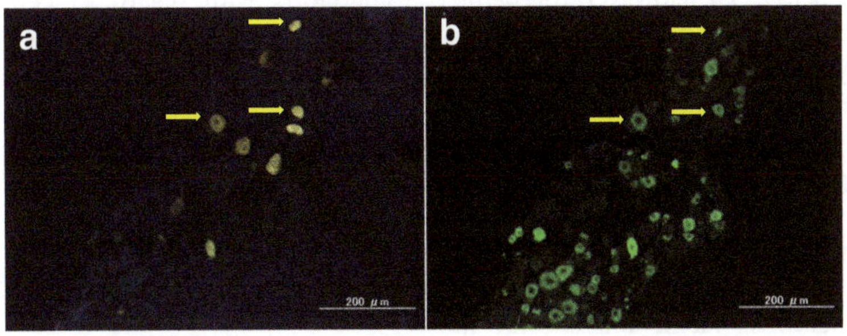

Fig. 4 Representative FG-labeled (**a**) and CGRP-IR (**b**) DRG neurons. **a** and **b** are the same section. The arrow indicates FG- and CGRP-double labeled DRG neurons

changes within four weeks [16]. We therefore used the MIA injection model as a knee OA model in this study.

Regarding knee pain behavior, several authors reported that knee pain models exhibited mechanical allodynia using the von Frey test [13, 16]. In addition, Shelton DL et al. report NGF induced mechanical allodynia in autoimmune arthritis [26]. Therefore, evaluating knee pain using the von Frey test seems to be appropriate for basic research using animal models. However, there is doubt about whether these models of knee pain simulate clinical situations, because knee OA patients do not typically complain of mechanical allodynia in their foot. Recently, gait analysis studies have focused on behavioral studies to evaluate pain behavior. The CatWalk system was initially developed to evaluate motor function, such as that modified in a spinal cord injury model, a Parkinson's disease model, or an olivocerebellar degeneration model [19, 27–29]. Recently, this system has been applied to various models to evaluate behavior associated with pain, such as mechanical allodynia models [30]. We also previously evaluated low back pain behavior using the CatWalk system, and concluded that rat models of low back pain exhibit changes in rat gait, including a long standing time and short strides [21, 31]. Recently several authors applied the CatWalk system to evaluate behavior associated with knee pain. Ferland et al. reported that the MIA-induced knee pain model shows gait changes, including a short Duty cycle and a small Swing Speed. In our previous preliminary study, the MIA-induced knee pain model exhibited a small duty cycle, small swing speed, and small print area. (un-published date) Therefore, in this study, we compared the ratio of ipsi and contralateral hind paw values for the three variables, namely duty cycle, swing speed, and print area among the three groups to evaluate the effect of anti-NGF therapy.

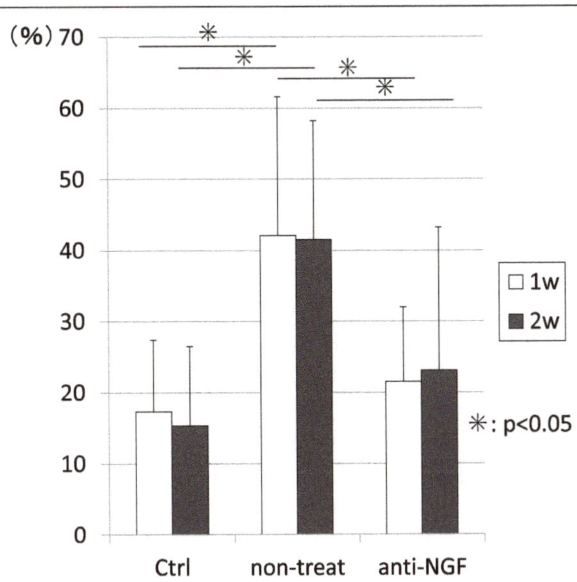

Fig. 5 Percentages of FG and CGRP double labeling of DRGneurons among all FG labeled DRG neurons. (**p* < 0.05, compared among the three groups using a non-repeated measures ANOVA with Bonferroni's *post-hoc* correction)

Regarding the up-regulation of CGRP in the sensory nervous system, we previously evaluated potential pain-like states by evaluating the up-regulation of pain-related neuropeptides such as CGRP and substance P in the sensory nervous system using a combination of immunohistochemistry and retrograde tracing instead of evaluating pain behavior [22]. CGRP-IR DRG neurons have been reported to be NGF-dependent DRG neurons involved in pain perception related to inflammation [32], suggesting that CGRP is a marker of inflammatory pain. We previously reported that MIA injection to the knee joint induced the up-regulation of CGRP in DRGs [16]. These results suggest that the animals in the group receiving MIA injection to their knee joints were in a state of knee pain.

We focused on NGF as target for the treatment for knee OA pain based on our previous report that MIA injection induced the up-regulation not only inflammatory cytokines but also NGF in the knee joints [16]. Regarding the efficacy of anti-NGF therapy for knee OA pain, NGF is generally involved in chronic inflammatory or neuropathic pain states [33]. Several basic and clinical research had been reported the efficacy of anti-NGF therapy for knee OA pain [34, 35]. However, the pathological mechanism of knee OA pain was not fully understood. NGF is physically produced in articular structures and expressed in both normal and OA synovial tissues, but is increased in synovial inflammation, especially upon synovial tissue exposure to inflammatory cytokines including TNF-alpha [36, 37]. Thus, the up-regulation of inflammatory cytokines in OA knee joints promoted NGF production, which induced the up-regulation of CGRP in the sensory nervous system and chronic inflammatory or neuropathic pain states. Ashraf S et al. report that NGF injection into knee OA joints results in gait disturbance as compared to NGF injection into non-OA joints. This group used two models of knee OA, including an MIA injection model and a meniscal transection model [38]. Further, McNamee KE et al. report NGF expression is correlated with knee pain but that TNF alpha is not up-regulated in the late stages of OA [39]. These findings indicate inflammatory cytokines including TNF might only develop during the pain state, but that NGF might play a role in maintaining as well as in development of the pain state in knee OA patients. Therefore, NGF represents a possible important therapeutic target in the treatment of knee OA pain. In preclinical studies, newly developed tanezumab and its murine precursor muMab-911 have effectively targeted the NGF pathway in various chronic and inflammatory pain models [40]. In addition, phase I and II clinical trials for osteoarthritic pain and chronic lower back pain have demonstrated efficacy for the compound, as well as a good safety and tolerability profile [41]. In the present study, anti-NGF therapy suppressed the impairment gait and up-regulation of CGRP in DRG neurons. These findings may explain the pathological mechanism of knee OA pain.

There were some limitations in this study. First, we should have used tanezumab and its murine precursor muMab-911 for this study. We also did not evaluate differences in efficacy between muMab-911 and anti-NGF antibody, which we used in this study. Second, we did not evaluate the efficacy of positive control including non-steroid anti-inflammatory drugs for knee OA pain. Third, we also evaluated the efficacy of only a one-time injection of anti-NGF antibody. In the future, it will be necessary to evaluate the effect of repeated injections for knee pain. Fourth, we did not evaluate the histopathology of the knee joint. In clinical trials of the monoclonal NGF antibody tanezumab for knee and hip OA pain, osteonecrosis was reported as a side effect [42]. Therefore, further study focusing on side effects of anti-NGF therapy is necessary. Fifth, we did not include a power calculation to justify the group sizes. Further, due to ethical concerns related to using the animals, we combined our behavioral and immunohistochemical evaluations. Therefore, with regard to behavioral evaluation, some experiments ended after 4 weeks and others ended after 5 weeks.

Conclusions

MIA injection into the knee joint induced gait impairment and the up-regulation of CGRP in DRG neurons in a knee OA pain model in mice. Further, intraperitoneal injection of anti-NGF antibody suppressed gait impairment and the up-regulation of CGRP in DRG neurons. These finding indicate that anti-NGF therapy might be valuable in the treatment of OA pain in the knee.

Abbreviations

CGRP: Calcitonin gene related peptide; DRG: dorsal root ganglion; FG: FluoroGold; IR: immunoreactive; MIA: monoiodeacetate; NGF: nerve growth factor; OA: osteoarthritis

Acknowledgments

Not applicable.

Funding

MM was supported by Mitsui Sumitomo Insurance Welfare Foundation.

Authors' contributions

MM conceived this study and carried out the behavioral studies and immunohistochemical studies, participated in its design and coordination and drafted the manuscript, TI carried out behavioral studies and immunohistochemical studies and drafted the manuscript, HK MS and GI made animal models and helped to revise the manuscript, YS, YO, SO carried out behavioral studies and participated in the design of the study, KU carried out statistical analysis and revised the manuscript, KT and MT participated in the design of the study and SO conceived the study and participated in its design and coordination. All authors have read and approved the final manuscript.

Consent for publication

Not applicable.

Competing interests

This work was supported by Mitsui Sumitomo Insurance Welfare Foundation. The authors declare that they have no competing interests.

Author details

[1] Department of Orthopaedic Surgery, Kitasato University, School of Medicine, 1-15-1, Kitasato, Minami-ku, Sagamihara city, Kanagawa 252-0374, Japan.

[2]Department of Orthopaedic Surgery, Graduate School of Medicine, Chiba University, Chiba, Japan.

References

1. Vaishya R, Pariyo GB, Agarwal AK, Vijay V. Non-operative management of osteoarthritis of the knee joint. J Clin. Orthop Trauma. 2016;7(3):170–6.
2. Miyagi M, Ishikawa T, Kamoda H, Suzuki M, Inoue G, Sakuma Y, Oikawa Y, Uchida K, Suzuki T, Takahashi K, Takaso M, Ohtori S. The efficacy of nerve growth factor antibody in a mouse model of neuropathic cancer pain. Exp. Anim 2016; 65 (4):337-343.
3. Mendell LM. Neurotrophins and sensory neurons: role in development, maintenance and injury. A thematic summary. Philos.Trans.R.Soc.Lond B Biol. Sci. 1996;351(1338):463–7.
4. Lewin GR, Mendell LM. Nerve growth factor and nociception. Trends Neurosci. 1993;16(9):353–9.
5. Lewin GR, Rueff A, Mendell LM. Peripheral and central mechanisms of NGF-induced hyperalgesia. EurJ Neurosci. 1994;6(12):1903–12.
6. Ramer MS, Bisby MA. Adrenergic innervation of rat sensory ganglia following proximal or distal painful sciatic neuropathy: distinct mechanisms revealed by anti-NGF treatment. Eur. J Neurosci. 1999;11(3):837–46.
7. Ro LS, Chen ST, Tang LM, Jacobs JM. Effect of NGF and anti-NGF on neuropathic pain in rats following chronic constriction injury of the sciatic nerve. Pain. 1999;79(2–3):265–74.
8. Wild KD, Bian D, Zhu D, Davis J, Bannon AW, Zhang TJ, Louis JC. Antibodies to nerve growth factor reverse established tactile allodynia in rodent models of neuropathic pain without tolerance. J Pharmacol.Exp.Ther. 2007; 322(1):282–7.
9. Ochiai N, Ohtori S, Sasho T, Nakagawa K, Takahashi K, Takahashi N, Murata R, Takahashi K, Moriya H, Wada Y, Saisu T. Extracorporeal shock wave therapy improves motor dysfunction and pain originating from knee osteoarthritis in rats. Osteoarthritis. Cartilage. 2007;15(9):1093–6.
10. Muramatsu Y, Sasho T, Saito M, Yamaguchi S, Akagi R, Mukoyama S, Akatsu Y, Katsuragi J, Fukawa T, Endo J, Hoshi H, Yamamoto Y, Takahashi K. Preventive effects of hyaluronan from deterioration of gait parameters in surgically induced mice osteoarthritic knee model. Osteoarthritis. Cartilage. 2014;22(6):831–5.
11. Bendele AM. Animal models of osteoarthritis. J Musculoskelet. Neuronal. Interact. 2001;1(4):363–76.
12. Daans M, Luyten FP, Lories RJ. GDF5 deficiency in mice is associated with instability-driven joint damage, gait and subchondral bone changes. Ann. Rheum.Dis. 2011;70(1):208–13.
13. Combe R, Bramwell S, Field MJ. The monosodium iodoacetate model of osteoarthritis: a model of chronic nociceptive pain in rats? Neurosci.Lett. 2004;370(2–3):236–40.
14. Guingamp C, Gegout-Pottie P, Philippe L, Terlain B, Netter P, Gillet P. Mono-iodoacetate-induced experimental osteoarthritis: a dose-response study of loss of mobility, morphology, and biochemistry. Arthritis Rheum. 1997;40(9): 1670–9.
15. Guzman RE, Evans MG, Bove S, Morenko B, Kilgore K. Mono-iodoacetate-induced histologic changes in subchondral bone and articular cartilage of rat femorotibial joints: an animal model of osteoarthritis. Toxicol.Pathol. 2003;31(6):619–24.
16. Orita S, Ishikawa T, Miyagi M, Ochiai N, Inoue G, Eguchi Y, Kamoda H, Arai G, Toyone T, Aoki Y, Kubo T, Takahashi K, Ohtori S. Pain-related sensory innervation in monoiodoacetate-induced osteoarthritis in rat knees that gradually develops neuronal injury in addition to inflammatory pain. BMCMusculoskeletDisord. 2011;12:134.
17. Ferland CE, Laverty S, Beaudry F, Vachon P. Gait analysis and pain response of two rodent models of osteoarthritis. Pharmacol.Biochem.Behav. 2011; 97(3):603–10.
18. Ferreira-Gomes J, Adaes S, Castro-Lopes JM. Assessment of movement-evoked pain in osteoarthritis by the knee-bend and CatWalk tests: a clinically relevant study. J Pain. 2008;9(10):945–54.
19. Hamers FP, Lankhorst AJ, van Laar TJ, Veldhuis WB, Gispen WH. Automated quantitative gait analysis during overground locomotion in the rat: its application to spinal cord contusion and transection injuries. J Neurotrauma. 2001;18(2):187–201.
20. Nwosu LN, Mapp PI, Chapman V, Walsh DA. Relationship between structural pathology and pain behaviour in a model of osteoarthritis (OA). Osteoarthritis. Cartilage. 2016;24(11):1910–7.
21. Miyagi M, Ishikawa T, Kamoda H, Orita S, Kuniyoshi K, Ochiai N, Kishida S, Nakamura J, Eguchi Y, Arai G, Suzuki M, Aoki Y, Toyone T, Takahashi K, Inoue G, Ohtori S. Assessment of gait in a rat model of myofascial inflammation using the CatWalk system. Spine (Phila Pa 1976). 2011;36(21):1760–4.
22. Miyagi M, Ishikawa T, Orita S, Eguchi Y, Kamoda H, Arai G, Suzuki M, Inoue G, Aoki Y, Toyone T, Takahashi K, Ohtori S. Disk injury in rats produces persistent increases in pain-related neuropeptides in dorsal root ganglia and spinal cord glia but only transient increases in inflammatory mediators: pathomechanism of chronic diskogenic low back pain. Spine (Phila Pa 1976). 2011;36(26):2260–6.
23. Myers SL, Brandt KD, O'Connor BL, Visco DM, Albrecht ME. Synovitis and osteoarthritic changes in canine articular cartilage after anterior cruciate ligament transection. Effect of surgical hemostasis. Arthritis Rheum. 1990; 33(9):1406–15.
24. Marijnissen AC, van Roermund PM, TeKoppele JM, Bijlsma JW, Lafeber FP. The canine 'groove' model, compared with the ACLT model of osteoarthritis. Osteoarthritis. Cartilage. 2002;10(2):145–55.
25. Janusz MJ, Bendele AM, Brown KK, Taiwo YO, Hsieh L, Heitmeyer SA. Induction of osteoarthritis in the rat by surgical tear of the meniscus: inhibition of joint damage by a matrix metalloproteinase inhibitor. Osteoarthritis. Cartilage. 2002;10(10):785–91.
26. Shelton DL, Zeller J, Ho WH, Pons J, Rosenthal A. Nerve growth factor mediates hyperalgesia and cachexia in auto-immune arthritis. Pain. 2005; 116(1–2):8–16.
27. Cendelin J, Voller J, Vozeh F. Ataxic gait analysis in a mouse model of the olivocerebellar degeneration. Behav. Brain Res. 2010;210(1):8–15.
28. Chuang CS, Su HL, Cheng FC, Hsu SH, Chuang CF, Liu CS. Quantitative evaluation of motor function before and after engraftment of dopaminergic neurons in a rat model of Parkinson's disease. J Biomed.Sci. 2010;17:9.
29. Koopmans GC, Deumens R, Honig WM, Hamers FP, Steinbusch HW, Joosten EA. The assessment of locomotor function in spinal cord injured rats: the importance of objective analysis of coordination. J Neurotrauma. 2005;22(2): 214–25.
30. Vrinten DH, Hamers FF. CatWalk' automated quantitative gait analysis as a novel method to assess mechanical allodynia in the rat; a comparison with von Frey testing. Pain. 2003;102(1–2):203–9.
31. Miyagi M, Ishikawa T, Kamoda H, Suzuki M, Sakuma Y, Orita S, Oikawa Y, Aoki Y, Toyone T, Takahashi K, Inoue G, Ohtori S. Assessment of pain behavior in a rat model of intervertebral disc injury using the CatWalk gait analysis system. Spine (Phila Pa 1976). 2013;38(17):1459–65.
32. Averill S, McMahon SB, Clary DO, Reichardt LF, Priestley JV. Immunocytochemical localization of trkA receptors in chemically identified subgroups of adult rat sensory neurons. Eur. J Neurosci. 1995;7(7):1484–94.
33. Pezet S, McMahon SB. Neurotrophins: mediators and modulators of pain. Annu.Rev.Neurosci. 2006;29:507–38.
34. Ishikawa G, Koya Y, Tanaka H, Nagakura Y. Long-term analgesic effect of a single dose of anti-NGF antibody on pain during motion without notable suppression of joint edema and lesion in a rat model of osteoarthritis. Osteoarthritis. Cartilage. 2015;23(6):925–32.
35. Schnitzer TJ, Marks JAA. Systematic review of the efficacy and general safety of antibodies to NGF in the treatment of OA of the hip or knee. Osteoarthritis. Cartilage. 2015;23(Suppl 1):S8–17.
36. Manni L, Lundeberg T, Fiorito S, Bonini S, Vigneti E, Aloe L. Nerve growth factor release by human synovial fibroblasts prior to and following exposure to tumor necrosis factor-alpha, interleukin-1 beta and cholecystokinin-8: the possible role of NGF in the inflammatory response. Clin.Exp.Rheumatol. 2003;21(5):617–24.
37. Takano S, Uchida K, Miyagi M, Inoue G, Fujimaki H, Aikawa J, Iwase D, Minatani A, Iwabuchi K, Takaso M. Nerve growth factor regulation by TNF-alpha and IL-1beta in synovial macrophages and fibroblasts in osteoarthritic mice. J Immunol Res. 2016;2016:5706359.
38. Ashraf S, Mapp PI, Burston J, Bennett AJ, Chapman V, Walsh DA. Augmented pain behavioural responses to intra-articular injection of nerve growth factor in two animal models of osteoarthritis. Ann.Rheum.Dis. 2014; 73(9):1710–8.
39. McNamee KE, Burleigh A, Gompels LL, Feldmann M, Allen SJ, Williams RO, Dawbarn D, Vincent TL, Inglis JJ. Treatment of murine osteoarthritis with TrkAd5 reveals a pivotal role for nerve growth factor in non-inflammatory joint pain. Pain. 2010;149(2):386–92.
40. Xu L, Nwosu LN, Burston JJ, Millns PJ, Sagar DR, Mapp PI, Meesawatsom P, Li L, Bennett AJ, Walsh DA, Chapman V. The anti-NGF antibody muMab 911

both prevents and reverses pain behaviour and subchondral osteoclast numbers in a rat model of osteoarthritis pain. Osteoarthritis. Cartilage. 2016; 24(9):1587–95.

41. Cattaneo A. Tanezumab, a recombinant humanized mAb against nerve growth factor for the treatment of acute and chronic pain. Curr.Opin.Mol. Ther. 2010;12(1):94–106.
42. Balanescu AR, Feist E, Wolfram G, Davignon I, Smith MD, Brown MT, West CR. Efficacy and safety of tanezumab added on to diclofenac sustained release in patients with knee or hip osteoarthritis: a double-blind, placebo-controlled, parallel-group, multicentre phase III randomised clinical trial. Ann.Rheum.Dis. 2014;73(9):1665–72.

5

Serum and synovial fluid cytokine profiling in hip osteoarthritis: distinct from knee osteoarthritis and correlated with pain

Guomin Ren[1], Ian Lutz[2], Pamela Railton[3], J. Preston Wiley[1,4], Jenelle McAllister[4], James Powell[1,2] and Roman J. Krawetz[1,2,5*]

Abstract

Background: Inflammation is associated with the onset and progression of osteoarthritis in multiple joints. It is well known that mechanical properties differ between different joints, however, it remains unknown if the inflammatory process is similar/distinct in patients with hip vs. knee OA. Without complete understanding of the role of any specific cytokine in the inflammatory process, understanding the 'profile' of inflammation in a given patient population is an essential starting point. The aim of this study was to identify serum cytokine profiles in hip Osteoarthritis (OA), and investigate the association between cytokine concentrations and clinical measurements within this patient population and compare these findings to knee OA and healthy control cohorts.

Methods: In total, 250 serum samples (100 knee OA, 50 hip OA and 100 control) and 37 synovial fluid samples (8 knee OA, 14 hip OA and 15 control) were analyzed using a multiplex ELISA based approach. Synovial biopsies were also obtained and examined for specific cytokines. Pain, physical function and activity within the hip OA cohort were examined using the HOOS, SF-36, HHS and UCLA outcome measures.

Results: The three cohorts showed distinct serum cytokine profiles. EGF, FGF2, MCP3, MIP1α, and IL8 were differentially expressed between hip and knee OA cohorts; while FGF2, GRO, IL8, MCP1, and VEGF were differentially expressed between hip OA and control cohorts. Eotaxin, GRO, MCP1, MIP1β, VEGF were differentially expressed between knee OA and control cohorts. EGF, IL8, MCP1, MIP1β were differentially expressed in synovial fluid from a sub-set of patients from each cohort. Specifically within the hip OA cohort, IL-6, MDC and IP10 were associated with pain and were also found to be present in synovial fluid and synovial membrane (except IL-6) of patients with hip OA.

Conclusion: OA may include different inflammatory subtypes according to affected joints and distinct inflammatory processes may drive OA in these joints. IL6, MDC and IP10 are associated with hip OA pain and these proteins may be able to provide additional information regarding pain in hip OA patients.

Keywords: Osteoarthritis, Inflammation, Pain, Hip

Background

Approximately 1 in 8 individuals are afflicted with Osteoarthritis (OA) and although it is more common in older populations, it is becoming a serious health and economical concern in young, active individuals [1, 2]. Therefore, it is essential to further understand the factors involved in the onset and progression of the disease, so that more efficient diagnostics and treatments can be developed.

While much of the research focus in OA has been directed towards the knee, it is necessary to examine if the pathways and mechanisms in knee OA are conserved in other joints. For example, in the hip, recent literature have provided insight into mechanical causes of hip OA including impingement and dysplasia [3], while others have focused on potential genetic predispositions with or without mechanical risk factors [4]. This suggests that, as

* Correspondence: rkrawetz@ucalgary.ca
[1]McCaig Institute for Bone and Joint Health, Faculty of Medicine, University of Calgary, 3330 Hospital Drive NW, Calgary, Alberta T2N 4N1, Canada
[2]Department of Surgery, University of Calgary, Calgary, Alberta, Canada
Full list of author information is available at the end of the article

in knee OA, there could be potentially many avenues of hip OA onset that eventually result in patients with diverse etiology converging later in the disease trajectory. Our previous work in knee OA looking at systemic and local inflammatory profiles suggests that inflammatory profiles are distinct in patients with knee OA from those without OA [5] and therefore that this approach may be able to discriminate systemic inflammatory differences between patients with knee vs. hip OA.

More generally, there have been a number of studies and many biochemical markers that have been identified in knee OA [6–10]. Historically groups have focused on cartilage metabolism markers including which demonstrate changes in concentration and fragment species with the onset and progression of OA [11–14]. Inflammation is known to be present in OA and the changes in individual inflammatory markers have been correlated with both severity and progression and OA [15, 16]. Regardless of the type of biochemical marker examined however, knee OA and hip OA are almost always grouped together or only one joint is examined within a given study [17]. Most of the common OA biochemical markers (collagen fragments, cartilage oligomeric matrix protein (COMP), etc.) have been tested on both knee and hip cohorts, but only a very few studies looked at both joints and run comparisons [17]. The uncontrolled variances (such as different definition of OA, cohort characteristic, experimental method) across studies make the results almost incomparable. Among the studies that contain both cohorts, the comparisons of biochemical markers between knees and hips are largely ignored [18, 19]. It is well known that mechanical properties differ between joints (knee vs. hip) [20, 21], but as far as we are aware only two studies have directly compared between cohorts of hip and knee OA patients: the effectiveness of bone metabolism for OA prognostic [22] and the difference of association between COMP and OA symptoms [23]. However, neither of them compared the absolute concentration of biochemical markers between two phenotypes.

In addition to biochemical markers, it is also important to gain a better understanding of pain in OA. Pain is the leading disabling symptom of OA [24]. According to the American College of Rheumatology (ACR) criteria for OA, pain is a necessary condition for clinical diagnosis of OA, with the support by other sufficient conditions such as age, radiographic evidences or physical examinations. OA pain is hard to quantify from patient to patient based on a number of confounding factors [25] and its inconsistency with other symptoms such as radiographic findings is not yet well understood. Recent studies have greatly improved our understanding of pain at the molecular level [26], and new biochemical markers have also been reported to be correlated with severity of OA pain in the past decade (Additional file 1: Table S1). Cytokines play an important role in the pain signal pathway from lesions to higher brain processing centers [27]. While cytokines can change the sensitivity of peripheral receptors to nociceptive input by a variety of mechanisms in experimental animal models [28–30], very few human studies have reported correlations between cytokines and OA pain. The chemokine sub-family of cytokines is also of specific interest in patients with arthritis since these small molecules are capable of recruiting additional immune and/or stem/progenitor cells to sites of injury and/or increased inflammation.

With our incomplete understanding of the role of any specific cytokine in the inflammatory process, understanding the 'profile' of inflammation in a given patient population is an essential starting point. Therefore, the primary aim of this study was to examine system and local inflammatory profiles in hip OA patients, using knee OA and non-OA control as comparator groups to identify if differences exist between hip and knee OA. Furthermore in the hip OA cohort, it was attempted to determine if there were any cytokine (s) that correlated with pain symptoms, as well as other clinical measurements.

Methods

Subjects and clinical evaluation

This study protocol was approved by the University of Calgary Human Research Ethics Board (REB15–0880). Participants (Table 1) provided written consent. In all patient cohorts a previous diagnosis of metabolic disease/disorder, diabetes and/or abdominal obesity excluded the individual from the current study. For all cohorts, prescription anti-inflammatory medication use within the past 3 months also excluded the individual from the current study. Individuals from all cohorts presented in this study are a sub-set of a larger on-going cohort study at the University of Calgary and were selected based on the inclusion/exclusion criteria for this study. Sample sizes were based off our previous reported study [5].

Control (n = 100; mean age 40.0 ± 9.5 years)

Individuals showed no clinical signs of OA or RA (based on ACR criteria), and were questioned (and potentially excluded) regarding personal (intraarticular joint injury, inflammatory arthritis, autoimmune diseases) and family (inflammatory arthritis including any autoimmune diseases) histories.. Individuals (e.g. faculty, staff, students, volunteers) were recruited from the sports medicine program and human performance laboratory.

Knee osteoarthritis (n = 100; mean age 60.4 ± 10 years)

Inclusion criteria required a diagnosis of OA performed at the OA clinic (University of Calgary) based on clinical

Table 1 Demographics of 3 cohorts

Characteristic	Knee OA ($n = 100$)	Hip OA ($n = 50$)	Control ($n = 100$)
Gender (% female)	46	42	75
Age (SD)	60.2 (10.4)	59.0 (9.5)	40.0 (9.5)
K/L 0	0	0	100
K/L 1	72	0	0
K/L 2	1	0	0
K/L 3	28	14	0
K/L 4	0	36	0
Serum Sample	100	50	100
Synovial Fluid Sample	8	14	15[a]
Synovium Sample	5	5	5[a]

[a]these sample are collected from cadaveric donations

symptoms of 3 months or greater with radiographic (standing AP radiographs) evidence (Kellgren and Lawerence (K/L) grading: all radiographs were graded by a sports medicine physician and registered nurse first assistant: inter-reader reliability/kappa, $\kappa = 0.84$) of changes associated with OA in accordance with ACR criteria. A K/L grade of at least 1 was required for inclusion into the knee OA cohort. A previous diagnosis of hip, hand or spine OA resulted in exclusion and a clinical assessment was undertaken to identify potential undiagnosed OA in these joint was undertaken at the time of recruitment.

Hip osteoarthritis (n = 50; mean age 59 ± 9.5 years)

Inclusion criteria was based on a diagnosis of hip OA determined by patient symptoms, clinical exam and radiographic (K/L) evidence (all radiographs were graded by an orthopedic surgeon and registered nurse first assistant: $\kappa = 0.87$) in accordance with ACR criteria. A K/L grade of at least 1 was required for inclusion into the hip OA cohort. A previous diagnosis of knee, hand or spine OA resulted in exclusion and a clinical assessment was undertaken to identify potential undiagnosed OA in these joint was undertaken at the time of recruitment. Two major etiologies were impingement ($n = 35$) and dysplasia ($n = 7$).

Clinical assessment of hip OA cohort

Patients were asked to consent to complete the following questionnaires at the time of surgery (Birmingham hip resurfacing or total hip replacement):

1. The Harris Hip score (HHS) [31]. The score has a maximum of 100 points (best possible outcome) covering pain (1 item, 0–44 points), function (7 items, 0–47 points), absence of deformity (1 item, 4 points), and range of motion (2 items, 5 points).
2. Hip disability and osteoarthritis outcome score (HOOS) [32]. It consists of 40 items assessing 5 subscales including pain, symptoms, activity limitations daily living, function in sport and recreation and hip related quality of life. Standardized answer options are given in 5 Likert-boxes with scores from 0 to 4 (no, mild, moderate, severe and extreme).
3. Short form 36 (SF36) [33]. It consists 8 sections including vitality, physical functioning, bodily pain, general health perceptions, physical role functioning, emotional role functioning, social role functioning, mental health. Each measurement is scale from 0 (worst) to 100 (best).
4. The University of California Los Angeles (UCLA) activity score [34]. The evaluation has 10 descriptive activity levels ranging from wholly inactive and dependent on others (level 1), to regular participation in impact sports (level 10).

The questionnaires were the most common ones in the literature concerning hip function and symptoms, and all of them had shown a good reliability.

Sample collection

Serum samples were collected at rest by standard venipuncture with untreated vacuum tubes. Serum was immediately aliquoted and stored at -80 °C until required for analysis. All samples analyzed were only thawed once (at the time of analysis).

Synovial fluid (knee and hip OA cohorts) was aspirated from the knee joint by the attending orthopedic surgeon or sports medicine physician. Control synovial fluid samples were obtained from the Southern Alberta Tissue Donation Program. Criteria for control cadaveric donations were an age of 40 years or older, no history of arthritis, joint injury or surgery (including visual inspection of the cartilage surfaces during recovery), no prescription anti-inflammatory medications, no co-morbidities (such as diabetes/cancer), and availability within 4 h of death. Synovial fluid samples were collected without the use of lavage. The samples centrifuged at 3000 g for 15 min after blood has clotted at 4 °C and stored at -80 °C. All samples analyzed were only thawed once (at the time of analysis).

Synovium tissue collection

Control tissue samples were obtained from the Southern Alberta Tissue Donation Program based on the sample criteria for cadaveric donations as listed above. Synovial biopsies from OA subjects were taken during surgery.

Multiplexed arrays

Sample analysis was performed by Eve Technologies (Calgary, AB Canada) using the Milliplex MAP Human Cytokine/Chemokine Panel (Millipore), according to the manufacturer's instructions. All samples (serum and synovial fluid) were assayed at least in duplicate and prepared standards were included in all runs. The following proteins were examined by Luminex in this study: EGF, Eotaxin, FGF2, Flt3L, Fractalkine, GCSF, GMCSF, GROα, IFNα2, IFNγ, IL1α, IL1β, IL1rα, IL2, IL3, IL4, IL5, IL6, IL7, IL8, IL9, IL10, IL12 (p40), IL12 (p70), IL13, IL15, IL17A, IL18, IP10, MCP1, MCP3, MDC, MIP1α, MIP1β, PDGFAA, PDGFAB/BB, RANTES, sCD40L, TGFα, TNFα, TNFβ, VEGFA. The sensitivities of these makers range from 0.1–10.1 pg/mL (average 2.359 pg/ml) and the inter-array accuracies range from 3.5% – 18.9% coefficient of variation (average 10.7%).

Immunohistochemistry

Immunofluorescence was performed on synovium specimens with fluorescent-conjugated antibodies were obtained as follows: PE Mouse Anti-Human MDC/CCL22 (Cat. No. 565950, BD), PE Mouse Anti-Human IP-10 (Cat. No. 555049, BD), FITC Rat Anti-Human IL-6 (Cat. No. 554544, BD).

Statistical methods

The normality of each cytokines was assessed by QQ plots. Because many of the cytokine concentrations were not normally distributed, both t-test and Mann–Whitney–Wilcoxon (MWW) tests were utilized. T-test and MWW were performed to compare the ages and BMI between groups. Principle component analysis (PCA) was used to reduce the dimensionality of the cytokine dataset and the first 3 components were used for 3-D scatter plot.

For hip OA cohort, T-test and MWW were used to compare the means of cytokines with pain scores, BMI between two subgroups-impingement and dysplasia. PCA was run to extract two factors from 10 HOOS pain questions. Pairwise associations between cytokines and clinical questionnaire scores were assessed using Spearman's rank correlation test. First, we tested the correlation between 7 cytokines which have been reported correlated with osteoarthritis pain previously [27] and pain levels (evaluated by HOOS pain sub scores and SF36 body pain score). Then, we screened all the associations between every single cytokines and the log transformed ratios of any two cytokines and clinical variables (i.e., age, gender, BMI and clinical questionnaire scoring). *P*-values were adjusted by two different multiple testing correction procedures: Bonferroni procedure with familywise error rate of 0.05 ($\alpha \approx 0.001$) and Benjamini–Hochberg procedure with a false discovery rate of 0.20.

For both hip and knee OA cohorts, multivariable linear regression was applied to test the potential confounding effects including age, gender, K/L grade and affected joint (hip or knee) on cytokine profiles. Statistical analyses were performed using Python version 2.7 with scipy package (for screening associations between all cytokines and clinical questionnaire scores) and SPSS 20.0 (SPSS, Inc., Chicago IL). $P < 0.05$ (two-sided) was considered statistically significant, except for the tests whose *p*-values were adjusted by multiple testing correction. The 3-D scatter plots of PCA were generated by SPSS 20.0. The bar graphs were generated by GraphPad Prism 6 (Graphpad Software. San Diego, CA).

Results

Inflammatory profile between hip and knee OA cohorts

To uncover any differences in systemic inflammatory signaling in patients with hip OA vs knee OA or normal controls a multiplex approach was utilized in where we would quantify the levels of 42 cytokines (including lymphokines, interferons, colony stimulating factors and chemokines, outlined in methods section) that are involved in many signaling pathways regulating inflammation and disease. Significant differences in serum cytokines levels were identified when comparing cohorts (hip OA vs. knee OA vs. control). While 5 cytokines were differentially expressed between knee and hip OA cohorts (Fig. 1), 3 cytokines (GRO: growth-regulated oncogene aka C-X-C motif ligand 1/CXCL1, MCP1: monocyte chemoattractant protein aka C-C motif ligand 2/CCL2 and VEGF: vascular endothelial growth factor) were conserved in both hip and knee OA cohorts when compared to the control cohort (Fig. 1). Overall, 10 cytokines were differentially expressed between all three cohorts. The first 3 components of PCA (explained 64.5% of total variance) clearly separated 3 cohorts (Fig. 1).

Synovial fluid cytokine profiles were also found to be distinct across 3 cohorts. Synovial fluid and serum shared common cytokines that were differentially expressed between cohorts: EGF (epidermal growth factor) differed between hip OA and knee OA; IL8 (interleukin 8) was different between hip OA and control; MCP1, MIP1β (macrophage inflammatory protein aka C-C motif ligand 3/CCL3) differed between knee OA and control (Fig. 2).

Previous studies showed age, gender and severity of OA might have effects on cytokine expression [35, 36]. Therefore, a multivariable linear regression model was applied to access the correlations between cytokines and potential confounding variables (age, gender and K/L grade of OA and affected joint) in OA cohorts (Table 2). For cytokines that were significantly different between hip and knee OA cohorts, none were found to be related

a

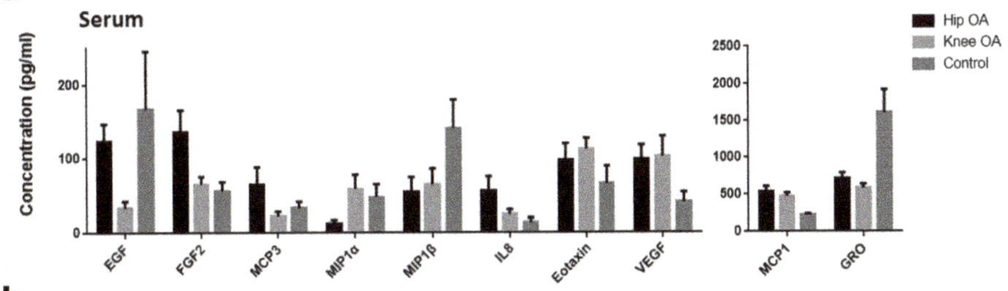

b

	Hip OA	Knee OA
Knee OA	EGF*, FGF2, MCP3, MIP1α, IL8,	
Control	FGF2, GRO, IL8*, MCP1/CCL2, VEGF	Eotaxin, GRO, MCP1/CCL2*, MIP1β*, VEGF

c

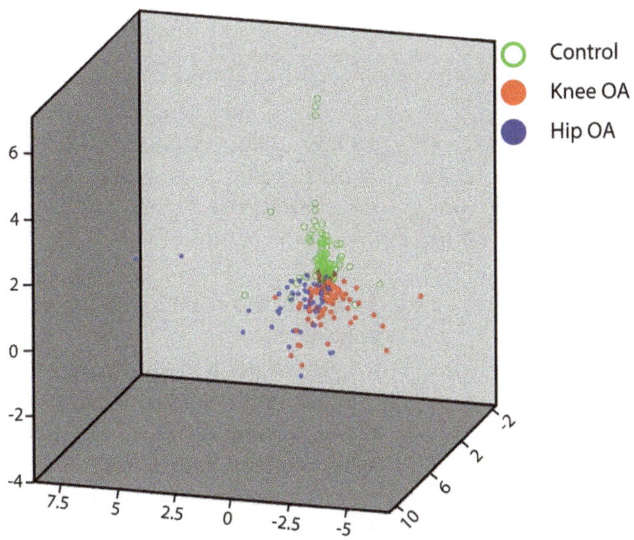

Fig. 1 Comparison of cytokine profiles in serum in control, hip OA and knee OA cohorts. The serum concentrations of cytokines that were found to be significantly differently between the cohorts examined (**a**). The significantly different cytokines in each cohort are present in more detail in (**b**) after Bonferroni correction ($p < 0.0012$) (* = Significantly different in both serum and synovial fluid). Scatter plot of first 3 components of PCA of cytokine profiles of 3 cohorts demonstrates that the serum cytokine profiles are capable of discriminating the 3 different cohorts (**c**)

to age, gender or K/L grade, suggesting there were minimal effects of these variables confounding the cytokine profiles observed. After adjusting for confounding variables, EGF, FGF2 (fibroblast growth factor 2), MCP3 (aka C-C motif ligand 7/CCL7), and IL8 remained different between hip and knee OA.

Correlations between cytokines and clinical data in hip OA cohort

To determine if any clinical outcome measures were associated with the cytokine profile of hip OA patients, the pain, physical function and activity limitations of hip OA cohort were assessed using the HOOS, SF-36, HHS and UCLA scores.

First the discriminativity of all clinical measurements was examined by comparing each measurement between different severity of OA (different K/L grade). Six subscores showed a difference between K/L grade 3 and 4 groups (significant threshold was corrected by Benjamini–Hochberg procedure with a false discovery rate of 0.20) (Additional file 1: Table S2). These scores included the HOOS pain 5 (walking on a flat surface, p-value = 0.037), HOOS pain 6 (going up or down stairs, p-value = 0.034), SF36 GH (general-health, p-value = 0.023), SF36 MH (mental health, p-value = 0.007), SF36 PCS (physical component summary, p-value = 0.018) and SF36 MCS (mental component summary, p-value = 0.024). None were significant after Bonferroni testing correction.

Previously reported OA pain related cytokines (TNFα, IL1β, IL6, IL15, IL10, MCP1 and Fractalkine) [27] were also examined within our hip OA cohort dataset (Additional file 1: Table S3). Only IL6 was found to be significant when correlated with HOOS pain score factor 2 (correlation = 0.319, P-value = 0.024). When testing all

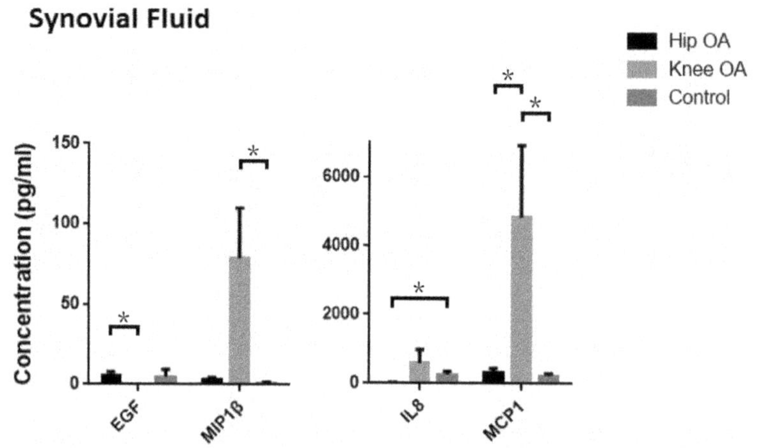

Fig. 2 Differently expressed cytokines in synovial fluid in control, hip OA and knee OA cohorts. Of the cytokines examined in the serum that were significantly different between the hip OA, knee and control cohorts; EGF, MCP1, MIP1β and IL8 protein levels were also found to be significantly different between the synovial fluid samples obtained from the cohorts. Bonferroni correction (*$p < 0.001$)

36 cytokines, 2 cytokines were found to be correlated with pain severity: MDC (macrophage-derived chemokine aka C-C motif chemokine 22/CCL22) was negatively correlated with BPSF36 (body pain SF36, correlation = – 0.302, *p*-value = 0.033), IP10 was positively correlated with HOOS pain (correlation = 0.294, *p*-value = 0.038) and HOOS pain 8 (standing upright, correlation = 0.390, *p*-value = 0.005) (Fig. 3).

Table 2 Multivariable linear regression result of associations between cytokines and age, gender, K/L grade and affected joint (e.g. knee vs. hip)

Cytokines	Covariates	Sig.	95% CI	
			Lower	Upper
EGF	Age	0.396	−1.440	0.573
	Gender	0.177	−34.025	6.343
	K/L Grade	0.437	−7.964	18.331
	Affected Joint*	< 0.001	−37.895	−14.098
FGF2	Age	0.370	−1.761	0.659
	Gender	0.195	−40.270	8.269
	K/L Grade	0.803	−13.809	17.809
	Affected Joint *	0.003	−36.048	−7.434
MCP3	Age	0.778	−0.751	1.001
	Gender	0.238	−28.085	7.046
	K/L Grade	0.909	−12.108	10.776
	Affected Joint *	0.005	−25.219	−4.508
MIP1α	Age	0.863	−1.426	1.197
	Gender	0.298	−40.207	12.400
	K/L Grade	0.572	−22.039	12.228
	Affected Joint	0.130	−3.555	27.458
IL8	Age	0.799	−0.881	0.680
	Gender	0.544	−20.479	10.832
	K/L Grade	0.731	−8.422	11.973
	Affected Joint *	0.049	−18.501	−0.042

*$p < 0.05$

Synovium examination from control, hip OA and knee OA cohorts

To determine if the cytokines that were correlated with hip pain could be originating from the joint environment, the expression of MDC, IL6 and IP10 were examined in synovial membrane biopsies from a sub-set of the hip OA ($n = 5$), knee OA ($n = 5$) and control cohorts ($n = 5$) (Fig. 4). MDC and IP10 positive cells were observed in the synovium of patients with hip OA. IL6 positive cells were not regularly observed in the synovium of hip OA patients, but were observed in the synovium of patients with knee OA. MDC, IL6 or IP10 positive cells were not observed within the synovium of patients without OA. To further narrow down the potential source of the MDC, IL6 and IP10, synovial fluid and serum samples were examined in a sub-set of patients. High levels of MDC were observed in the serum of all cohorts, however, only patients with hip OA maintained high levels of MDC within their synovial fluid (Fig. 4 and Additional file 1: Figure S1). While IP10 was present in serum at lower levels, high levels were observed in the synovial fluid of hip OA patients alone. IL6 levels were present at low levels in serum and synovial fluid of all cohorts examined (Fig. 4 and Additional file 1: Figure S1). It is important to note that although multiple comparisons were not undertaken for this experiment, we chose to present the data (Fig. 4) with the same multiple comparison correction as the previous results for consistency. However, a non-multiple comparison corrected version of the same data is presented in Additional file 1: Figure S1.

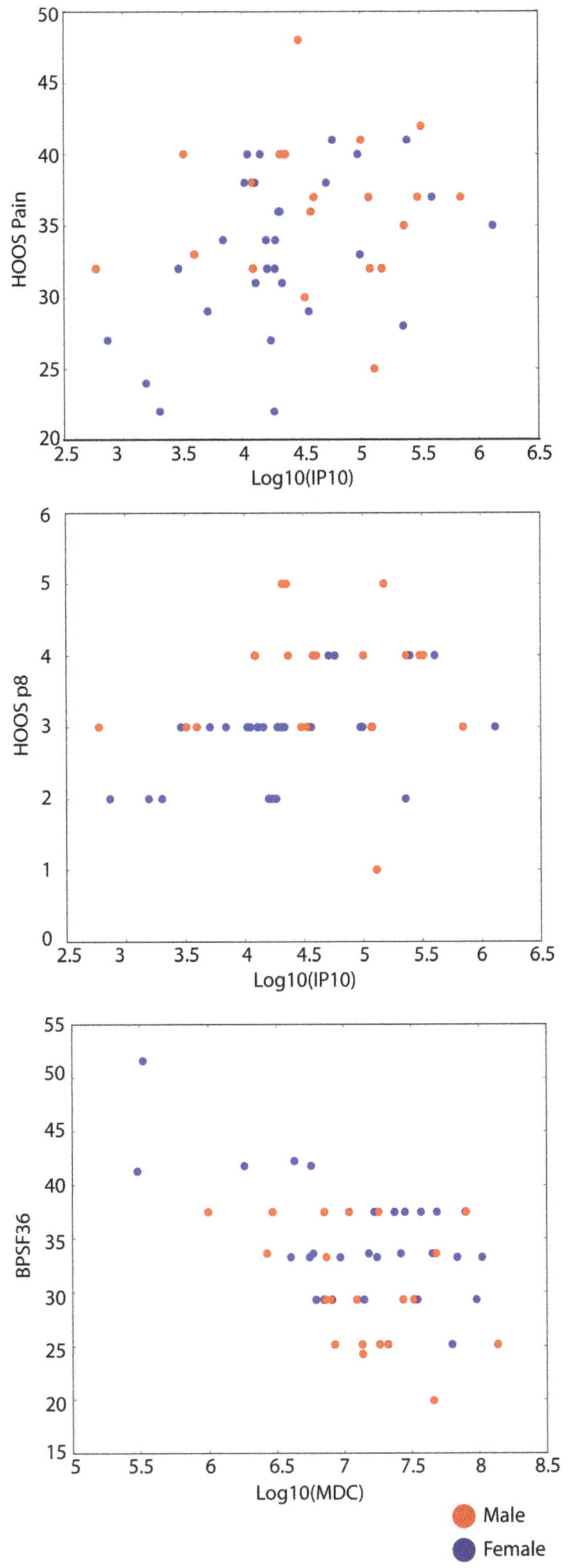

Fig. 3 Scatter plot of two cytokines and correlated pain scores. Left: IP10 (log transferred) was positively correlated with HOOS pain score (correlation = 0.294, p-value = 0.038). Middle: IP10 (log transferred) was positively correlated with HOOS pain question 8 (correlation = 0.390, p-value = 0.005). Right: MDC (log transferred) was negatively correlated with SF36 body pain score (correlation = – 0.302, p-value = 0.033)

Discussion

To our knowledge, few papers have discriminated which joint the OA is affecting when comparing OA with control groups. In this study, we have found that 4 cytokines (EGF, FGF2, MCP3, IL8) are expressed differently in knee OA patients versus hip OA patients after controlling for age, gender and K/L grade. Interestingly, when we compared these two OA cohorts with the control cohort, the picture became even more complex. EGF levels were similar between the hip OA and control cohorts but both differed from the knee OA cohort. MCP3 was similar between the knee OA and control cohorts but differed from the hip OA cohort. The scatter plot of first 3 components of PCA of the 3 cohorts (hip OA, knee OA and control) showed that, neither Hip OA nor Knee OA is "closer" to the control. The center of gravity of the 3 cohorts represents a triangle shape (Fig. 1). This infers that the three cohorts have their own characteristic cytokine profiles (though knee OA and hip OA cohorts are more similar to each other than either is to the control cohort). This may suggest that, at least for serum cytokines, OA may have distinct inflammatory profiles with subtypes that vary according to the affected joint. Failing to treat them as separate groups may be one of the reasons that the accuracy of biochemical markers in OA varies among studies [37]. This may partially explain why none of the biochemical markers that have been studied to date have been approved for diagnosis or prognosis of OA. Another possible reason might be the heterogenetic and multifactorial nature of OA itself. The existence of subgroups in OA might invalidate any statistical single biochemical marker comparison which considers OA as one group-one biochemical marker is not enough to classify all of these subgroups. Previous studies have looked into subgrouping OA before statistical analyses [38]. For instance, by using serum metabolomics data of OA patients, Zhang et al. identified at least 3 distinct subgroups which were not associated with any known confounders including age, sex, BMI and comorbidities [39]. The current study suggests that hip and knee OA cohorts may not be as similar in terms of the disease as previously thought and this has implications that OA in other joints (hands, spine, etc.) may also cloud diagnostic efforts, however, this hypothesis will require further study and validation.

In specific regards to the inflammatory cytokines examined in the current study, it is believed that aging brings about changes in the expression of many

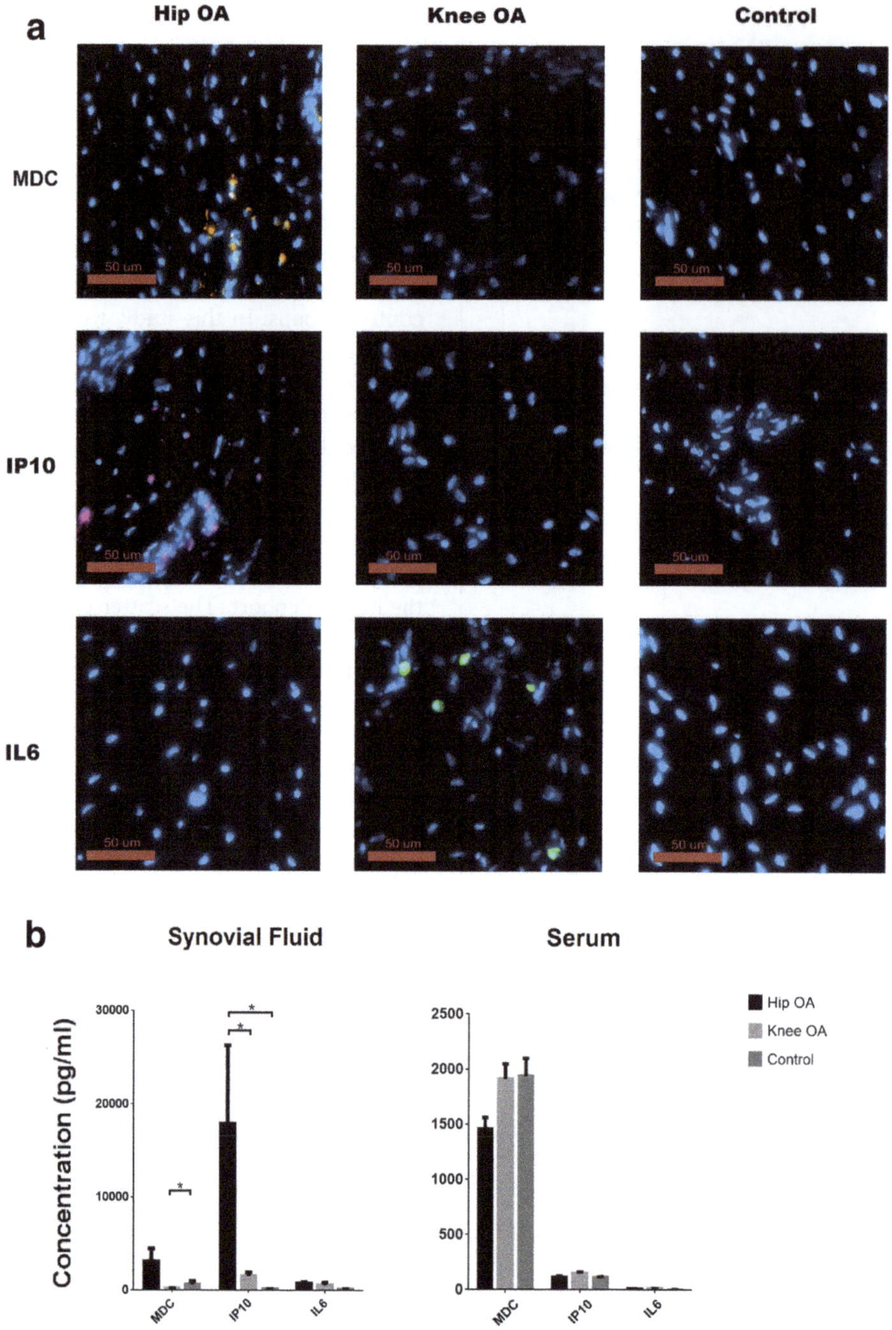

Fig. 4 Presence of MDC, IL6 and IP10 in Hip OA, Knee OA and control synovium, synovial fluid and serum. Representative images demonstrating the presence of MDC (orange) positive (MDC: 3/5 hip OA, 0/5 knee OA, 0/5 control) and IP10 (purple) positive (3/5 hip OA, 0/5 knee OA, 0/5 control) cells in synovium of Hip OA patients. IL-6 (green) positive cells within the synovium were not observed in the Hip OA cohort, but observed with the knee OA cohort (1/5 hip OA, 4/5 knee OA, 0/5 control) (**a**). Serum and synovial fluid levels of MDC, IL6 and IP10 were also examined in the three cohorts (**b**). Bonferroni correction (*$p < 0.001$)

cytokines. Aged-related changes in the immune system may elevate the concentrations of cytokines which some have postulated may ultimately lead to chronic inflammation [40]. This being said, in our dataset none of the cytokines are statistically significantly correlated with age. This might be due to the fact that most patients have passed their middle-age and the age distribution of these two cohorts are relatively concentrated (mean = 59.9, SD = 10.1). Although the control cohort is significant younger than the two OA cohorts (mean = 40.0, SD = 9.5). A limitation of the current study is that we unfortunately do not have the linked age information for each patient sample in the control cohort (only the cohort level details) and therefore we are not able to run a correlation analysis. Additionally, many factors can confound cytokine concentrations, such as statistical errors and mismatched cohort characteristics (such as races, disease history, diet and etc.). While, it can be unrealistic to find two exactly matched cohorts, these mismatch factors may lead to changes in serum cytokine concentrations in an unpredictable way and highly controlled cohort studies will be required to address these discrepancies.

TNFα, IL1, IL6 and IL17 have been reported to be correlated with development of neuropathic pain in various animal models [27, 41]; however, except for IL6, which had weak correlation with PCA factor 2 of 10 HOOS pain questions, none of these proteins were significantly correlated with pain level scores in our dataset. We have tested the correlation between our two different pain level scores-SF36 body pain and HOOS pain sub-score, they are significantly correlated (correlation = 0.569, p-value < 0.0001). This suggests the method that we chose to evaluate osteoarthritis pain levels was reliable between questionnaires. Among all 36 cytokines, we found that MDC and IP10 were correlated with pain in the hip OA cohort. IP10 (CXCL10) belongs to CXC chemokine family. It is expressed by a variety of cell types. When IP10 binds to CXCR3, this can result in activation and recruitment of leukocytes, and also regulate cell growth and apoptosis [42]. In specific regard to pain, IP10 has been reported to be involved in breast cancer-induced bone pain by activation of microglia in rat models [43]. In our study, IP10 was positively correlated with pain in patients with hip OA. It is possible that IP10 could be inducing OA pain through a similar pathway by activation of microglia in the joint environment. MDC (CCL22) belongs to the CC chemokine family and it is expressed mainly by macrophages and dendritic cells. MDC recruits Th2, Th17 and regulatory T cells through the binding of trafficking receptor CCR4 [44, 45]. To our knowledge, no publication has directly looked at MDC and pain.

The concentrations of these cytokines in synovial fluid were consistent with the immuno-histochemistry results; with MDC and IP10 higher in synovial fluid than in serum, and were higher in hip OA than knee OA or control cohorts. This strongly suggests that within the hip OA cohort, MDC and IP10 are being produced within the joint environment and then may diffuse into serum through the synovial fluid. In the knee OA cohort however, MDC and IP10 were not present within the joint (synovium or synovial fluid) and therefore any detectable levels of these in the serum are most likely being generated in other tissues in the body. While, the concentration of IL6 was higher in hip and knee OA cohorts than controls, IL6 was not found in hip synovium. This suggests that there might be other tissues in the joint (cartilage, ligaments, etc) that produce IL6 in the hip OA cohort. The relationship between serum and synovial fluid cytokine levels are still poorly understood with previous studies demonstrating little correlation [46] or high correlation [47] between systemic vs. local levels. However, the biological basis behind these correlations (or lack thereof) remain unknown, and further study will be required on specific markers to determine if the choice of sample local will impact the usefulness of the result obtained.

Conclusions

These findings validate previous studies that cytokines are differently expressed in OA patients [15]; and suggest that while cytokine profiles are generally similar between hip and knee OA, that there are specific differences that may be related to differential disease processes within a given joint. Furthermore, 3 cytokines (IL6, MDC and IP10) were identified that correlated with hip OA. These results set the ground work for future studies that will be required to understand: if cytokines play distinct roles in in the onset/pathogenesis of OA in different joints; and what is the pathway and/or mechanism by which the identified cytokines regulate OA pain.

Abbreviations

ACR: American College of Rheumatology; BMI: Body mass index; COMP: Cartilage oligomeric matrix protein; EGF: Epidermal growth factor; FGF2: Fibroblast growth factor 2; GRO: Growth-regulated protein; HHS: Harris Hip score; HOOS: Hip disability and osteoarthritis outcome score; IL: Interleukin; IP: Interferon gamma-induced protein; K/L: Kellgren and Lawerence; MCP: Monocyte chemoattractant protein; MDC: Macrophage-derived chemokine; MIP: Macrophage inflammatory protein; MWW: Mann–Whitney–Wilcoxon test; OA: Osteoarthritis; PCA: Principle component analysis; SF36: Short Form 36; Th: T Helper; TNF: Tumor necrosis factor; UCLA: University of California Los Angeles activity score; VEGF: Vascular endothelial growth factor

Acknowledgments

The authors would like to thank Mark Fritzler of Eve Technologies for assistance with Luminex analysis.

Funding

This work was funded by grants through the Alberta Innovates Health Solutions (AIHS) Osteoarthritis Team Grant to JPW and RJK, Canada Foundation for Innovation (CFI) RJK, Grace Glaum Professorship to RJK and Canada Research Chairs (CRC) Program to RJK. GR is supported by an Arthritis Society Studentship. The funders had no role in study design, data collection and analysis, decision to publish, or preparation of the manuscript.

Authors' contributions
GR, PR, JPW, JP and RJK contributed to the conception and design of the study. GR, IL, PR, and JM performed the collection and/or assembly of data. GR, IL, and PR performed data analysis and interpretation. JPW, JP and RJK provided study materials and/or patients. GR drafted the article. GR, IL, PR, JPW and RJK provided critical revision of the article for important intellectual content. RJK had final approval of manuscript. JP and RJK provided financial support. All authors have read and approved the manuscript.

Consent for publication
All patient information has been de-identified.

Competing interests
Roman Krawetz is a member of the editorial board of BMC Musculoskeletal Disorders. The authors have no further conflicts of interest to disclose regarding the present study.

Author details
[1]McCaig Institute for Bone and Joint Health, Faculty of Medicine, University of Calgary, 3330 Hospital Drive NW, Calgary, Alberta T2N 4N1, Canada. [2]Department of Surgery, University of Calgary, Calgary, Alberta, Canada. [3]Charles Sturt University, Sydney, Australia. [4]Sports Medicine Centre, Faculty of Kinesiology, University of Calgary, Calgary, Alberta, Canada. [5]Department of Anatomy and Cell Biology, University of Calgary, Calgary, Alberta, Canada.

References
1. Lawrence RC, Felson DT, Helmick CG, Arnold LM, Choi H, Deyo RA, Gabriel S, Hirsch R, Hochberg MC, Hunder GG, et al. Estimates of the prevalence of arthritis and other rheumatic conditions in the United States. Part II. Arthritis Rheum. 2008;58(1):26–35.
2. Wright EA, Katz JN, Cisternas MG, Kessler CL, Wagenseller A, Losina E. Impact of knee osteoarthritis on health care resource utilization in a US population-based national sample. Med Care. 2010;48(9):785–91.
3. Ganz R, Leunig M, Leunig-Ganz K, Harris WH. The etiology of osteoarthritis of the hip: an integrated mechanical concept. Clin Orthop Relat Res. 2008; 466(2):264–72.
4. Sandell LJ. Etiology of osteoarthritis: genetics and synovial joint development. Nat Rev Rheumatol. 2012;8(2):77–89.
5. Heard BJ, Rosvold JM, Fritzler MJ, El-Gabalawy H, Wiley JP, Krawetz RJ. A computational method to differentiate normal individuals, osteoarthritis and rheumatoid arthritis patients using serum biomarkers. J R Soc Interface. 2014;11(97):20140428.
6. Rousseau J, Garnero P. Biological markers in osteoarthritis. Bone. 2012;51(2): 265–77.
7. Poole AR. Biochemical/immunochemical biomarkers of osteoarthritis: utility for prediction of incident or progressive osteoarthritis. Rheum Dis Clin N Am. 2003;29(4):803–18.
8. Van Spil W, Jansen N, Bijlsma J, Reijman M, DeGroot J, Welsing P, Lafeber F. Clusters within a wide spectrum of biochemical markers for osteoarthritis: data from CHECK, a large cohort of individuals with very early symptomatic osteoarthritis. Osteoarthr Cartil. 2012;20(7):745–54.
9. Balakrishnan L, Nirujogi RS, Ahmad S, Bhattacharjee M, Manda SS, Renuse S, Kelkar DS, Subbannayya Y, Raju R, Goel R, et al. Proteomic analysis of human osteoarthritis synovial fluid. Clin Proteomics. 2014;11(1):6.
10. Hunter DJ, Nevitt M, Losina E, Kraus V. Biomarkers for osteoarthritis: current position and steps towards further validation. Best Pract Res Clin Rheumatol. 2014;28(1):61–71.
11. Erhart-Hledik J, Favre J, Asay J, Smith R, Giori N, Mündermann A, Andriacchi T. A relationship between mechanically-induced changes in serum cartilage oligomeric matrix protein (COMP) and changes in cartilage thickness after 5 years. Osteoarthr Cartil. 2012;20(11):1309–15.
12. Heard BJ, Martin L, Rattner JB, Frank CB, Hart DA, Krawetz R. Matrix metalloproteinase protein expression profiles cannot distinguish between normal and early osteoarthritic synovial fluid. BMC Musculoskelet Disord. 2012;13(1):126.
13. van Spil WE, Drossaers-Bakker KW, Lafeber FP. Associations of CTX-II with biochemical markers of bone turnover raise questions on its tissue origin: data from CHECK, a cohort study of early osteoarthritis. Ann Rheum Dis. 2013;72(1):29–36.
14. Bernard NJ. Osteoarthritis: circulating miRNAs-early osteoarthritis biomarkers? Nat Rev Rheumatol. 2014;10(4):197.
15. Mabey T, Honsawek S. Cytokines as biochemical markers for knee osteoarthritis. World J Orthod. 2015;6(1):95.
16. Kapoor M, Martel-Pelletier J, Lajeunesse D, Pelletier JP, Fahmi H. Role of proinflammatory cytokines in the pathophysiology of osteoarthritis. Nat Rev Rheumatol. 2011;7(1):33–42.
17. Saberi Hosnijeh F, Runhaar J, van Meurs JB, Bierma-Zeinstra SM. Biomarkers for osteoarthritis: can they be used for risk assessment? A systematic review. Maturitas. 2015;82:36.
18. Schett G, Kiechl S, Bonora E, Zwerina J, Mayr A, Axmann R, Weger S, Oberhollenzer F, Lorenzini R, Willeit J. Vascular cell adhesion molecule 1 as a predictor of severe osteoarthritis of the hip and knee joints. Arthritis Rheum. 2009;60(8):2381–9.
19. Rego-Perez I, Fernandez-Moreno M, Deberg M, Pertega S, Fenandez-Lopez C, Oreiro N, Henrotin Y, Blanco FJ. Mitochondrial DNA haplogroups modulate the serum levels of biomarkers in patients with osteoarthritis. Ann Rheum Dis. 2010;69(5):910–7.
20. Reijman M, Pols HA, Bergink AP, Hazes JM, Belo JN, Lievense AM, Bierma-Zeinstra SM. Body mass index associated with onset and progression of osteoarthritis of the knee but not of the hip: the Rotterdam study. Ann Rheum Dis. 2007;66(2):158–62.
21. Bennell KL, Hunt MA, Wrigley TV, Hunter DJ, FJ MM, Hodges PW, Li L, Hinman RS. Hip strengthening reduces symptoms but not knee load in people with medial knee osteoarthritis and varus malalignment: a randomised controlled trial. Osteoarthr Cartil. 2010;18(5):621–8.
22. Van Spil WE, Welsing PM, Bierma-Zeinstra SM, Bijlsma JW, Roorda LD, Cats HA, Lafeber FP. The ability of systemic biochemical markers to reflect presence, incidence, and progression of early-stage radiographic knee and hip osteoarthritis: data from CHECK. Osteoarthr Cartil. 2015;23:1388.
23. Tseng S, Reddi AH, Di Cesare PE. Cartilage Oligomeric Matrix Protein (COMP): a biomarker of arthritis. Biomark Insights. 2009;4:33–44.
24. Felson DT. The sources of pain in knee osteoarthritis. Curr Opin Rheumatol. 2005;17(5):624–8.
25. Somers TJ, Keefe FJ, Godiwala N, Hoyler GH. Psychosocial factors and the pain experience of osteoarthritis patients: new findings and new directions. Curr Opin Rheumatol. 2009;21(5):501–6.
26. Sofat N, Ejindu V, Kiely P. What makes osteoarthritis painful? The evidence for local and central pain processing. Rheumatology. 2011;50(12):2157–65.
27. Miller RE, Miller RJ, Malfait AM. Osteoarthritis joint pain: the cytokine connection. Cytokine. 2014;70(2):185–93.
28. Miller RE, Tran PB, Das R, Ghoreishi-Haack N, Ren D, Miller RJ, Malfait AM. CCR2 chemokine receptor signaling mediates pain in experimental osteoarthritis. Proc Natl Acad Sci U S A. 2012;109(50):20602–7.
29. Boettger MK, Hensellek S, Richter F, Gajda M, Stockigt R, von Banchet GS, Brauer R, Schaible HG. Antinociceptive effects of tumor necrosis factor alpha neutralization in a rat model of antigen-induced arthritis: evidence of a neuronal target. Arthritis Rheum. 2008;58(8):2368–78.
30. Ebbinghaus M, Uhlig B, Richter F, von Banchet GS, Gajda M, Brauer R, Schaible HG. The role of interleukin-1beta in arthritic pain: main involvement in thermal, but not mechanical, hyperalgesia in rat antigen-induced arthritis. Arthritis Rheum. 2012;64(12):3897–907.
31. Harris W. Traumatic arthritis of the hip after dislocation and acetabular fractures: treatment by mold arthroplasty. An end-result study using a new method of result evaluation. J Bone Joint Surg Am. 1969;51(4):737.
32. Klassbo M, Larsson E, Mannevik E. Hip disability and osteoarthritis outcome score. An extension of the Western Ontario and McMaster Universities Osteoarthritis Index. Scand J Rheumatol. 2003;32(1):46–51.
33. Jenkinson C, Wright L, Coulter A. Criterion validity and reliability of the SF-36 in a population sample. Qual Life Res. 1994;3(1):7–12.
34. Zahiri CA, Schmalzried TP, Szuszczewicz ES, Amstutz HC. Assessing activity in joint replacement patients. J Arthroplast. 1998;13(8):890–5.
35. Pietschmann P, Gollob E, Brosch S, Hahn P, Kudlacek S, Willheim M, Woloszczuk W, Peterlik M, Tragl KH. The effect of age and gender on cytokine production by human peripheral blood mononuclear cells and markers of bone metabolism. Exp Gerontol. 2003;38(10):1119–27.
36. Vangsness CT Jr, Burke WS, Narvy SJ, RD MP, Fedenko AN. Human knee

synovial fluid cytokines correlated with grade of knee osteoarthritis–a pilot study. Bull NYU Hosp Jt Dis. 2011;69(2):122–7.
37. Hosnijeh FS, Runhaar J, van Meurs JB, Bierma-Zeinstra SM. Biomarkers for osteoarthritis: can they be used for risk assessment? A systematic review. Maturitas. 2015;82(1):36–49.
38. Castaneda S, Roman-Blas JA, Largo R, Herrero-Beaumont G. Osteoarthritis: a progressive disease with changing phenotypes. Rheumatology (Oxford). 2014;53(1):1–3.
39. Zhang W, Likhodii S, Zhang Y, Aref-Eshghi E, Harper PE, Randell E, Green R, Martin G, Furey A, Sun G, et al. Classification of osteoarthritis phenotypes by metabolomics analysis. BMJ Open. 2014;4(11):e006286.
40. Michaud M, Balardy L, Moulis G, Gaudin C, Peyrot C, Vellas B, Cesari M, Nourhashemi F. Proinflammatory cytokines, aging, and age-related diseases. J Am Med Dir Assoc. 2013;14(12):877–82.
41. Leung L, Cahill CM. TNF-alpha and neuropathic pain–a review. J Neuroinflammation. 2010;7:27.
42. Lee EY, Lee ZH, Song YW. The interaction between CXCL10 and cytokines in chronic inflammatory arthritis. Autoimmun Rev. 2013;12(5):554–7.
43. Bu H, Shu B, Gao F, Liu C, Guan X, Ke C, Cao F, Hinton AO Jr, Xiang H, Yang H, et al. Spinal IFN-gamma-induced protein-10 (CXCL10) mediates metastatic breast cancer-induced bone pain by activation of microglia in rat models. Breast Cancer Res Treat. 2014;143(2):255–63.
44. Lim HW, Lee J, Hillsamer P, Kim CH. Human Th17 cells share major trafficking receptors with both polarized effector T cells and FOXP3+ regulatory T cells. J Immunol. 2008;180(1):122–9.
45. Andrew DP, Chang M-s, McNinch J, Wathen ST, Rihanek M, Tseng J, Spellberg JP, Elias CG. STCP-1 (MDC) CC chemokine acts specifically on chronically activated Th2 lymphocytes and is produced by monocytes on stimulation with Th2 cytokines IL-4 and IL-13. J Immunol. 1998; 161(9):5027–38.
46. Madson KL, Moore TL, Lawrence JM 3rd, Osborn TG. Cytokine levels in serum and synovial fluid of patients with juvenile rheumatoid arthritis. J Rheumatol. 1994;21(12):2359–63.
47. Kaneko S, Satoh T, Chiba J, Ju C, Inoue K, Kagawa J. Interleukin-6 and interleukin-8 levels in serum and synovial fluid of patients with osteoarthritis. Cytokines Cell Mol Ther. 2000;6(2):71–9.

6

Effect of vitamin E on oxidative stress level in blood, synovial fluid, and synovial tissue in severe knee osteoarthritis

Saran Tantavisut[1], Aree Tanavalee[1*], Sittisak Honsawek[2], Tanyawan Suantawee[2], Srihatach Ngarmukos[1], Sirichai Adisakwatana[3] and John J. Callaghan[4]

Abstract

Background: This study was performed to evaluate the antioxidative and anti-inflammatory effects of vitamin E on oxidative stress in the plasma, synovial fluid, and synovial tissue of patients with knee osteoarthritis.

Methods: Seventy-two patients with late-stage knee osteoarthritis scheduled for total knee arthroplasty were randomized to take oral placebo (Group A) or 400 IU of vitamin E (Group B) once a day for 2 months before undergoing surgery. The blood levels of endpoints indicating oxidative stress or antioxidant capacity, Knee Society Score (KSS), Western Ontario and McMaster Universities Osteoarthritis Index score (WOMAC), and adverse effects were compared before and after the intervention between the two groups. At surgery, these redox endpoints and histological findings were compared between the synovial fluid and synovial tissue.

Results: In blood samples, the pre-intervention of oxidative stress and antioxidative capacity were not different between Group A and Group B. In post-intervention blood samples, the Malondialdehyde (Group A 1.34 ± 0.10, Group B 1.00 ± 0.09, $p < 0.02$), Alpha tocopherol (Group A 15.92 ± 1.08, Group B 24.65 ± 1.47, $p < 0.01$) and Trolox equivalent antioxidant capacity (Group A 4.22 ± 0.10, Group B 5.04 ± 0.10, 0 < 0.01) were significantly different between Group A and Group B. In synovial fluid samples, the Malondialdehyde (Group A 1.42 ± 0.12, Group B 1.06 ± 1. 08, p 0.01), Alphatocopherol (Group A 4.51, Group B 7.03, $p < 0.01$), Trolox equivalent antioxidant capacity (Group A, 1.89 ± 0.06, Group B 2.19 ± 0.10) were significantly different between Group A and Group B. The pre-intervention WOMAC score and KSS score were not different between Group A and Group B. The post-intervention WOMAC score was significantly improved in all categories in Group B (Pain: Group A 27.26 ± 0.89, Group B 19.19 ± 1.43, $p < 0.01$; Stiffness: Group A 8.23 ± 0.79, Group B 5.45 ± 0.73, p 0.01; Function: Group A 94.77 ± 4.22, Group B 72.74 ± 6.55, $p < 0.01$). The post-intervention KSS score was significantly improved in all categories in Group B (Clinical: Group A 25.31 ± 14.33, Group B 33.52 ± 16.96, $p < 0.01$; Functional: Group A 41.43 ± 16.11, Group B 51. 61 ± 19.60, p 0.02). Significantly fewer synovial tissue cells were stained with nitrotyrosine and hematoxylin–eosin in Group B than in Group A. There were no differences in adverse effects or surgical complications between the groups.

Conclusion: Vitamin E is an effective antioxidant that can improve clinical symptoms and reduce oxidative stress conditions in patients with late-stage knee osteoarthritis.

(Continued on next page)

* Correspondence: areetana@hotmail.com
[1]Department of Orthopaedics, Faculty of Medicine, Chulalongkorn University, 1873 Rama 4 road, Pathumwan, Bangkok 10330, Thailand
Full list of author information is available at the end of the article

(Continued from previous page)

Keywords: Knee osteoarthritis, Oxidative stress, Antioxidant, Anti-inflammation, Vitamin E

Background

Although osteoarthritis (OA) of the knee is a major cause of chronic disability in the older population, full comprehension of the pathogenesis of this disease has proven elusive [1, 2]. Recent evidence demonstrates that oxidative stress, the condition wherein oxidant levels exceed those of antioxidative agents, is one of the inducing factors of OA [3–9]. Reactive oxygen species, including oxidants that are produced under physiological conditions in the human body and removed by cellular antioxidants, lead to structural and functional damage of cartilage cells. Several laboratory investigations of the relationship between oxidative stress and OA have been undertaken. Increased nitrite, a stable decomposition biochemical marker of the presence of nitric oxide, has been reported in the plasma and synovial fluid of patients with OA [5]. In addition, several oxidative damage end-products following intracellular molecular oxidative stress have been identified, such as malondialdehyde (MDA) and nitrotyrosine. Elevated levels of MDA have been reported in the plasma of patients with OA [6]. Notably, patients with knee OA have higher levels of plasma oxidative stress parameters but lower levels of plasma antioxidant parameters than those of healthy controls [8]. The combined antioxidant effects of these antioxidative agents have been described as the total antioxidant capacity. Assays of the ferric reducing antioxidant power (FRAP) and Trolox equivalent antioxidant capacity (TEAC) have been utilized in this manner to measure the total antioxidant status [8].

Vitamin E, a dietary antioxidant capable of augmenting the total cellular antioxidant capacity, reportedly has a positive effect on the symptomatic treatment of arthritis [10–15]. However, there is very little evidence from high quality trials that vitamin E modifies oxidative markers and symptoms in people with knee osteoarthritis [16, 17]. This is the first randomized controlled trial that focus on the effects of vitamin E in end stage knee OA and completely evaluates clinical symptoms, biochemistry and histology results. We hypothesized that a sustained duration of vitamin E administration will decrease the oxidative stress, inflammatory process and improve symptoms in patients with end stage knee OA. Therefore, the purpose of this study was to evaluate the antioxidative and anti-inflammatory effects of vitamin E on oxidative stress in the plasma, synovial fluid, and synovial tissue of patients with knee OA.

Methods

Study design

The level of evidence in this study is level I. This study was approved by the Institutional Review Board on Human Research of the Faculty of Medicine, Chulalongkorn University (reference number 412/52) and was conducted in compliance with the guidelines of the Declaration of Helsinki. Written informed consent was obtained from the patients prior to their participation in the study. This research project had been approved for registration at Thai Clinical Trials Registry (TCTR) since 2016-08-28 11:26:32 (Retrospective registered). The TCTR identification number is TCTR20160828001. This single-center, randomized, double-blinded, placebo-controlled trial was performed at our institution from 1 July 2011 through 31 July 2012. An independent safety monitoring board evaluated the patients' safety and conducted semiannual meetings during the trial.

Participants

Eligible patients were ≥18 years of age, clinically diagnosed with knee OA according to the criteria of the American College of Rheumatology [18], radiographically diagnosed with severe knee OA (grade 3–4) as defined by the Kellgren–Lawrence classification [19], and scheduled for total knee arthroplasty (TKA) within 2 months (60 ± 2 days) after enrollment. Patients were excluded if they had an established diagnosis of a bleeding disorder; currently used vitamin E-containing drugs or dietary supplements, anticoagulants, or antiplatelet therapy; or had a vitamin E allergy. The use of nonsteroidal anti-inflammatory drugs was not allowed during the study period. The participants were allowed to use only acetaminophen 500 mg 1–2 tablets (depending on participant's weight) every 6 h as needed for pain.

Randomization and blinding

Using sealed envelopes, participants were randomly assigned by independent outpatient unit nurses to one of two groups in a 1:1 ratio: those who received placebo per oral once daily for 2 months (Group A) and those who received 400 IU of vitamin E per oral once daily for 2 months (Group B). The placebo and its container have identical color, form and size as the vitamin E. The surgeons and care team, all investigators, participants, staff collecting data, statistician and staff performing assays were blinded from the randomization.

Outcome measurements

The primary outcome measurements are biochemistry and histology results. The secondary outcome measurements are clinical results. In both groups of participants, the modified Thai Western Ontario and McMaster Universities Osteoarthritis Index Score (WOMAC) [20], Knee Society Score (KSS), and blood samples were collected before participants took the first dose of the assigned treatment (baseline) and at 2 months of drug administration, just prior to the surgery (post-intervention). Adverse events and surgical complications were recorded from the first dose of the assigned treatment until 2 weeks postoperatively. All patients underwent TKA within 2 days after completion of the 2-month course of vitamin E or placebo. Our calculation showed that 33 participants in each treatment group would provide the study with ≥80% power to detect a mean between-group difference (calculated with a standard deviation of 1.6 from our pilot study and a two-sided type I error rate of 0.05). The estimated mean between group differences that could be detected is 1.21. Considering a drop-out rate of 10%, the total sample size required was 72 (36 in each arm).

Specimen collection and laboratory methods

A 5-ml venous blood sample was collected from the cubital vein of each patient at baseline and postintervention. All samples were centrifuged at 4000 rpm for 10 min and stored immediately at −80 °C until analysis. The synovial fluid was aspirated prior to opening of the knee. The synovial tissue was collected from the most inflamed and redness area of the anterior femoral fat pad during TKA. The synovial fluid was then instantly centrifuged to remove cells and joint debris. Similarly, both the synovial fluid and tissue specimens were stored at −80 °C until sample collection from the last patient had been completed. Multiple investigations of oxidative stress, vitamin E, and antioxidant capacity were performed as described below.

Determination of nitrite concentrations [21]

The nitrite concentrations in plasma and synovial fluid were measured with the Griess Reagent System (Promega, Madison, WI, USA) using sulfanilamide and N-1-napthylenediamine dihydrochloride under acidic (phosphoric acid) conditions. Formation of the azo compound was determined via its absorbance at 540 nm by spectrophotometry.

Determination of MDA concentration

The MDA concentrations in plasma and synovial fluid were determined by the reaction between MDA and 2-thiobarbituric acid (Sigma-Aldrich, St. Louis, MO, USA) at 95 °C [22]. MDA and 2-thiobarbituric acid react with each other to produce a pink chromogen with absorbance at 532 nm by spectrophotometry. Malondialdehyde tetrabutylammonium salt (Sigma-Aldrich) was used as standard MDA.

Determination of vitamin E concentration by reverse-phase high-performance liquid chromatography

Plasma or synovial fluid samples were extracted with ethanol (Merck, Darmstadt, Germany) and hexane (Merck). Alpha-tocopheryl acetate (Sigma-Aldrich) was used as internal standard. We used alpha tocopherol (258,024 Sigma) as an external standard to make a standard curve. Then we calculated vitamin E concentrations from that standard curve. After drying the hexane layer under nitrogen gas and resuspending it in methanol (Merck), the extract was injected into the high-performance liquid chromatography (HPLC) system. The stationary phase was established using a C18 column (Inertsil ODS-3; GL Sciences, Tokyo, Japan). The mobile phase was a mixture of isocratic methanol/water (98/2, *v*/v) at a flow rate of 1.5 ml/min. The HPLC peaks were detected with an ultraviolet detector at 292 nm [23].

Determination of total antioxidant capacity by FRAP

The total antioxidant capacity was measured by FRAP assay as described by Benzie and Strain [24]. This assay depends upon the reduction of ferric tripyridyltriazine complex (Sigma-Aldrich) to ferrous tripyridyltriazine form at low pH. After this reduction, the absorbance was determined at 593 nm. Ferrous sulfate (Sigma-Aldrich) was used as the standard.

Determination of total antioxidant capacity by TEAC assay [25, 26]

The TEAC assay is based on the samples' scavenging of the 2,2′-azinobis-(3-ethylbenzothiazoline-6-sulfonic acid) (Sigma-Aldrich) radical anion, which is converted into a colorless product. The decrease in absorption at 734 nm after 6 min of the addition of a test compound was used

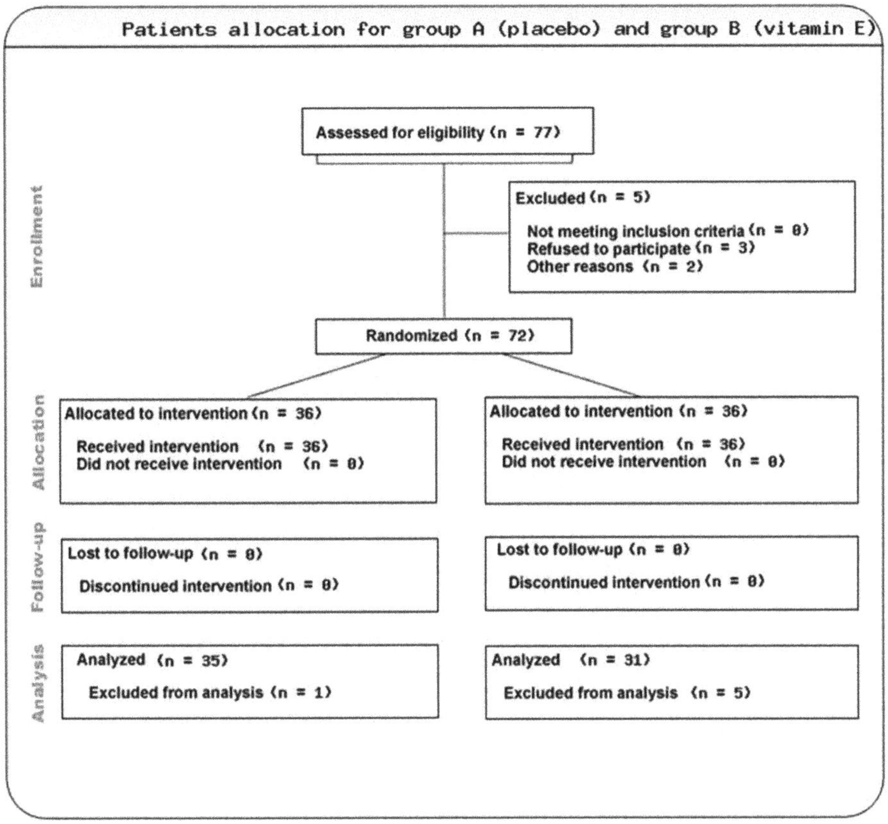

Fig. 1 The CONSORT flow diagram of the studied group

to calculate the TEAC values. Different concentrations of hydroxy-2,5,7,8-tetramethylchromane-2-carboxylic acid (Trolox) (Sigma-Aldrich) were used to create a calibration curve.

Determination of tissue nitrotyrosine concentration [27]

Synovial tissues were fixed in neutral buffered formalin, embedded in paraffin, and cut into 4-μm sections. Nitrotyrosine immunohistochemistry was performed using rabbit polyclonal anti-nitrotyrosine antibody (Upstate Biotechnology, Lake Placid, USA) as the primary antibody followed by anti-mouse/anti-rabbit immunoglobulins (Dako Envision System, Dako, Denmark) conjugated to peroxidase enzyme. For secondary antibody

Table 1 Baseline demographic data of patients

	Group A	Group B	*p* value
Number of patients	35	31	–
Age, years	69.20 ± 1.30	69.50 ± 1.30	0.87
Sex			
Male/female	9/26	2/29	–
Weight, kg	63.90 ± 1.60	60.10 ± 2.00	0.13
Height, cm	155.10 ± 1.30	154.80 ± 1.20	0.90
Body mass index, kg/m^2	26.60 ± 0.60	25.00 ± 0.40	0.09
Kellgren–Lawrence grading			
Grade 3	10	9	–
Grade 4	25	22	–

Data are presented as number of patients or mean ± standard deviation

Table 2 Western Ontario and McMaster Universities Osteoarthritis Index Score

	Group A (placebo)	Group B (vitamin E)	*p* value
Pain (50 points)			
Pre-intervention	25.20 ± 1.19	23.77 ± 1.69	0.49
Post-intervention	27.26 ± 0.89	19.19 ± 1.43	<0.01[a]
Δ (post −pre)	2.06 ± 0.88	−4.581 ± 1.11	<0.01[a]
Stiffness (20 points)			
Pre-intervention	7.80 ± 0.87	8.94 ± 1.02	0.39
Post-intervention	8.23 ± 0.79	5.45 ± 0.73	0.01[a]
Δ (post − pre)	0.43 ± 0.73	−3.48 ± 0.77	<0.01[a]
Function (170 points)			
Pre-intervention	90.06 ± 4.72	90.55 ± 7.12	0.95
Post-intervention	94.77 ± 4.22	72.74 ± 6.55	<0.01[a]
Δ (post − pre)	4.71 ± 3.81	−17.81 ± 4.23	<0.01[a]

Data are presented as mean ± standard deviation
P value represent the test between groups
[a]Statistically significant

Table 3 Clinical and functional Knee Society Scores

	Group A (placebo)	Group B (vitamin E)	*p* value
Clinical			
Pre-intervention	23.20 ± 14.52	22.48 ± 16.66	0.85
Post-intervention	25.31 ± 14.33	33.52 ± 16.96	<0.01[a]
Δ (post − pre)	2.11 ± 7.26	11.03 ± 8.561	<0.01[a]
Functional			
Pre-intervention	41.14 ± 16.05	41.94 ± 18.20	0.85
Post-intervention	41.43 ± 16.11	51.61 ± 19.60	0.02[a]
Δ (post − pre)	0.29 ± 1.312	9.68 ± 1.99	<0.01[a]

Data are presented as mean ± standard deviation
P value represent the test between groups
[a]Statistically significant

evaluation, the immunolabeling results of both groups were compared by direct visual inspection.

Determination of inflammatory infiltration of synovial tissue

Synovial tissues were fixed and embedded in paraffin then cut into 4-μm sections as above. Slides were stained with hematoxylin and eosin (H&E), and inflammatory cells were counted using a light microscope at 40× magnification (randomly selected 10 fields/specimen).

Statistical analysis

The baseline demographic data and patient characteristics were compared between the treatment groups. Categorical data were analyzed with the chi-square test or Fisher's exact test as appropriate. Continuous variables were analyzed using independent sample t-test or the Wilcoxon rank sum test. All *p* values were two-sided. A *p* value of ≤0.05 was considered to indicate statistical significance. All computations were carried out using GraphPad Prism 5.0.1 (GraphPad Software Inc., La Jolla, CA, USA).

Results

The CONSORT flow diagram of the studied cohort is shown in Fig. 1. At the time of analysis, six patients were excluded (one in Group A and five in Group B) because the operative date was delayed for more than 2 days from the scheduled date. The delay in surgery were because of personal reasons and not related to the trial or knee symptoms. Thus, there were 35 patients in Group A (placebo) and 31 patients in Group B (vitamin E). All participants were fully adherent to their interventions.

Baseline characteristics

The baseline comparative demographic data between the patients with knee OA in Group A (placebo) and Group B (vitamin E) are shown in Table 1. There were no significant differences in age, sex, or body mass index between the two groups. Sex was not a potential confounder in this study based on the absence of any differences in treatment response between males and females. Similarly, the baseline preoperative WOMAC score (Table 2) and KSS score (Table 3) were not significantly different between the two groups.

Oxidative stress, vitamin E, and antioxidant capacity in plasma and synovial fluid

The HPLC chromatogram is shown in Fig. 2. Changes in the oxidative stress level in plasma between before and after the intervention with each tested agent are shown in Table 4. The post-intervention nitrite concentration in Group B was lower than that in Group A, but the difference was not significant ($p = 0.19$); however, the post-intervention MDA level in Group B was significantly lower than that in Group A ($p = 0.02$). The post-intervention levels of vitamin E (alpha-tocopherol) and TEAC in Group A increased to a significantly lesser degree than those in Group B ($p < 0.01$ and <0.01, respectively). In contrast, the post-intervention changes in the antioxidant capacity

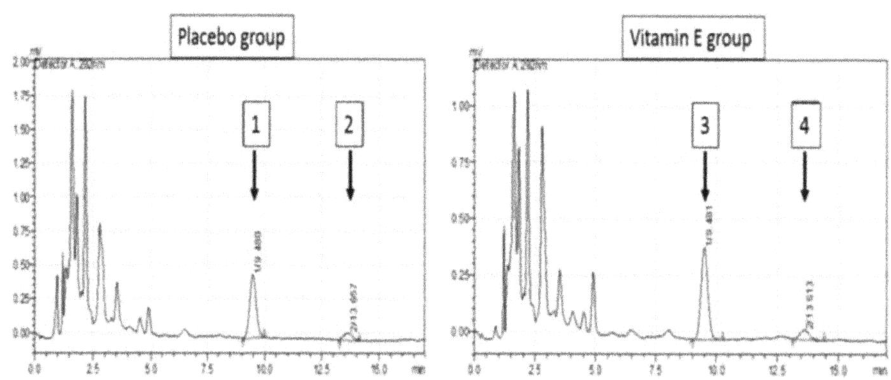

Fig. 2 The HPLC chromatogram from serum samples demonstrates "peak 2" and "peak 4" which represent alpha tocopheryl acetate (internal standard) in group A and group B respectively; "Peak 1" demonstrates alpha tocopherol in group A; "Peak 3" demonstrates alpha tocopherol in group B

Table 4 Oxidative stress and antioxidative capacity measurements from blood samples

	Group A (placebo)	Group B (vitamin E)	*p* value
Oxidative agents and products			
- Nitrite (μM)			
Pre-intervention	5.55 ± 0.57	5.60 ± 1.09	0.96
Post-intervention	5.63 ± 0.58	3.89 ± 1.25	0.19
Δ (post − pre)	0.08 ± 0.03	−1.70 ± 1.2	0.12
- Malondialdehyde (μM)			
Pre-intervention	1.32 ± 0.11	1.43 ± 0.07	0.43
Post-intervention	1.34 ± 0.10	1.00 ± 0.09	0.02[a]
Δ (post − pre)	0.01 ± 0.02	−0.79 ± 0.39	0.03[a]
Antioxidative agents			
- Alpha-tocophorol (μg/ml)			
Pre-intervention	15.50 ± 0.98	16.24 ± 0.99	0.59
Post-intervention	15.92 ± 1.08	24.65 ± 1.47	<0.01[a]
Δ (post − pre)	0.43 ± 0.33	8.41 ± 1.18	<0.01[a]
- FRAP (mM)			
Pre-intervention	923.30 ± 29.46	905.20 ± 35.16	0.69
Post-intervention	951.30 ± 29.03	1020 ± 40.22	0.17
Δ (post − pre)	28.01 ± 9.11	114.4 ± 35.19	0.01[a]
- TEAC (mM)			
Pre-intervention	4.26 ± 0.10	4.56 ± 0.14	0.08
Post-intervention	4.22 ± 0.10	5.04 ± 0.10	<0.01[a]
Δ (post − pre)	−0.04 ± 0.05	0.89 ± 0.45	0.03[a]

Data are presented as mean ± standard deviation
P value represent the test between groups
FRAP ferric reducing antioxidant power, *TEAC* Trolox equivalent antioxidant capacity
[a]Statistically significant

using the FRAP assay were not different between the two groups. The synovial fluid analysis results were similar to the serum analysis results, as shown in Table 5.

Correlation analysis of the differences between postoperative and preoperative (Delta, Δ) of oxidative stresses, antioxidative capacity and clinical outcomes in group B were performed. The results are shown in Table 6. The significant inverse correlation of Δ TEAC and Δ WOMAC score was found (p = 0.03). In addition, the significant inverse correlation of Δ TEAC and Δ MDA was also demonstrated.

Histological evaluation of synovial tissue

Immunohistochemical analyses of synovial tissue revealed that the nitrotyrosine staining in Group A was substantially more prominent than that in Group B (Fig. 3). In both groups, the staining was prominent at synovial lining cells, subsynovium area, synoviocytes and capillary endothelial cells. In addition, the H&E-stained slides showed significantly higher numbers of inflammatory cells in Group A than in Group B (Fig. 4).

Clinical outcomes

The post-intervention WOMAC score was significantly improved in all categories in Group B (Pain: Group A 27.26 ± 0.89, Group B 19.19 ± 1.43, $p < 0.01$; Stiffness: Group A 8.23 ± 0.79, Group B 5.45 ± 0.73, p = 0.01; Function: Group A 94.77 ± 4.22, Group B 72.74 ± 6.55, $p < 0.01$). The post-intervention KSS score was significantly improved in all categories in Group B (Clinical: Group A 25.31 ± 14.33, Group B 33.52 ± 16.96, $p < 0.01$; Functional: Group A 41.43 ± 16.11, Group B 51.61 ± 19.60, p = 0.02). There were no differences in adverse events or surgical complications between the two groups. The adverse events were diarrhea (2.9% in Group A, 6.5% in Group B), minor prolonged wound bleeding (2.8% in Group A, 3.2% in Group B), and nausea/vomiting (5.7% in Group A, 3.2% in Group B).

Discussion

Oxidative agents such as nitrite [2, 3, 28] and MDA [29], antioxidants such as vitamin E [30–32], and the total antioxidant capacity [32] as indicated by TEAC and FRAP have been investigated in patients with OA. In the present study, participants in Group B demonstrated lower levels of all oxidant endpoints in both the plasma and synovial fluid than did participants in group A; the differences were both statistically significant (MDA in

Table 5 Oxidative stress and antioxidative capacity measurements from synovial fluid

	Group A (placebo)	Group B (vitamin E)	*P* value
Oxidative agents and products			
- Nitrite (μM)	5.94 ± 1.09	5.24 ± 0.91	0.63
- Malondialdehyde (μM)	1.42 ± 0.12	1.06 ± 1.08	0.01[a]
Antioxidative agents			
- Alpha-tocopherol (μg/ml)	4.51 ± 0.31	7.03 ± 0.86	<0.01[a]
- FRAP (mM)	999.10 ± 39.51	1103 ± 44.77	0.09
- TEAC (mM)	1.89 ± 0.06	2.19 ± 0.1	0.01[a]

Data are presented as mean ± standard deviation
P value represent the test between groups
FRAP ferric reducing antioxidant power, *TEAC* Trolox equivalent antioxidant capacity
[a]Statistically significant

Table 6 Correlation analysis of the differences between preintervention and postintervention (Delta, Δ) of oxidative stresses, antioxidative capacity and clinical outcomes in the serum samples of group B

		Δ WOMAC	Δ KSS	Δ MDA	Δ TEAC	Δ Vit E	Δ Nitrite
Δ WOMAC	C*	1	−0.08	0.31	−0.40	−0.09	−0.02
	P**	-	0.69	0.09	0.03*	0.62	0.91
Δ KSS	C*	−0.08	1	−0.16	0.21	−0.10	−0.17
	P**	0.69	-	0.40	0.26	0.96	0.35
Δ MDA	C*	0.31	−0.16	1	−0.38	−0.22	−0.03
	P**	0.09	0.40	-	0.04*	0.24	0.89
Δ TEAC	C*	−0.40	0.21	−0.38	1	0.10	0.25
	P**	0.03	0.26	0.04	-	0.58	0.18
Δ Vit. E	C*	−0.09	−0.10	−2.2	0.10	1	0.09
	P**	0.62	0.96	0.24	0.58	-	0.61
Δ Nitrite	C*	−0.02	−0.17	−0.03	0.25	0.09	1
	P**	0.91	0.35	0.89	0.18	0.61	-

C* = Pearson correlation
P** = *p* value

plasma and synovial fluid) and statistically insignificant (nitrite). The nitric oxide is produced by the synovium and cells such as endothelial cells, polymorphonuclear leucocytes and macrophages. These cells are increased in inflamed synovial tissue. This phenomenon may explain the prominent nitrotyrosine stained in synovium lining and subsynovium tissue. The inflamed synovial tissue with intense nitric oxide production may obviously reaction to vitamin E leading to markedly decrease nitrotyrosine stain in group B tissue. The synovial fluid contains less amount of nitric oxide comparing with synovial tissue.

With respect to the antioxidant and total antioxidant capacity, the levels of vitamin E (alpha-tocopherol), FRAP, and TEAC in Group B were higher than those in Group A in both the plasma and synovial fluid. However, statistical significance between the two groups was found in the levels of vitamin E ($p = < 0.01$ in serum and $p = < 0.01$ in synovial fluid) and TEAC ($p < 0.01$ in serum and synovial fluid). These findings are in agreement with several previous studies [13, 14].

The changes in oxidative stress, the antioxidant level, and the total antioxidant capacity in the serum samples were in agreement with the changes in clinical outcomes: patients in Group B showed significant improvement in all entities of the WOMAC scores (pain, stiffness, and functional parts), as well as in the clinical and functional KSS, while there were no changes in these clinical scoring systems in Group A. The correlation analysis in this study also support that the increasing of TEAC significantly correlate with improvement of the WOMAC score. Vasanthi et al. [13], concluded that vitamin E has an analgesic effect by suppression of nitric oxide and protein kinase C, which might desensitize the central pain pathway. The improvement of both clinical scores in this research possibly be related to the analgesic effect from the vitamin E itself, increasing of antioxidant and decreasing of oxidative level.

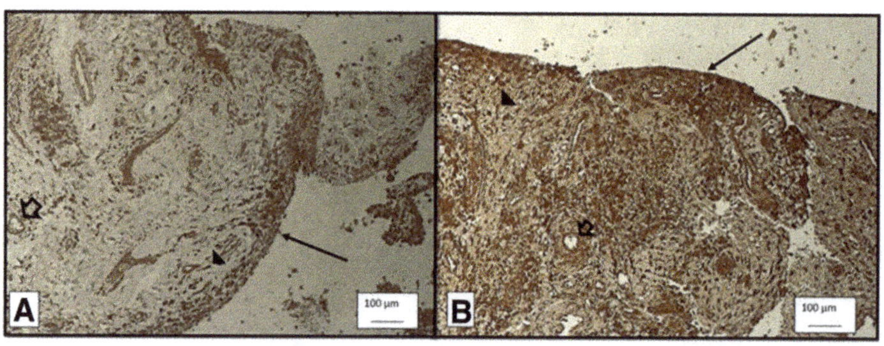

Fig. 3 Oxidative stress marker Nitrotyrosine stain under 10X light microscope in group A (**a**) and group B (**b**). The nitrotyrosine staining in Group A (3A) was substantially more prominent than that in Group B (3B). In both groups, the staining was prominent at synovial lining cells and subsynovium area (*arrow*), synoviocytes (*arrow head*) and capillary endothelial cells (*hollow arrow*)

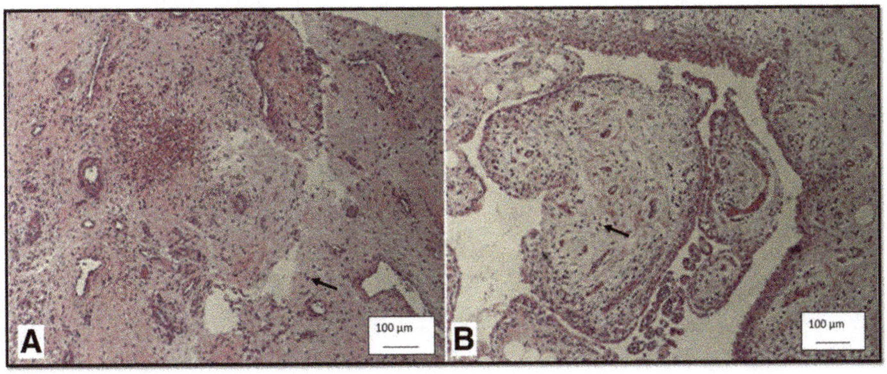

Fig. 4 The Hematoxylin and Eosin stain under 10X light microscope demonstrates inflammation cells which were stained in *blue* (*arrow*). The mean inflammation cells were 15.33 ± 1.19 cells/high power field in group A (**a**) and 9.47 ± 0.54 cells/high power field in group B (**b**) with statistical significance ($p < 0.01$)

Furthermore, the histological study using H&E staining of synovial tissue in the current study found significantly lower inflammation in samples of Group B than those of Group A. This finding is in agreement with several previous studies reporting that vitamin E, as a potent antioxidant, has anti-inflammatory effects on knee tissues [13, 33, 34]. Thus, the lower inflammation in Group B might have improved patient pain and played an important role in improving the WOMAC score and KSS in the present study.

The significantly increased level of vitamin E (alpha-tocopherol) in the serum and synovial fluid samples in this study suggests that 400 IU of vitamin E daily for 2 months is well distributed into both the blood system and target site within the knee joint without any serious side effects or complications related to treatment. In the present study, vitamin E demonstrated the ability to decrease oxidative stress and increase the total antioxidant power in patients with knee OA. Thus, vitamin E may have the potential to act as a disease-modifying agent for OA.

The strengths of the present study include its randomized design allowing for the evaluation of clinical outcomes, laboratory findings, and histological findings of all patients simultaneously after the intervention. Thus, the combination of the evaluated parameters provides high reliability. However, the major weakness of the present study was the relatively short-term vitamin E administration (2 months) in patients with severe knee OA that had developed over a lifetime. Further studies involving patients with less severe OA with a focus on the application time and duration of vitamin E supplementation should be performed to determine whether vitamin E is a viable nonsurgical intervention for this debilitating disease.

Conclusions

Vitamin E is an effective antioxidant that can safely improve clinical symptoms and reduce oxidative stress conditions in patients with late-stage knee osteoarthritis.

Abbreviations

FRAP: Ferric reducing antioxidant power; H&E stained: Hematoxylin and Eosin stained; HPLC: High-performance liquid chromatography; KSS: Knee society score; MDA: Malondialdehyde; OA: Osteoarthritis; TCTR: Thai Clinical Trials Registry; TEAC: Trolox equivalent antioxidant capacity; TKA: Total knee arthroplasty; WOMAC: The Western Ontario and McMaster Universities arthritis score

Acknowledgements

This research was supported by the Ratchadapiseksompotch Fund, Faculty of Medicine, Chulalongkorn University; the Thailand Research Fund; and the National Research Council of Thailand. We are grateful to Chulalongkorn Medical Research Center for kindly providing the facilities for the study. We also thank Mitchell Coleman from the University of Iowa, Iowa City, IA, USA for his expertise and time.

Authors' contributions

ST participated in the design of the study, data collection and draft the manuscript. AT participated in design of the study, interpretation of data. SH, TS and SA carried out the biochemistry studies and pathology study, participated in the sequence alignment and drafted the manuscript. SN participated in the design of the study and performed the statistical analysis. JJC coordination and helped to draft the manuscript. All authors read and approved the final manuscript.

Competing interests

The authors declare that they have no competing interests.

Author details

[1]Department of Orthopaedics, Faculty of Medicine, Chulalongkorn University, 1873 Rama 4 road, Pathumwan, Bangkok 10330, Thailand. [2]Department of Biochemistry, Faculty of Medicine, Chulalongkorn University, Bangkok, Thailand. [3]Faculty of Allied Health Sciences, Chulalongkorn University, Bangkok, Thailand. [4]Department of Orthopaedics, Faculty of Medicine, University of Iowa Hospitals and Clinics, Iowa City, IA, USA.

References

1. Martel-Pelletier J. Pathophysiology of osteoarthritis. Osteoarthr Cartil. 1999;7: 371–3.
2. Wieland HA, Michaelis M, Kirschbaum BJ, Rudolphi KA. Osteoarthritis—an untreatable disease? Nat Rev Drug Discov. 2005;4:331–44.
3. Jang D, Murrell GA. Nitric oxide in arthritis. Free Radic Biol Med. 1998;24: 1511–9.
4. Melchiorri C, Meliconi R, Frizziero L, Silvestri T, Pulsatelli L, Mazetti I, et al. Enhanced and coordinated in vivo expression of inflammatory cytokines and nitric oxide synthase by chondrocytes from patients with osteoarthritis. Arthritis Rheum. 1998;41:2165–74.
5. Karan A, Karan MA, Vural P, Erten N, Tascioglu C, Aksoy C. Synovial fluid nitric oxide levels in patients with knee osteoarthritis. Clin Rheumatol. 2003; 22:397–9.
6. Sarban S, Kocyigit A, Yazar M, Isikan UE. Plasma total antioxidant capacity, lipid peroxidation, and erythrocyte antioxidant enzyme activities in patients with rheumatoid arthritis and osteoarthritis. Clin Biochem. 2005;38:981–6.
7. Henrotin Y, Kurz B, Aigner T. Oxygen and reactive oxygen species in cartilage degradation: friend or foe? Osteoarthr Cartil. 2005;13:643–54.
8. Suantawee T, Tantavisut S, Adisakwattana S, Tanavalee A, Yuktanandana P, Anomasiri W, et al. Oxidative stress, vitamin E, and antioxidant capacity in knee osteoarthritis. J Clin Diagn Res. 2013;7:1855–9.
9. Cedergren J, Forslund T, Sundqvist T, Skogh T. Inducible nitric oxide synthase is expressed in synovial fluid granulocytes. Clin Exp Immunol. 2002;130:150–5.
10. McAlindon TE, Jacques P, Zhang Y, Hannan MT, Aliabadi P, Weissman B, et al. Do antioxidant micronutrients protect against the development and progression of knee osteoarthritis? Arthritis Rheum. 1996;39:648–56.
11. Wang Y, Prentice LF, Vitetta L, Wluka AE, Cicuttini FM. The effect of nutritional supplements on osteoarthritis. Altern Med Rev. 2004;9:275–96.
12. Edmonds SE, Winyard PG, Guo R, Kidd B, Merry P, Langrish-Smith A, et al. Putative analgesic activity of repeated oral doses of vitamin E in the treatment of rheumatoid arthritis. Results of a prospective placebo controlled double blind trial. Ann Rheum Dis. 1997;56:649–55.
13. Vasanthi B, Komathi J, Arun KD. Therapeutic effect of vitamin E in patients with primary osteoarthritis. Int J Recent Adv Pharm Res. 2012;2:46–50.
14. Bhattacharya I, Saxena R, Gupta V. Efficacy of vitamin E in knee osteoarthritis management of north Indian geriatric population. Ther Adv Musculoskelet Dis. 2012;4:11–9.
15. Haflah NHM, Jaarin K, Abdullah S, Omar M. Palm vitamin E and glucosamine sulphate in the treatment ofosteoarthritis of the knee. Saudi Med J. 2009; 30(11):1432–8.
16. Zhang W, Nuki G, Moskowitz RW, Abramson S, Altman RD, Arden NK, et al. OARSI recommendations for the management of hip and knee osteoarthritis Part III: changes in evidence following systematic cumulative update of research published through January 2009. Osteoarthr Cartil. 2010; 18:476–99.
17. Nelson AE, Allen KD, Golightly YM, Goode AP, Jordan JM. A systematic review of recommendations and guidelines for the management of osteoarthritis: the chronic osteoarthritis management initiative of the U.S. bone and joint initiative. Sem Arthritis Rheum. 2014;43:701–12.
18. Altman R, Asch E, Bloch D, Bole G, Borenstein D, Brandt K, et al. Development of criteria for the classification and reporting of osteoarthritis. Classification of osteoarthrotos of the knee. Diagnosis and therapeutic criteria committee of the American rheumatism association. Arthritis Rheum. 1986;29:1039–49.
19. Kellgren JH, Lawrence JS. Radiological assessment of osteo-arthrosis. Ann Rheum Dis. 1957;16:494–502.
20. Kuptniratsaikul V, Rattanachaiyanont M. Validation of a modified Thai version of the Western Ontario and McMaster (WOMAC) osteoarthritis index for knee osteoarthritis. Clin Rheumatol. 2007;26:1641–5.
21. Fiddler RN. Collaborative study of modified AOAC method of analysis for nitrite in meat and meat products. J Assoc Off Anal Chem. 1977;60:594–9.
22. Bastos AS, Loureiro AP, de Oliveira TF, Corbi SC, Caminaga RM, Junior CR, et al. Quantitation of malondialdehyde in gingival crevicular fluid by a high-performance liquid chromatography-based method. Anal Biochem. 2012; 423:141–6.
23. Merzouk S, Hichami A, Madani S, Mazouk H, Berrouiguet AY, Prost J, et al. Antioxidant status and levels of different vitamins determined by high performance liquid chromatography in diabetic subjects with multiple complications. Gen Physiol Biophys. 2003;22:15–27.
24. Benzie Iris FF, Strain JJ. The ferric reducing ability of plasma (FRAP) as a measure of "antioxidant power": the FRAP assay. Anal Biochem. 1996;293: 70–6.
25. Lien EJ, Ren S, Bui HH, Wang R. Quantitative structure-activity relationship analysis of phenolic antioxidants. Free Radic Biol Med. 1999;26:285–94.
26. Madhujith T, Izydorczyk M, Shahidi F. Antioxidant properties of pearled barley fractions. J Agric Food Chem. 2006;54:3283–9.
27. Sandhu JK, Robertson S, Birnboim HC, Goldstein R. Distribution of protein nitrotyrosine in synovial tissues of patients with rheumatoid arthritis and osteoarthritis. J Rheumatol. 2003;30:1173–81.
28. Ersoy Y, Ozerol E, Baysal O, Temel L, MacWalter RS, Meral U, et al. Serum nitrate and nitrite levels in patients with rheumatoid arthritis, ankylosing spondylitis, and osteoarthritis. Ann Rheum Dis. 2002;61:76–8.
29. Surapaneni KH, Venkataramana G. Status of lipid peroxidation, glutathione, ascorbic acid, vitamin E and antioxidant enzymes in patients with osteoarthritis. Indian J Med Sci. 2007;61:9–14.
30. Sutipornpalangkul W, Morales NP, Charoencholvanich K, Harnroongroj T. Lipid peroxidation, glutathione, vitamin E, and antioxidant enzymes in synovial fluid from patients with osteoarthritis. Int J Rheum Dis. 2009;12: 324–8.
31. Calvisi DF, Ladu S, Hironaka K, Factor VM, Thorgeirsson SS. Vitamin E down-modulates iNOS and NADPH oxidase in c-Myc/TGF-alpha transgenic mouse model of liver cancer. J Hepatol. 2004;41:815–22.
32. Tam LS, Li EK, Leung VY, Griffith JF, Benzie IF, Lim PL, et al. Effects of vitamins C and E on oxidative stress markers and endothelial function in patients with systemic lupus erythematosus: a double blind, placebo controlled pilot study. J Rheumatol. 2005;32:275–82.
33. Beharka AA, Wu D, Serafini M, Meydani SN. Mechanism of vitamin E inhibition of cyclooxygenase activity in macrophages from old mice: role of peroxynitrite. Free Radic Biol Med. 2002;32:503–11.
34. Singh U, Devaraj S, Jialal I. Vitamin E, oxidative stress, and inflammation. Annu Rev Nutr. 2005;25:151–74.

7

Accuracy of injection and short-term pain relief following intra-articular corticosteroid injection in knee osteoarthritis

G. Hirsch[1*], T. W. O'Neill[2,3], G. Kitas[1], A. Sinha[4] and R. Klocke[1,3]

Abstract

Background: Intra-articular corticosteroid injections (IACI) are effective treatments for pain in knee osteoarthritis (KOA) but treatment response varies. There is uncertainty as to whether structural factors such as accurate placement of IACI affect outcome. We examined this question in a pragmatic observational study, using ultrasound (US) to verify accuracy of IACI.

Methods: 105 subjects with KOA (mean age 63.1 years, 59% female) routinely referred for IACI underwent assessment of demographic factors, x-ray and US of the knee before aspiration and IACI (based on clinical landmarks) with 40 mg triamcinolone acetonide with lignocaine plus a small amount of atmospheric air by an independent physician. US demonstration of intra-articular mobile air, i.e. a positive air arthrosonogram, was used to determine accurate placement of injection. Both patients and injecting physicians were blind to the US findings. Pain at baseline, three and nine weeks post injection was assessed using the 500 mm WOMAC pain subscale and response defined as ≥ 40% reduction in pain from baseline. Inter-observer reliability of air-arthrosonogram assessment was good: κ 0.79 (three raters).

Results: Sixty-three subjects (60.6%) were responders at three weeks and 43 (45.7%) at nine weeks. Seventy-four subjects (70.5%) had a positive arthrosonogram. A positive air arthrosonogram did not associate with a higher rate of response to treatment (p 0.389 at three weeks, p 0.365 at nine weeks). There was no difference in US effusion depth, power Doppler signal or radiographic grade between responders and non-responders to the injection, but female gender associated with response at 3 weeks and previous injection with non-response at 9 weeks.

Conclusions: Accurate intra-articular injection of corticosteroid results did not result in superior outcome in terms of pain compared to inaccurate injection in symptomatic knee OA.

Keywords: Intra-articular steroid injection, Knee osteoarthritis, Ultrasound, Predictors of response

Background

Osteoarthritis (OA) is the most common form of arthritis worldwide and its prevalence is increasing [1]. Knee osteoarthritis is one of the most common and disabling forms of the condition and has significant clinical and public health impact [2]. In conjunction with other conservative measures to treat pain in knee OA, intra-articular corticosteroid injections (IACI) are commonly used in accordance with published guidance [3, 4]. Meta-analyses of placebo-controlled studies have confirmed that IACI provide effective pain relief for at least three weeks [5, 6], with some studies suggesting effects of 14 weeks or longer [6]. There is considerable variation between individuals in both the magnitude and duration of response and identifying predictors of response to treatment has been suggested a priority for research in the field [5]. Systematic reviews [7, 8] of previous studies addressing the subject have found insufficient evidence of associations between radiographic grade of arthritis [9, 10] or clinical evidence of

* Correspondence: g.hirsch@nhs.net
[1]Department of Rheumatology, Dudley Group for Health (DGH) NHS Foundation Trust, Russells Hall Hospital, Dudley, West Midlands DY1 2HQ, UK
Full list of author information is available at the end of the article

inflammation [10, 11] and response to IACI. One potentially relevant, but so far insufficiently investigated factor that may plausibly govern response to IACI is accuracy of the injection. While the knee joint is perceived as being easy to inject with a high degree of accuracy, up to a third of routine injections based on anatomical landmarks may fail to enter the joint cavity [12, 13]; it remains unclear whether localisation of the steroid injection to within the knee joint cavity influences outcome.

The aim of this study was to determine whether accuracy of intra-articular placement of the injection, assessed by ultrasound, associates with improved outcome in terms of pain relief following routine IACI, based on clinical landmarks, in knee osteoarthritis.

Methods

Subjects

This was a prospective observational cohort study of a series of subjects with symptomatic knee OA who had been recommended by their treating physician to have an intra-articular steroid injection as part of their routine care. The setting was a single teaching district general hospital in the West Midlands of the UK. Potential participants were identified from orthopaedic and rheumatology clinics based in the hospital.

Men and women were eligible if they satisfied the following criteria: i) aged 40 years and over, ii) evidence of osteoarthritis of the knee according to ACR criteria [14], iii) baseline pain of 100/500 mm or higher on the Western Ontario and McMaster Universities Osteoarthritis Index, version 3 (WOMAC) pain subscale [15], and iv) symptoms judged by the referring clinician as meriting IACI. Subjects were excluded if they had received an intra-articular or intramuscular steroid injection within the preceding twelve weeks or were taking oral prednisolone at a dose of 7.5 mg or higher or, a had a diagnosis of fibromyalgia or complex widespread pain, active RA or other inflammatory arthritis

Baseline assessment

Subjects who consented to the study underwent baseline assessment, immediately prior to treatment. They completed an interviewer-assisted questionnaire which included information about their age, past medical history and whether or not they had received previous knee injection. They also completed the WOMAC questionnaire [15]. This uses five 100 mm visual analogue scales (VAS) to assess knee pain and produces scores with a potential range of 0-500, with higher scores denoting higher levels of pain. Height and weight were assessed in a standard fashion. The baseline assessment also included psychological scales, the details of which will be reported in a separate manuscript. Subjects had radiographs (antero-posterior, lateral and patellofemoral 'skyline' views) of their index knee unless already performed within the previous 6 months. High-sensitivity CRP (hsCRP) was measured using an enzyme immunoassay (MP Biomedicals, Solon, Ohio, US).

Radiographs were graded by agreement by two observers (GH and RK), blinded to clinical details, using a standard atlas [16] which allows grading from 0 to 3 [0, normal; 3, severe changes] for individual features of osteophyte and joint space narrowing at both the tibiofemoral and patellofemoral joint (PFJ) including skyline views of the patellofemoral joint. In this grading system, which has been validated previously [17], grade 1 osteophyte is considered equivalent to Kellgren-Lawrence grade 2 [16]. The highest grade for each feature at any site was used for further analysis. In addition, subjects underwent ultrasound assessment with a 5–13 MHz linear US probe (VF13-5; Antares, Siemens Healthcare Diagnostics, Camberley, Surrey, UK) prior to injection for synovial effusion thickness and semi-quantative synovial power Doppler signal estimation as described previously [18, 19]. All ultrasound procedures in the study were performed by GH, a rheumatologist trained and with two years' experience in MSK US [18].

Intervention

The intervention was performed by one of several clinicians who were not involved with any of the other study procedures, including ultrasound. Using their usual preferred anatomical approach and injection technique and under guidance of clinical examination and landmarks only, the clinician positioned the patient and they aspirated and injected the joint under aseptic precautions with a 21 G needle and a standard mixture of 40 mg triamcinolone acetonide, 4 ml 1% lignocaine and 2 ml atmospheric air.

Assessment of accuracy of intra-articular placement of injection

While the independent clinician performed the injection, the sonographer placed the US probe over the knee joint during the injection to determine placement of the injection. Blinding was maintained: the study subject and injecting clinician were not informed about the US findings. Air provides an effective US contrast medium through its features of being strongly hyperechoic, exhibiting posterior acoustic shadowing, buoyancy and mobility in fluid. We defined an accurate injection by the presence of a positive air arthrosonogram (see Fig. 1), i.e. the presence of any mobile air visible within the joint cavity at the supra-patellar pouch. The technique was adapted from Qvistgaard et al [20] and applied as follows: at the time of injection, the US probe was applied by GH to the midline suprapatellar pouch in the transverse plane and a video clip recorded. Immediately after the injection, a systematic US of all suprapatellar

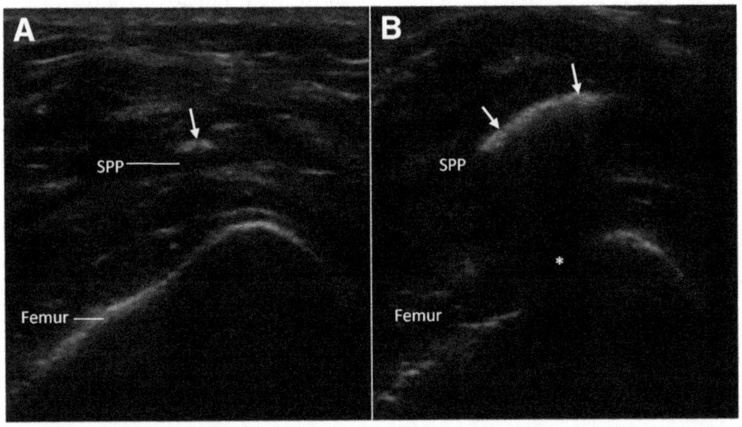

Fig. 1 A transverse ultrasound section of the mid supra-patellar pouch area of the right knee during the very early (**a**) and later (**b**) phase of injection, showing a positive air arthrosonogram. There is an emerging area of intra-articular air bubbles (arrows), initially faintly (**a**) and then more clearly visible (**b**), with posterior acoustic shadowing (*). Varying transducer pressure demonstrated the echogenic layer to be displaceable and display buoyancy, consistent with intra-articular placement of the injection. SPP denotes suprapatellar pouch

pouch areas was performed, starting at the site of injection in order to identify a positive air-arthrosonogram. Representative video clips were recorded, as was the sonographer's immediate impression of whether air-arthrosonogram was present. A positive air-arthrosonogram at any of these sites was used for further analysis. Following intervention, participants were advised to rest the joint as much as possible for 24 h, in line with normal departmental practice.

Assessment of response

Participants completed the WOMAC pain subscale in clinic at three weeks post injection and again at nine weeks by postal questionnaire. We classified participants as responders at each time point, if their pain scores reduced by 40% or more from baseline, which has been estimated both a clinically important and perceptible change following intervention in knee OA [21].

Analysis

Descriptive statistics were used to summarise the subject characteristics. We determined at both 3 and 9 weeks whether subjects were responders or non-responders. We looked for differences in subject characteristics by response status at 3 and 9 weeks using t-tests for continuous data and either Fisher's exact test/Chi-Squared tests for categorical data. Where subjects had omitted individual WOMAC questionnaire items, these were replaced with mean values for the relevant subscale, as far as was permitted according to the manual. Factors considered as potential confounders for adjustment in a multivariable analysis included included gender, baseline pain, radiographic grade, previous injection, body mass index. Inter-observer reliability of the air-arthrosonogram technique was calculated by presenting a sample of 26 stored video clips from the study to three observers (GH, AS, RK; the latter being a consultant radiologist and rheumatologist, respectively, with over ten years experience in musculo-skeletal ultrasound each. An equal number of clips were selected from each set of originally classified as positive or negative air arthrograms, respectively, at random. The studies were viewed in random order, independently, by the observers, who then scoring each as showing either positive or negative air-arthrosonogram. Inter-observer agreement was calculated for each pair of observers as a kappa values and the mean value calculated for the three pairs of observers. All analyses were conducted using SPSS version 20.

Results

Subjects

A total of 105 patients were recruited to the study (Table 1). Their mean age was 63.1 years and 62 (59%) were female. Mean Body Mass Index (BMI) was 30.8 kg/m^2. Baseline pain level was 266 (SD 95.5)/500 mm. 104 subjects contributed outcome data at three weeks and 94 (89.5%) at nine weeks. One participant submitted incomplete WOMAC pain scores at 3 weeks. Of the 11 participants who did not contribute to outcome data at nine weeks, one was withdrawn due to an intercurrent episode of crystal arthritis, one questionnaire was lost in the post and 9 failed to return questionnaires. Those who failed to provide data at nine weeks were younger, more likely to be male and had higher CRP values than those providing full data, but there was no difference in accuracy of injections and response rate at 3 weeks between these two groups (see Table 2).

Accuracy of injection

Mean inter-observer agreement for air-arthrosonogram status was good, with mean kappa value between three

Table 1 Baseline characteristics and responder status of study population

Characteristics	n = 105
Age [years] [mean (SD)]	63.1 (11.3)
Female [n (%)]	62 (59%)
BMI [mean (SD)]	30.8 (5.5)
Previous injection [n (%)]	60 (57%)
Baseline WOMAC Pain [mean(SD)]	266 (95.5)
US effusion depth [mm] [Mean (SD)]	3.74 (2.27)
PD grade [median (IQR)]	0 (0,1)
Osteophyte grade [median (IQR)]	2 (1, 3)
JSN grade [median (IQR)]	2 (1,2)
hs CRP [mg/L] [median (IQR)]	4.4 (1.7,7.1)
Positive US arthrogram [n (%)]	74 (70.5%)
Responders at 3 weeks [n (%)]	63 (60.6%)
Responder at 9 weeks [n (%)]	43 (45.7%)

Abbreviations: *BMI* body mass index, *PD* power Doppler, *JSN* joint space narrowing, *hsCRP* high-sensitivity CRP, *US* ultrasound

raters of 0.79. 98 (69.5%) injections were considered to be accurate as determined by the presence of air on the arthrosonogram at the time of injection.

Predictors of response

The overall positive response rate was 61% at three weeks and 46% at nine weeks. A positive arthrosonogram did not predict responder status at 3 or 9 weeks; in fact at both time points, response rates were higher in those with negative than those with positive arthrosonogram (e.g. 75% vs 64%, $p = 0.365$ at nine weeks) (Table 3), although these results were not statistically significant. There were no statistically significant differences in baseline clinical, radiographic, sonographic and serological characteristics between responders and non-responders with two exceptions: Female gender associated with response at three weeks ($p = 0.045$) and previous injection with non-response at nine weeks ($p = 0.021$) (Table 3).

A post-hoc analysis of absolute change in pain scores from baseline in groups with positive vs negative arthrosonogram showed no difference: -114.0 vs -123.4. mm, p 0.724 at three weeks; and -58.8 vs -96.5 mm, p 0.185 at nine weeks (data not shown in table).

Table 2 Characteristics of subjects completing the study compared with those who failed to complete the study

	3 weeks (n = 104)		
Characteristics	Completer (n = 94)	Non completion (n = 11)	P
Age [years] [mean (SD)]	64.3 (11.4)	57.1 (8.3)	0.043
Female [n (%)]	59 (62.8%)	3 (27.3%)	0.047
BMI [mean(SD)]	30.7 (5.3)	31.7 (7.5)	0.549
Previous injection [n (%)]	56 (59.6%)	4 (36.4%)	0.199
Baseline Pain [mean (SD)]	264.5 (97.1)	275.4 (84.3)	0.724
US effusion depth [mm] [mean (SD)]	3.7 (2.3)	3.8 (1.7)	0.924
PD grade [median (IQR)]	0 (0,1)	0 (0,1)	0.702
Osteophyte grade [median (IQR)]	2 (1,3)	2 (1,3)	0.977
JSN grade [median (IQR)]	2 (1,2)	2 (1,2)	0.538
hsCRP [mg/L] [median (IQR)]	5.58 (1.5,6.5)	7.80 (3.8, 10.1)	0.021
Positive US arthrogram [n (%)]	66 (70.2%)	8 (72.7%)	1.00
Responder at 3 weeks [n (%)]	56 (60.2)	7 (63.6)	1.00

Discussion

In this prospective observational study we have shown that in knee osteoarthritis accurate intra-articular placement of a corticosteroid injection, as determined by positive air-arthrosonogram, did not improve the rate of clinically significant response or mean pain reduction at three or nine weeks post injection, compared to a group in whom a negative arthrosonogram suggested that placement of injection was predominantly extra-articular. A recent systematic review [13] found that on average only 77% of knee injections enter accurately the intra-articular cavity when using clinical landmarks as guidance for injection. It is therefore plausible to assume that accuracy of injection may potentially explain the variability of response to IACI in knee OA. While there is little doubt that guidance by US improves accuracy of intra-articular placement of injection, there remains uncertainty, however, as to how whether this affects outcome [13]. In a small randomized placebo-controlled study of 38 patients with knee OA, Sambrook et al found no difference in outcome between intentional intra-articular vs peri-patellar injection of methylprednislone between one and 12 weeks post injection. This remains the only study that we are aware of that used clinical guidance of injection to address the role of intra- vs extra-articular corticosteroid injection in knee OA on outcome. The fact that no difference was observed in that study may have been due to the fact that correct intra-articular placement was not verified by further imaging (i.e. some intended intra-articular injections may still have ended up extra-articularly) and/or lack of power (i.e. insufficient study sample) to show a difference. Sibbitt et al [22] examined the effect of ultrasound (US)-guidance vs clinically guided IACI in a randomised study of 94 subjects with knee OA. No information on accuracy of the injection with either method is provided, but subjects undergoing US-guided injection were approximately twice as likely to have a positive response at 2 weeks (defined as a pain VAS of < 2 cm). A second

Table 3 Baseline characteristics of responders vs non-responders (n = 105)

	3 weeks (n = 104)			9 weeks (n = 94)		
Characteristics	Responder (n = 63)	Non-responder (n = 41)	*P*	Responders (n = 43)	Non-Responder (n = 51)	*P*
Age [years] [mean (SD)]	64.4(10.6)	61.8(11.9)	0.258	64.1(11)	64.5(11)	0.890
Female [n (%)]	42 (67%)	19 (46%)	0.045	31 (72%)	28 (55%)	0.093
BMI [mean(SD)]	31.3(5.4)	30.0(5.8)	0.265	30.9(4.8)	30.4(5.8)	0.658
Previous injection [n (%)]	33 (52%)	26 (63%)	0.314	20 (47%)	36 (71%)	0.021
Baseline Pain [mean (SD)]	256(87)	279(107)	0.240	243(91)	282(99)	0.057
US effusion depth [mm] [mean (SD)]	3.57(2.1)	4.07(2.6)	0.280	3.29(1.9)	4.14(2.59)	0.080
PD grade [median (IQR)]	0(0,1)	0(0,1)	0.790	0(0,1)	0(0,1)	0.376
Osteophyte grade [median (IQR)]	2(1,3)	2(1,3)	0.870	2(1,2)	2(1,3)	0.540
JSN grade [median (IQR)]	2(1,2)	2(1,2)	0.796	2(1,2)	2(1,2)	0.461
hsCRP [mg/L] [median (IQR)]	3.5(1.5,6.8)	4.6(2.2,8.6)	0.147	3.0(1.5,5.7)	4.5(1.7,8.6)	0.857
Positive US arthrogram [n (%)]	42 (67%)	30 (73%)	0.389	27 (64%)	38 (75%)	0.365

See legend to Table 1 for abbreviations

smaller study of essentially similar design by the same group showed similar findings. Both studies have not tried to control for any treatment effect likely to be conferred by the use of ultrasound itself, in other words: having an injection under ultrasound than without may have significant beneficial effect per se without any relationship to improved accuracy. That this is likely to be relevant is suggested by work by Cunnington et al [23] who used sham-US to compare US-guided injection vs clinically-guided injections in a variety of joints in a large study of 184 subjects with inflammatory arthritis: whilst, as expected US-guided injections were more accurate than clinically guided with sham-US, there was no difference in outcome (both pain and function) between the two groups. Furthermore, and more relevant to this study, function (but not pain) at six (but not two) weeks was the only parameter that showed positive correlation with accuracy of injection. A trial studying US-guided vs 'sham-US' clinically-guided injection has been terminated and is to date unreported (ClinicalTrials.gov Identifier: NCT01032720; accessed 15 June 2015).

We chose outcome assessment at three and nine weeks, as these time points reflect the period during which benefit of treatment has been suggested in previous systematic reviews of placebo-controlled trials [5, 6].

Our study showed further interesting observations: participants who had previous experience of injection were less likely to report response to treatment than those undergoing their first injection at nine weeks (p 0.021), but not three weeks. This seems to concur with the anecdotal clinical observation that the effect of subsequent IACI in knee OA is less than of first injections. In line with most [11, 24–26], but not all studies [9, 10], we found no association between radiographic severity and rate of response, despite scoring separately for individual features of knee osteoarthritis. In accordance with other investigators [27, 28], we found no relationship between response and sonographic effusion or synovial power Doppler, despite using a sonographic assessment that included measures from the medial, mid and lateral aspect of the supra-patellar pouch rather than single view data.

The main strength of our study is that it was based on routine practice of IACI, using clinical guidance and subjects referred for IACI by their clinician as part of routine clinical management. As such we believe the results are applicable to a general population. However, we have seen a better response rates than placebo-controlled studies [5] probably due to contextual, non-specific treatment effects. Conversely, in trying to reflect a 'real-world' treatment environment, we did not limit the use of other interventions including analgesics, walking sticks and physiotherapy, which could have affected patient outcomes.

This study has a number of limitations: As an observational study, it remains possible that an adequately powered, placebo-controlled trial might disclose an effect of accuracy of injection on outcome. We did not perform a formal power calculation based on arthrogram status for this observational trial and one could argue that our sample size is too small to show an effect of accuracy or other structural factors on outcome However, the reported rate of response was numerically higher in those with a negative air-arthrosonogram at both three and nine weeks, suggesting that a larger sample would be unlikely to show superiority of response rate in those with a positive vs those with a negative arthrogram. We did not use a second imaging method (e.g. MRI or limited CT) to validate our method to verify accurate intra-articular injection as previously described by Qvistgaard et al [20]. We therefore acknowledge that there are limitations in the air-arthrosonogram technique as an indicator of intra- vs extra-articular placement of injection, even though our interobserver reliability was good. Our accuracy data on the basis of the air-arthrosonogram method of 70% are also broadly in line with those reported in a recent systematic review [13]. We therefore do not believe that the technique resulted in significant systemic misclassification.

Beyond the question of relevance of precise intra- vs extra-knee joint cavity placement, the question remains as to whether an injection close to the synovium (e.g. the fat-pad of the knee) can be shown to be of equivalent effectiveness on outcome. Our study suggests this possibility, but due to its lack of precise visualisation of injectate localisation in those with a negative arthrosonogram, we are unable to draw any firm conclusions on this possibility. Our findings suggest that accurate intra-articular injection is neither a guarantor nor a pre-requisite of response at 3 and 9 weeks and provides support the current practice of IACI in knee OA using clinical landmarks and palpation. Whilst US may well have a treatment effect of its own and recognised to be useful to assist for aspiration or technically difficult injections, there is to date no convincing indication that the improved accuracy it confers to the injection matters to outcome of pain relief in this setting.

Conclusion

Our 'real-life', observational study suggests that IACI based on routine, clinically guided practice leads to relief of knee pain in osteoarthritis in the short- and medium-term in patients with uncertain placement of injection, as well as those in whom injections could be demonstrated to be in the intra-articular space. This casts doubt over the relevance of accuracy of intra-articular injection placement to clinical outcome in this setting.

Abbreviations

ACR: American college of rheumatology; BMI: Body mass index; IACI: Intra-articular corticosteroid injections; IQR: inter-quartile range; JSN: Joint space narrowing; KOA: knee osteoarthritis; PD: Power doppler; RA: Rheumatoid arthritis; SD: Standard deviation; US: ultrasound; VAS: Visual analogue score; WOMAC: Western Ontario and McMaster Universities Osteoarthritis Index

Acknowledgements

We thank Mr Tom Clare and Mr Matthew Waites, Consultant Orthopaedic Surgeons, and all medical Rheumatology Staff of DGH NHS FT for referring patients and performing injections for this study. We are also grateful to Dr Peter Nightingale, Wolfson Computer Laboratories, Queen Elizabeth Hospital, Birmingham, UK, for statistical advice.

Funding

Dudley Group NHS Foundation Trust provided GH with an unrestricted grant that enabled this research.

Authors' contributions

GH design and preparation of study, collection of data, analysis, preparation and review of manuscript, TO'N design and preparation of study, analysis of data, preparation and review of manuscript, GK design and preparation of study, analysis of data, preparation and review of manuscript, AS design of study, collection of data, review of manuscript, RK design and preparation of study, collection of data, analysis, preparation and review of manuscript. All authors have read and approved the final manuscript.

Authors information

Nil additional.

Competing interests

The authors declare that they have no competing interests.

Consent for publication

Not applicable.

Author details

[1]Department of Rheumatology, Dudley Group for Health (DGH) NHS Foundation Trust, Russells Hall Hospital, Dudley, West Midlands DY1 2HQ, UK. [2]Faculty of Medical and Human Sciences, Arthritis Research UK Centre for Epidemiology, Institute of Inflammation and Repair, Manchester Academic Health Science Centre, University of Manchester, Manchester, UK. [3]NIHR Manchester Musculoskeletal Biomedical Research Unit, Central Manchester NHS Foundation Trust, Manchester Academic Health Science Centre, Manchester, UK. [4]Department of Radiology, DGH NHS Foundation Trust, Russells Hall Hospital, Dudley, West Midlands, UK.

References

1. Cross M, Smith E, Hoy D, Nolte S, Ackerman I, Fransen M, et al. The global burden of hip and knee osteoarthritis: estimates from the Global Burden of Disease 2010 study. Ann Rheum Dis. 2014;73(7):1323–30.
2. Gupta S, Hawker GA, Laporte A, Croxford R, Coyte PC. The economic burden of disabling hip and knee osteoarthritis (OA) from the perspective of individuals living with this condition. Rheumatology. 2005;44(12):1531–7.
3. Jordan KM, Arden NK, Doherty M, Bannwarth B, Bijlsma JWJ, Dieppe P, et al. EULAR Recommendations 2003: an evidence based approach to the management of knee osteoarthritis: Report of a Task Force of the Standing Committee for International Clinical Studies Including Therapeutic Trials (ESCISIT). Ann Rheum Dis. 2003;62(12):1145–55.
4. National Institute for Health and Care Excellence. Osteoarthrtis: care and management in adults. CG177th ed. London: National Institute for Health and Care Excellence; 2014.
5. Bellamy N, Campbell J, Welch V, Gee T, Bourne R, Wells G. Intraarticular corticosteroid for treatment of osteoarthritis of the knee. Cochrane Database Syst Rev. 2006;19(2), CD005328.
6. Arroll B, Goodyear-Smith F. Corticosteroid injections for osteoarthritis of the knee: meta-analysis. BMJ. 2004;328(7444):869.
7. Maricar N, Callaghan MJ, Felson DT, O'Neill TW. Predictors of response to intra-articular steroid injections in knee osteoarthritis; a systematic review. Rheumatology. 2012;52(6):1022–32.
8. Hirsch G, Kitas G, Klocke R. Intra-articular corticosteroid injection in osteoarthritis of the knee and hip: Factors predicting pain relief; systematic review. Semin Arthritis Rheum. 2013;42:451–73.
9. Smith MD, Wetherall M, Darby T, Esterman A, Slavotinek J, Roberts-Thomson P, et al. A randomized placebo-controlled trial of arthroscopic lavage versus lavage plus intra-articular corticosteroids in the management of symptomatic osteoarthritis of the knee. Rheumatology. 2003;42(12):1477–85.
10. Arden N. A randomised controlled trial of tidal irrigation vs corticosteroid injection in knee osteoarthritis: the KIVIS study. Osteoarthr Cartil. 2008;16:733–9.
11. Gaffney K, Ledingham J, Perry JD. Intra-articular triamcinolone hexacetonide in knee osteoarthritis: factors influencing the clinical response. Ann Rheum Dis. 1995;54(5):379–81.

12. Jones A, Regan M, Ledingham J, Pattrick M, Manhire A, Doherty M. Importance of placement of intra-articular steroid injections. Br Med J. 1993;307(6915):1329–30.
13. Maricar N, Parkes MJ, Callaghan MJ, Felson DT, O'Neill TW. Where and how to inject the knee: a systematic review. Semin Arthritis Rheum. 2013;43(2): 195–203.
14. Altman R, Asch E, Bloch D, Bole G, Borenstein D, Brandt K, et al. The American College of Rheumatology criteria for the classification and reporting of osteoarthritis of the knee. Arthritis Rheum. 1986;29:1039–49.
15. Bellamy N, Buchanan WW, Goldsmith CH, Campbell J, Stitt LW. Validation study of WOMAC - A health-status instrument for measuring clinically important patient relevant outcomes to antirheumatic drug therapy in patients with osteoarthritis of the hip or knee. J Rheumatol. 1988;15(12):1833–40.
16. Burnett S, Hart D, Cooper C, Spector TD. A radiographic atlas of osteoarthritis. London: Springer; 1994.
17. Cicuttini FM, Baker J, Hart J, et al. Choosing the best method for radiographic assessment of the patellofemoral joint. Ann Rheum Dis. 1996;55:134–6.
18. Hirsch G, O' Neill T, Kitas G, Klocke R. Distribution of effusion in knee arthritis as measured by high-resolution ultrasound. Clin Rheumatol. 2012;31(8):1243–6.
19. D'Agostino MA, Conaghan P, Le Bars M, Baron G, Grassi W, Martin-Mola E, et al. EULAR report on the use of ultrasonography in painful knee osteoarthritis. Part 1: Prevalence of inflammation in osteoarthritis. Ann Rheum Dis. 2005;64(12):1703–9.
20. Qvistgaard E, Kristoffersen H, Terslev L, Danneskiold-Samsoe B, Torp-Pedersen S, Bliddal H. Guidance by ultrasound of intra-articular injections in the knee and hip joints. Osteoarthr Cartil. 2001;9(6):512–7.
21. Tubach F, Ravaud P, Baron G. Evaluation of clinically relevant changes in patient reported outcome measures in patients with knee and hip osteoarthritis: the minimal clinically important improvement. Ann Rheumeumatic Dis. 2005;64(1):29–33.
22. Sibbitt WLJ, Band PA, Kettwich LG, Chavez-Chiang NR, DeLea SL, Bankhurst AD. A Randomized Controlled Trial Evaluating the Cost-Effectiveness of Sonographic Guidance for Intra-Articular Injection of the Osteoarthritic Knee. J Clin Rheumatol. 2011;17(8):409–15.
23. Cunnington J, Marshall N, Hide G, Bracewell C, Isaacs J, Platt P, et al. A Randomized, Double-Blind, Controlled Study of Ultrasound-Guided Corticosteroid Injection Into the Joint of Patients With Inflammatory Arthritis. Arthritis Rheum. 2010;62(7):1862–9.
24. Dieppe P, Sathapatayavongs B, Jones H, Bacon P, Ring E. Intra-articular steroids in osteoarthritis. Rheumatol Rehabil. 1980;19:212–7.
25. Leopold SS, Redd BB, Warme WJ, Wehrle PA, Pettis PD, Shott S. Corticosteroid compared with hyaluronic acid injections for the treatment of osteoarthritis of the knee - A prospective, randomized trial. J Bone Joint Surg Am Vol. 2003;85A(7):1197–203.
26. Raynauld J-P. Safety and efficacy of long term intra-articular steroid injections of the knee. A randomised double blind placebo controlled trial. Arthritis Rheum. 2003;48(2):370–7.
27. Pendleton A, Millar A, O'Kane D, Wright G, Taggart A. Can sonography be used to predict the response to intra-articular corticosteroid injection in primary osteoarthritis of the knee? Scand J Rheumatol. 2008;37:395–7.
28. Bevers K, Zweers MC, Vriezekolk JE, Bijlsma JWJ, den Broeder AA. Are ultrasonographic signs of inflammation predictors for response to intra-articular glucocorticoids in knee osteoarthritis? Clin Exp Rheumatol. 2014;32(6):930–4.

Change in physical activity level and clinical outcomes in older adults with knee pain: a secondary analysis from a randomised controlled trial

Jonathan G. Quicke*, Nadine E. Foster, Peter R. Croft, Reuben O. Ogollah and Melanie A. Holden

Abstract

Background: Exercise interventions improve clinical outcomes of pain and function in adults with knee pain due to osteoarthritis and higher levels of physical activity are associated with lower severity of pain and higher levels of physical functioning in older adults with knee osteoarthritis in cross-sectional studies. However, to date no studies have investigated if change in physical activity level during exercise interventions can explain clinical outcomes of pain and function. This study aimed to investigate if change in physical activity during exercise interventions is associated with future pain and physical function in older adults with knee pain.

Methods: Secondary longitudinal data analyses of a three armed exercise intervention randomised controlled trial. Participants were adults with knee pain attributed to osteoarthritis, over the age of 45 years old ($n = 514$) from Primary Care Services in the Midlands and Northwest regions of England.
Crude and adjusted associations between absolute change in physical activity from baseline to 3 months (measured by the self-report Physical Activity Scale for the Elderly (PASE)) and i) pain ii) physical function (Western Ontario and McMaster Universities Osteoarthritis Index) and iii) treatment response (OMERACT-OARSI responder criteria) at 3 and 6 months follow-up were investigated using linear and logistic regression.

Results: Change in physical activity level was not associated with future pain, function or treatment response outcomes in crude or adjusted models at 3 or 6 months ($P > 0.05$). A 10 point increase in PASE was not associated with pain $\beta = -0.01$ (-0.05, 0.02), physical function $\beta = -0.09$ (-0.19, 0.02) or likelihood (odds ratio) of treatment response 1.02 (0.99, 1.04) at 3 months adjusting for sociodemographics, clinical covariates and the trial intervention arm. Findings were similar for 6 month outcome models.

Conclusions: Change in physical activity did not explain future clinical outcomes of pain and function in this study. Other factors may be responsible for clinical improvements following exercise interventions. However, the PASE may not be sufficiently responsive to measure change in physical activity level. We also recommend further investigation into the responsiveness of commonly used physical activity measures.

Keywords: Osteoarthritis, Knee, Pain, Physical activity, Exercise, Geriatrics

* Correspondence: j.g.quicke@keele.ac.uk
Arthritis Research UK Primary Care Centre, Research Institute for Primary Care and Health Sciences, Keele University, Keele, Staffordshire ST5 5BG, UK

Background

Knee pain attributable to osteoarthritis (OA) is both common and disabling in older adults [1]. Exercise and physical activity (PA), including lower limb muscle strengthening and aerobic exercise (for example walking, cycling and swimming) are core recommended treatments in OA clinical guidelines [1–3]. Such interventions are associated with, on average, small to medium effect sizes in terms of reduction in pain and improvements in physical function compared to non-exercise control groups [4–6], although improvements may not be maintained over the longer-term. In order to optimise the effectiveness of exercise interventions, it is important to understand the active components that contribute to improved clinical outcomes [7].

Higher levels of physical activity have been shown to be associated with lower severity of pain and higher physical function in older adults with knee pain in cross-sectional studies [8]. It is plausible that changes in participants' physical activity level as a result of exercise interventions may explain changes in pain and physical functioning either directly or indirectly. For example, increase in levels of moderate and vigorous cardiovascular intensity physical activity are associated with weight loss in longitudinal cohorts with or at risk of knee OA [9] which is associated with reduced pain and improved function in those who are overweight [10]. However, to date, no studies have investigated the association between change in physical activity level and clinical outcomes of pain and function. The aim of this study, therefore, was to investigate if change in physical activity level is associated with future pain, physical function and overall response to treatment [11] in older adults with knee pain.

Methods

Design

This study involved secondary analyses of data from a multi-centre, pragmatic, three-parallel group, randomised controlled trial (RCT) of three physical therapist-led exercise interventions (The Benefits of Effective Exercise for knee Pain-BEEP trial ISRCTN 93634563) [12]. Longitudinal data from all three groups at baseline, three months (following treatment in two of three groups) and six months (following treatment in all groups) were combined, with a priori adjustment for intervention group allocation. Ethical approval was provided by the North West 1 Research Ethics Committee, Cheshire, UK (REC reference 10/H1017/45). Full detail of the RCT is available elsewhere [12] but a concise summary is provided below for context.

Participants

Participants were adults with knee pain attributable to OA from the BEEP trial (n = 514). Inclusion criteria were a clinical diagnosis of knee OA made by either a general practitioner or a primary care research nurse based on age (being 45 years old or older), the presence of pain and/or stiffness in one or both knees [1] and the exclusion of knee pain due to other sources, such as those who had pain due to trauma or recent injury, potentially serious pathology other than OA (such as malignancy or rheumatoid arthritis) and those who had undergone previous total knee replacements. Those with exercise contraindications (such as those with unstable cardiovascular disorders, severe hypertension or congestive heart failure) and those unable to travel to physical therapy treatment centres were also excluded [12].

Participants were recruited from 65 general practices in the midlands and northwest regions of England from: i) records of general practitioner consulters with knee pain in the last year, ii) those referred to physical therapy with knee pain and, iii) adults registered at participating general practices who responded to a questionnaire and reported knee pain [12].

Trial intervention arms

The three physical therapist-delivered exercise intervention arms were: usual care (UC), individually tailored exercise (ITE) and targeted exercise adherence (TEA). All participants received an advice and information booklet in addition to an exercise programme delivered one-to-one for up to three (UC and ITE) and six months (TEA). Additional intervention detail is provided in Additional file 1: Table S1.

Outcomes

Pain and physical function

Knee pain severity and physical function were assessed using the Western Ontario and McMaster Universities Osteoarthritis Index (WOMAC) pain and function subscales [13]. The pain subscale comprises five items measuring self-reported pain during various activities and gives a total score ranging from 0 (no pain) to 20 (maximum pain). The physical function subscale comprises 17 items and measures the self-reported difficulty an individual has with a broad range of physical functions giving a total score ranging from 0 (no disability) to 68 (maximum disability). Both subscales have been widely used in knee OA studies and their clinimetric properties have been widely investigated elsewhere [13–15].

Treatment response

Clinically important response to treatment was assessed using the Outcome Measures in Rheumatology Clinical Trials clinical responder criteria (OMERACT-OARSI responder criteria) [11, 16]. This internationally agreed measure combines outcome data on pain and physical function from the WOMAC scales with patient's global assessment of change (recorded using a 6 point Likert Scale) [11, 16]. Treatment responders are classified as those who either make a large improvement in pain or function (≥50% improvement and absolute change ≥20 in a 0–100 scale) or a small improvement (≥20% improvement and absolute change≥10 in a 0–100 scale) in two out of three of pain, physical function or global assessment of change (at follow-up compared to baseline).

Determinants

Change in physical activity

Absolute change in physical activity from baseline to three month follow-up (referred to henceforth as *"change in physical activity"*) was calculated by subtracting baseline physical activity score from follow-up physical activity score at three months using the self-report Physical Activity Scale for the Elderly (PASE) [17]. The PASE scale (scored from 0 to over 400 with higher scores indicating higher levels of physical activity) measures physical activity in the previous week summed from questions regarding the frequency and duration of household, leisure time and work physical activity. It has demonstrated construct validity in terms of correlation with 6 min walk test (r = 0.35) and knee strength (0.41) in older adults with knee pain [18] and test-retest reliability in older adults (intra-class correlation 0.75) [17]. The PASE scale has been used in previous longitudinal studies of knee pain and OA [19–21].

Potential confounders

A range of sociodemographic and clinical covariates measured within the BEEP dataset may be potential confounders of the relationship between change in physical activity and clinical outcomes due to their association with both physical activity [8] and clinical outcome [22, 23]. These included age, gender, Body Mass Index (BMI), individual socioeconomic status [24], employment status, comorbidities (categorised into none, one and two or more), depression measured by the Personal Health Questionnaire (PHQ 8) [25], anxiety measured by the generalized Anxiety Disorder Questionnaire (GAD-7) [26], and widespread pain measured by the Manchester Widespread Pain criteria [27].

Analyses

All analyses were carried out using STATA version 13.1 [28] and all primary longitudinal analyses utilised a multiply imputed dataset. Multiple imputation (25 imputations) using chained equations was used to adjust for the effect of missing data by maximising sample size and reducing the possible bias associated with loss to follow-up and missing data [29] since there was between 12 and 22% missing clinical outcome data at 3 and 6 months. A wide range of sociodemographic and clinical variables available within the BEEP dataset, including the outcome variables, were used in the imputation model [30].

Descriptive statistics

Baseline characteristics (complete case) together with longitudinal descriptive statistics (at baseline, three and six months) of physical activity, change in physical activity (measured by the PASE) and clinical outcomes of pain, physical function (WOMAC) and treatment response (OMERACT-OARSI responder criteria) were summarised using means and standard deviations (SD) or frequency and percentage as appropriate.

Analyses to investigate the association between change in physical activity and clinical outcome

Associations between change in physical activity and clinical outcomes of pain, physical function and treatment response at three and six months were determined using linear and logistic regression. Both univariable and multivariable models were fitted. ANCOVA type multivariable models were used where the clinical outcome variable of interest (pain or function) at 6 months (and subsequently 12 months) were adjusted for baseline clinical severity (pain in the pain and treatment response models, and function in the function model), potential confounders and the trial intervention arm. The a priori decision to hold the intervention arm within multivariable models was made to account for any between trial arm treatment effects (although similar clinical improvements were found in all groups). Additional methodological detail regarding adjusted model building is provided in the Additional file 2.

Sensitivity analyses

Sensitivity analyses on missing data was performed by use of complete case analysis (CCA), which restricts the analysis to subjects with complete data on the variables involved in the analysis. CCA assumes that missing cases are missing completely at random and makes the assumption that results would be similar to intended sample results [31].

Results

Descriptive statistics

Table 1 describes the baseline characteristics of the 514 BEEP trial participants. The sample was 51% female with a participant mean (SD) age of 62.8 (9.7) years. Mean WOMAC pain score (SD) was 8.4 (3.5) and physical function score was 28.1 (12.2) suggesting that on average participants had moderate levels of clinical severity. Mean physical activity score, measured by the PASE, was 177 (83.3) (see Table 2).

Table 1 Baseline characteristics

Characteristic	Total (*n* = 514)
Age, *n* (%), years	
45–49	52 (10)
50–59	153 (30)
60–69	183 (36)
70–79	99 (19)
≥80	27 (5)
Female, *n* (%)	262 (51)
BMI, *n* (%), *	
Underweight/ normal	97 (20)
Overweight	208 (42)
Obese	192 (39)
Currently employed n (%) *	214 (42)
Socioeconomic category, *n* (%) *	
Professional	166 (43)
Intermediate	94 (25)
Routine and manual work	124 (32)
Comorbidities, *n* (%)	
None	164 (32)
1 comorbidity	180 (35)
2 or more comorbidities	170 (33)
PHQ 8, 0–24, mean (SD) *	4.0 (+/− 4.7)
WOMAC, mean (SD)	
Pain, 0–20, *	8.4 (+/− 3.5)
Function, 0–68, *	28.1 (+/− 12.3)
Stiffness, 0–8, *	3.7 (+/− 1.7)
Knee pain duration, *n* (%), years *	
≤ 1	125 (25)
More than1 but < 5	198 (39)
More than 5 but < 10	94 (19)
10+	91 (18)
Widespread pain *n* (%) *	79 (15)

Footnote: Baseline descriptive statistics based on complete cases; * = subject to missing data (hence individual item frequencies may not add to total sample). Missing data was 2% in primary clinical variables, less than 10% in all remaining variables except socioeconomic category which was 25% missing. Body Mass Index: less than 25 = underweight/ normal, 25 or more but less than 30 = overweight, 30 or more = obese. Comorbidities included (in descending order of frequency) Hypertension, Asthma, Diabetes, Angina, Heart attack and Heart failure
Abbreviations: *BMI* Body Mass Index, *PHQ* 8 Personal Health Depression Questionnaire (higher scores indicate lower mood), *SD* Standard deviation; Widespread pain = Manchester Widespread Pain [27]; *WOMAC* Western Ontario and McMaster Universities Osteoarthritis Index

The proportion of the baseline sample lost to follow up was 17% at three months and 11% at six months. For information, participants lost to follow-up had slightly worse pain and function at baseline, higher levels of depression and anxiety at baseline and were less likely to have used facilities for physical activity in the last 7 days [30]. Mean PASE increased to 192.1 (87.9) at three month follow-up and then remained relatively stable at six month follow-up 190.5 (89.3). Clinical outcome scores of pain and function improved over time with 45% classified as treatment responders at three months and 52% at six months follow-up. At three months, mean WOMAC pain and function were 6.7 (3.6) and 23.6 (12.5) respectively, changing to 6.3 (3.9) and 21.7 (13.7) at six month follow-up (see Table 2).

Table 2 Physical activity and clinical outcome longitudinal summary statistics

Variables (range)	Baseline	3 months	6 months
PASE (0–400+)	177.0 (83.3)	192.1 (87.9)	190.5 (89.3)
WOMAC pain (0–20)	8.4 (3.5)	6.7 (3.6)	6.3 (3.9)
WOMAC function (0–68)	28.1 (12.2)	23.6 (12.5)	21.7 (13.7)
OMERACT-OARSI response (%)	NA	45	52

Footnote: Multiple imputed data (combined results from 25 imputed datasets). All values are mean scores (standard deviation) except OMERACT-OARSI response which are given in percentages. All scores indicate higher levels of the variable except WOMAC function with higher scores indicating lower functioning
Abbreviations: *OMERACT-OARSI* Outcome Measures in Rheumatology Clinical Trials-Osteoarthritis Research Society International, *PASE* Physical Activity Scale for the Elderly, *WOMAC* Western Ontario and McMaster Universities Osteoarthritis Index

The mean PASE change score between baseline and three months was an increase of 15.1 with substantial individual variation as indicated by a standard deviation of 87.4. Change scores for physical activity and clinical outcomes are reported in Table 3.

Associations between change in physical activity and clinical outcome

Univariable models showed change in physical activity was not significantly associated with any of the three clinical outcomes of pain, physical function (Tables 4 and 5) or treatment response at both three and six months ($p > 0.05$) (Table 6).

Change in physical activity remained non-significantly associated with clinical outcomes in all multivariable clinical outcome models adjusting for age, continuous BMI, pain duration, depression, the trial intervention

Table 3 Physical activity, pain and function change scores

Change variable	Mean score baseline to 3 months(SD)	Mean score baseline to 6 months(SD)
Change in PASE	15.1 (87.4)	13.5 (86.9)
Change in WOMAC pain	−1.6 (3.2)	−2.1 (3.5)
Change in WOMAC function	−4.5 (10.1)	−6.4 (11.8)

Footnote: Multiple imputed data (combined results from 25 imputed datasets); all change scores calculated by subtracting the score at baseline from the score at three or six month follow up; Higher change in PASE scores indicate higher physical activity at follow up compared to baseline; Negative change in WOMAC pain and function scores indicate reduced pain and higher function at follow-up compared to baseline
Abbreviations: *PASE* Physical Activity Scale for the Elderly, *WOMAC* Western Ontario and McMaster Universities Osteoarthritis Index

Table 4 The association between change in physical activity level and pain and function at three months follow-up

	WOMAC pain at 3 months		WOMAC function at 3 months	
	Unadjusted β (95% CI)	**Adjusted β (95% CI)**	**Unadjusted β (95% CI)**	**Adjusted β (95% CI)**
Change in physical activity				
PASE 10 point increase#	0.01 (-0.03, 0.05)	-0.01 (-0.05, 0.02)	0.00 (-0.14, 0.15)	-0.09 (-0.19, 0.02)
Potential confounders				
Age	0.06** (0.02, 0.09)	0.05** (0.03, 0.08)	0.23** (0.12, 0.35)	0.15** (0.06, 0.24)
Continuous BMI	0.13** (0.08, 0.19)	0.06* (0.01, 0.10)	0.55** (0.35, 0.74)	0.21* (0.05, 0.37)
WOMAC pain baseline	0.60** (0.52, 0.67)	0.52** (0.44, 0.60)	1.93** (1.66, 2.21)	
WOMAC function baseline	0.16** (0.14, 0.18)		0.68** (0.61, 0.75)	0.60** (0.53, 0.68)
Pain duration				
(reference <1 year)				
>1 year and <5 years	1.13** (0.31, 1.94)	1.06** (0.39, 1.72)	3.26* (0.34, 6.18)	2.67* (0.40, 4.94)
>5 years and <10 years	2.09** (1.11, 3.07)	1.60** (0.80, 2.41)	5.64** (2.20, 9.08)	3.82 **(1.15, 6.50)
>10 years	2.07** (1.07, 3.06)	1.48** (0.66, 2.31)	4.93** (1.46, 8.01)	3.42* (0.69, 6.15)
PHQ8 depression	0.19** (0.12, 0.26)	0.11** (0.05-0.17)	0.68** (0.45, 0.91)	0.23* (0.03, 0.42)
Intervention arm				
(reference usual physio)				
Individually tailored exercise	0.26 (-0.53, 1.05)	0.04 (-0.59, 0.67)	-0.04 (-2.82, -2.74)	-0.38 (-2.50, 1.74)
Targeted exercise adherence	0.27 (-0.52, 1.06)	0.12 (-0.50, 0.75)	1.56 (-1.21, 4.33)	0.47 (-1.63, 2.57)

Key: White = Unadjusted Models; Blue = Adjusted pain at 3 months model; Gold = Adjusted physical function at 3 months model

Footnotes: Multiple imputed data; multiple linear regression adjusted models selected via backwards elimination holding treatment arm and change in physical activity in the model. * = statistically significant β coefficient $P < 0.05$; ** = statistically significant β coefficient $P < 0.01$. Higher WOMAC scores indicate higher pain and worse function. Higher PASE score indicates higher level of physical activity, #absolute change in PASE calculated by subtracting the baseline score from the score at three months. Higher PHQ8 depression scores indicate worse depression

Abbreviations: *β* Unstandardized coefficients, *BMI* Body Mass Index; CI=Confidence Interval, *PASE* Physical Activity Scale for the Elderly, *PHQ8* Personal Health Questionnaire, *WOMAC* Western Ontario and McMaster Osteoarthritis Index

arm and baseline pain/function ($P > 0.05$) (see Tables 4, 5 and 6). An increase of 10 PASE points between baseline and three months had a non-statistically significant, adjusted association with WOMAC pain at three (β = − 0.01 (95% Confidence Interval − 0.05, 0.02)) and six (β = − 0.02 (− 0.06, 0.02)) months. Interpreting these best estimate β coefficients, for every increase in physical activity of ten points on the PASE, WOMAC pain score decreased by 0.01 at three months and 0.02 at six months. These results are not statistically significant since the 95% confidence intervals cross zero. Similarly, an increase of 10 points on the PASE scale

Table 5 The association between change in physical activity level and pain and function at six months follow-up

	WOMAC pain at 6 months		WOMAC function at 6 months	
	Unadjusted β (95% CI)	**Adjusted β (95% CI)**	**Unadjusted β (95% CI)**	**Adjusted β (95% CI)**
Change in Physical activity				
PASE 10 point increase#	-0.00 (-0.05, 0.04)	-0.02 (-0.06, 0.02)	0.00 (-0.16, 0.17)	-0.09 (-0.22, 0.04)
Potential confounders				
Age	0.06** (0.03, 0.10)	0.05** (0.02-0.08)	0.28** (0.16, 0.40)	0.19** (0.09, 0.29)
WOMAC pain baseline	0.64** (0.56, 0.73)	0.59** (0.51, 0.67)	1.97** (1.66, 2.27)	
WOMAC function baseline	0.17** (0.015, 0.20)		0.66** (0.57, 0.74)	0.59** (0.50, 0.67)
Pain duration				
(reference <1 year)				
>1 year and <5 years	1.08* (0.19, 1.97)	0.96* (0.22, 1.69)	4.22** (1.15, 7.30)	3.53** (1.01, 6.05)
>5 years and <10 years	2.57** (1.52, 3.62)	2.03** (1.17, 2.90)	8.50** (4.83, 12.17)	6.65** (3.63, 9.67)
>10 years	2.17** (1.09, 3.25)	1.46** (0.56, 2.35)	6.31** (2.61, 10.01)	4.57** (1.52, 7.62)
PHQ8 depression	0.18** (0.10, 0.25)	0.10** (0.04, 0.16)	0.73** (0.48, 0.98)	0.36** (0.14, 0.58)
Intervention arm				
(reference usual physio)				
Individually tailored exercise	0.02 (-0.86, 0.90)	-0.25 (-0.96, 0.47)	0.86 (-2.14, 3.87)	0.51 (-1.89, 2.90)
Targeted exercise adherence	-0.12 (-0.98, 0.74)	-0.26 (-0.95, 0.44)	0.08 (-2.93, 3.09)	-0.72 (-3.13, 1.69)

Key: White = Unadjusted Models; Blue = Adjusted pain at 6 months model; Gold = Adjusted physical function at 6 months model

Footnotes: Multiple imputed data, multiple linear regression adjusted models selected via backwards elimination holding treatment arm and change in physical activity in the model. Regression coefficients shown are rounded to two decimal places and a score of − 0.00 is used to indicate a very small yet negative confidence interval coefficient. * = statistically significant β coefficient $P < 0.05$; ** = statistically significant β coefficient $P < 0.01$. Higher WOMAC scores indicate higher pain and worse function. Higher PASE score indicates higher level of physical activity, #absolute change in PASE calculated by subtracting the baseline score from the score at three months. Higher PHQ8 depression scores indicate worse depression

Abbreviations: *β* Unstandardized coefficients, *BMI* Body Mass Index, *CI* Confidence Interval, *PASE* Physical Activity Scale for the Elderly, *PHQ8* = Personal Health Questionnaire, *WOMAC* Western Ontario and McMaster Osteoarthritis Index

Table 6 The association between change in physical activity level and treatment response at three and six months follow-up

	OMERACT OARSI response at 3 months		OMERACT OARSI response at 6 months	
	Unadjusted OR (95% CI)	Adjusted Model OR (95% CI)	Unadjusted OR (95% CI)	Adjusted Model
Change in PA				
PASE 10 point increase#	1.01 (0.99, 1.04)	1.02 (0.99, 1.04)	1.01 (0.98, 1.03)	1.01 (0.98, 1.04)
Potential confounders				
WOMAC pain baseline	1.11** (1.05, 1.18)	1.15** (1.08, 1.23)	1.08** (1.03, 1.14)	1.12** (1.06, 1.19)
Age	0.97** (0.95, 0.99)	0.97** (0.94, 0.99)	0.98* (0.96, 1.00)	0.97** (0.95, 0.99)
Pain duration				
(reference <1 year)				
>1 year and <5 years	0.49** (0.30, 0.80)	0.46** (0.28, 0.78)	0.57* (0.35, 0.93)	0.56* (0.34, 0.93)
>5 years and <10 years	0.36** (0.20, 0.66)	0.31** (0.17, 0.59)	0.30** (0.17, 0.54)	0.27** (0.15, 0.50)
>10 years	0.64 (0.35, 1.17)	0.59 (0.32, 1.10)	0.45** (0.25, 0.80)	0.41** (0.22, 0.74)
PHQ8 depression	0.98 (0.95, 1.02)	0.95* (0.91, 0.99)	0.98 (0.94, 1.02)	0.95* (0.91, 0.99)
Intervention arm				
(reference usual physio)				
Individually tailored exercise	1.08 (0.70, 1.68)	1.05 (0.66, 1.68)	1.06 (0.68, 1.66)	1.04 (0.65, 1.67)
Targeted exercise adherence	1.02 (0.64, 1.62)	0.95 (0.58, 1.56)	1.22 (0.78, 1.92)	1.15 (0.71, 1.86)

Key: White = Unadjusted Models; Blue = Adjusted OMERACT-OARSI treatment response models

Footnotes: Multiple imputed data, multiple logistic regression adjusted models selected via backwards elimination holding treatment arm and change in physical activity in the model. Higher WOMAC scores indicate higher pain. * = statistically significant OR P < 0.05; ** = statistically significant OR P < 0.01. Higher PASE score indicates higher level of physical activity, #absolute change in PASE calculated by subtracting the baseline score from the score at three months. Higher PHQ8 depression scores indicate worse depression

Abbreviations: β Unstandardized coefficients, *CI* Confidence Interval, *OMERACT OARSI* Osteoarthritis Research Society International set of responder criteria for osteoarthritis clinical trials, *PASE* Physical Activity Scale for the Elderly, *PHQ8* Personal Health Questionnaire, *WOMAC* Western Ontario and McMaster Osteoarthritis Index; yr. = year

had a non-statistically significant adjusted association with function at three $\beta = -0.09$ (− 0.19, 0.02) and six months $\beta = -0.09$ (− 0.22, 0.04) and, treatment response at three months OR = 1.02 (0.99, 1.04) and six months OR = 1.01 (0.98, 1.04). Interpreting the treatment response best estimate odds ratios, for every increase in physical activity of ten points on the PASE, participants had a 2% increase in the odds of being able to be classified as a treatment responder using the OMERACT-OARSI criteria at three month follow-up and 1% increase in odds at six month follow-up but these findings were not statistically significant since the 95% confidence interval odds ratios cross one.

Complete case sensitivity analyses, investigating the adjusted association between a 10 point increase in PASE and clinical outcomes of WOMAC pain and function at 3 and 6 months produced similar non-statistically significant associations (results not shown).

Discussion

Main findings

This study investigated whether change in physical activity was associated with future clinical outcomes of pain and physical function in older adults with knee pain attributable to OA. This question is novel and important since change in physical activity may explain clinical improvements following exercise interventions and inform future interventions. The main finding from this RCT was that change in physical activity level was not associated with future pain, physical functioning or treatment response at either three or six month follow-up. Small β coefficients were expected given the difference in scale between the PASE (0–400+) and WOMAC pain and function scores (0–20 and 0–68 respectively) (since the PASE scale is larger by approximately a factor of 20 than the WOMAC pain scale). However, even taking this in to account and allowing for a 10 point change in PASE, the magnitude of associations were very small, non-statistically significant and do not appear to be of clinical importance (Tables 4, 5 and 6). For example, extrapolating from the β coefficients, changing physical activity by a full standard deviation (83 points on the PASE) would be associated with less than a 1 point change in WOMAC pain or function at either three or six months. Similarly, large changes in physical activity would only have a very small effect on the odds of being an OMERACT-OARSI responder.

The null association findings (Tables 4, 5 and 6) suggest that change in overall general physical activity level, as measured by the PASE, does not explain clinical outcome following exercise intervention within the BEEP trial and that other variables may be responsible for the observed improvements in pain and function (see Table 2). For example, lower limb strengthening [32] or psychosocial factors (such as outcome expectations, attention and monitoring, the interest and empathy expressed by physiotherapists and the credibility of the intervention) may contribute to improvements in pain and function [33, 34].

There is also a separate or further explanation for the null findings. Measuring change in physical activity using the self-report PASE involves a number of limitations that may increase the chance of a Type II error (i.e. rejecting an association between change in physical activity and clinical outcome if one exists). Although the PASE has been highlighted as a promising measure of physical activity in older adults with OA [35], all self-report measures of physical activity can either over- or under- estimate actual physical activity level [36] since they are at risk of recall bias (through errors in memory and activity recall), misclassification of physical activity intensity and duration [15, 37], and social desirability bias by participants [38]. Furthermore, modelling change in physical activity is methodologically challenging and using an absolute change score between two time-points may compound measurement errors and reduce regression coefficient precision, biasing our findings towards the null [39].

The PASE minimal detectable change statistic (87), which measures the threshold for a "real" change that with 95% confidence is beyond measurement error [40], is considerably larger than the mean change detected in the BEEP dataset (15.1). This suggests that the mean change in PASE scores detected during the exercise interventions was relatively small, potentially affected by measurement error and perhaps insufficient to influence clinical outcomes or alternatively that the PASE may have inadequate responsiveness in older adults with joint pain.

To the authors' knowledge, this is the first study to explicitly investigate the association between change in physical activity level and clinical outcomes of pain and function in older adults with knee pain attributable to OA. However, similar studies have investigated the association between change in physical activity level and disability in those with low back pain [41] and pain severity and physical function outcomes in those with fibromyalgia [42, 43]. Similar to our findings, no association was found in the back pain study using either self-report or accelerometer measured physical activity [41], however, associations were found between change in physical activity and future clinical outcomes in the two fibromyalgia studies [42, 43]. Whilst the aetiological differences between knee pain attributed to OA and fibromyalgia are likely to be substantial and prevent direct comparison, these findings do suggest it is possible to detect associations if they exist between self-report change in physical activity and clinical outcomes despite the previously discussed challenges in measuring change in physical activity.

Strengths and limitations

The strengths of this study were the ability to investigate both univariable and adjusted associations between change in physical activity and future clinical outcomes at two separate time-points. The use of multiple imputation helped preserve sample size, reducing the risk of bias due to loss to follow-up [29] whilst the sensitivity analysis added strength to the primary findings by exploring the dataset under different missing data assumptions.

The main study limitation, relating to the challenges in measuring change in physical activity, has been discussed above. With our available data we were unable to investigate levels of different types of physical activity, for example, time spent in strengthening or different cardiovascular intensities of exercise. Different types of physical activity may have had different effects on outcome. Another concern for our analysis is temporal bias. Temporal bias occurs when the inference about proper temporal sequence of cause and effect is erroneous [44]. Attempts were made to measure the exposure of interest- change in physical activity level (baseline to three months) prior to the clinical outcomes (at three and six months). Nevertheless, change in pain or physical function may have occurred prior to any change in physical activity, meaning we cannot be sure about the direction of any potential cause and effect. In handling missing data using multiple imputation for our analysis, we made the assumption that our data was "missing at random" (MAR) [29] since we deemed it likely that missing values could be estimated from observed values. If any missing data was "missing not at random" (MNAR) i.e. there are systematic differences between missing and observed values even after the observed data are taken into account then our multiple imputed analysis would be at risk of bias [29].

Finally, before generalising our findings it is important to remember this sample population were older adults with knee pain attributed to clinically diagnosed OA from a RCT of exercise interventions. Other populations of older adults with knee pain, for example, those who did not consent to exercise interventions may have different clinical outcomes with changing their physical activity levels.

Implications

Although change in physical activity was not shown to be associated with clinical outcomes of pain and physical function, insufficiently active older adults with knee pain can still be advised to increase their physical activity levels as able, in order to achieve the associated general health benefits [45–48] with the reassurance that modest increases in physical activity are not associated with increasing pain or deterioration in function at a group level.

In order to select the most appropriate physical activity measure for longitudinal studies measuring change in physical activity in older adults with knee pain, future research could investigate and compare the reliability and responsiveness of the PASE alongside other recommended measures of physical activity such as the International Physical Activity Questionnaire (IPAQ) [37] and direct measures such as pedometry and accelerometry.

The inclusion criteria for this trial sample was based on older adults with knee pain regardless of baseline level of physical activity. Future studies could investigate specific subgroups of older adults with knee pain, such as those who are inactive, who may plausibly respond differently to increases in physical activity than all adults with knee pain or those currently meeting guideline recommended activity levels.

Conclusions

Change in physical activity level was not associated with future pain, physical function or the proportion of participants who could be classified as treatment responders in this secondary analysis of a randomised trial dataset. Hence other factors may be responsible for improvements in these clinical outcomes following exercise interventions. Accurately measuring change in physical activity in older adults with knee pain remains a challenge and the PASE, although useful for capturing population snap shots of physical activity level, may not be sufficiently responsive to detect changes over time in this clinical population. We recommend the further investigation of responsiveness in commonly utilised measures of physical activity for older adults with joint pain including the PASE to aid future longitudinal studies assessing change in physical activity.

Abbreviations

BEEP: Benefits of Effective Exercise for Knee Pain; BMI: Body Mass Index; GAD-7: Generalised Anxiety Disorder-7; IPAQ: International Physical Activity Questionnaire; ISRCTN: International Standard Registered Clinical/soCial sTudy Number; ITE: Individually Tailored Exercise; MDC: Minimal Detectable Change; NIHR: National Institute for Health Research; OA: osteoarthritis; OMERACT-OARSI: Outcome Measures in Rheumatology Clinical Trials-Osteoarthritis Research Society International; OR: odds ratio; PA: Physical activity; PASE: Physical Activity Scale for the Elderly; PHQ 8: Personal Health Questionnaire 8; RCT: Randomised controlled trial; REC: Research Ethics Committee; TEA: Targeted Exercise Adherence; UC: Usual Care; WOMAC: Western Ontario and McMaster Universities Osteoarthritis Index

Acknowledgments

We would like to thank all the participants and staff involved with the BEEP trial, including Elaine Nicholls for data cleaning of the BEEP dataset and statistical input with the multiple imputation of missing data.

Funding

JQ was funded for this work by a Keele University Acorn PhD studentship. He is now funded by a National Institute for Health Research (NIHR) Academic Clinical Lectureship in Physiotherapy, awarded as part of Professor Christian Mallen's NIHR Research Professorship (NIHR-RP-2014-026). Neither funder had involvement in the study design, collection, data analysis, writing or publishing of this paper.

NF was supported through an NIHR Research Professorship (NIHR-RP-011-015) and is a NIHR Senior Investigator.

MH was supported through an NIHR School for Primary Care Research post-doctoral fellowship.

The views expressed in this publication are those of the authors and not necessarily those of the NHS, the NIHR or the Department of Health.

Authors' contributions

JQ was the overall lead for the work and was involved at all stages of the paper. JQ, NF, PC, RO and MH were involved with the conception of the design. JQ and RO were involved in data analysis. All authors were involved in the interpretation of the data, drafting of the article and final approval of the submitted version.

Authors' information

The lead author can be contacted by email:j.g.quicke@keele.ac.uk or at Primary Care and Health Sciences, David Wetherall Building, Keele University, Keele, Staffordshire, United Kingdom, ST5 5BG.

Consent for publication

All authors provided their consent for this publication.

Competing interests

The authors declare that they have no competing interests.

References

1. National Institute for Health and Care Excellence. Osteoarthritis: care and management in adults. NICE guideline 177, London. 2014.
2. Fernandes L, Hagen KB, Bijlsma JWJ, Andreassen O, Christensen P, Conaghan PG, et al. EULAR recommendations for the non-pharmacological core management of hip and knee osteoarthritis. Ann Rheum Dis. 2013; 72(7):1125–35.
3. McAlindon TE, Bannuru RR, Sullivan MC, Arden NK, Berenbaum F, Bierma-Zeinstra SM, et al. OARSI guidelines for the non-surgical management of knee osteoarthritis. Osteoarthr Cartil. 2014;22(3):363–88.
4. Uthman OA, van der Windt DA, Jordan JL, Dziedzic KS, Healey EL, Peat GM, et al. Exercise for lower limb osteoarthritis: systematic review incorporating trial sequential analysis and network meta-analysis. Br Med J. 2013;347:f5555.
5. Juhl C, Christensen R, Roos EM, Zhang W, Lund H. Impact of exercise type and dose on pain and disability in knee osteoarthritis: a systematic review and meta-regression analysis of randomized controlled trials. Arthritis Rheumatology. 2014;66(3):622–36.
6. Fransen M, McConnell S, Harmer AR, Van der Esch M, Simic M, Bennell KL. Exercise for osteoarthritis of the knee: a Cochrane systematic review. British Journal of Sports Medicine. 2015;bjsports – 2015–095424.
7. Runhaar J, Luijsterburg P, Dekker J, Bierma-Zeinstra SMA. Identifying potential working mechanisms behind the positive effects of exercise therapy on pain and function in osteoarthritis; a systematic review. Osteoarthr Cartil. 2015;23(7):1071–82.
8. Stubbs B, Hurley M, Smith T. What are the factors that influence physical activity participation in adults with knee and hip osteoarthritis? A systematic review of physical activity correlates. Clin Rehabil. 2015;29(1):80–94.
9. Pellegrini CA, Song J, Chang RW, Semanik PA, Lee J, Ehrlich-Jones L, Pinto D, Dunlop DD. Change in physical activity and sedentary time associated with 2-year weight loss in obese adults with osteoarthritis. J Phys Act Health. 2016;13(5):461–6.
10. Messier SP, Mihalko SL, Legault C, Miller GD, Nicklas BJ, DeVita P, et al. Effects of intensive diet and exercise on knee joint loads, inflammation, and

clinical outcomes among overweight and obese adults with knee osteoarthritis: the IDEA randomized clinical trial. JAMA. 2013;310(12):1263.
11. Pham T, Van Der Heijde D, Lassere M, Altman RD, Anderson JJ, Bellamy N, et al. Outcome variables for osteoarthritis clinical trials: the OMERACT-OARSI set of responder criteria. J Rheumatol. 2003;30(7):1648–54.
12. Foster NE, Healey EL, Holden MA, Nicholls E, Whitehurst DG, Jowett S, et al. A multicentre, pragmatic, parallel group, randomised controlled trial to compare the clinical and cost-effectiveness of three physiotherapy-led exercise interventions for knee osteoarthritis in older adults: the BEEP trial protocol (ISRCTN: 93634563). BMC Musculoskelet Disordors. 2014;15(1):254.
13. Bellamy N, Buchanan WW, Goldsmith CH, Campbell J, Stitt LW. Validation study of WOMAC: a health status instrument for measuring clinically important patient relevant outcomes to antirheumatic drug therapy in patients with osteoarthritis of the hip or knee. J Rheumatol. 1988 Dec;15(12):1833–40.
14. McConnell S, Kolopack P, Davis AM. The western Ontario and McMaster universities osteoarthritis index (WOMAC): a review of its utility and measurement properties. Arthritis Rheumatology. 2001;45(5):453–61.
15. Trudeau J, Van Inwegen R, Eaton T, Bhat G, Paillard F, Ng D, et al. Assessment of pain and activity using an electronic pain diary and actigraphy device in a randomized, placebo-controlled crossover trial of celecoxib in osteoarthritis of the knee. Pain Practice. 2015;15(3):247–55.
16. Pham T, van der Heijde D, Altman RD, Anderson JJ, Bellamy N, Hochberg M, et al. OMERACT-OARSI initiative: osteoarthritis research society international set of responder criteria for osteoarthritis clinical trials revisited. Osteoarthr Cartil. 2004;12(5):389–99.
17. Washburn RA, Smith KW, Jette AM, Janney CA. The physical activity scale for the elderly (PASE): development and evaluation. J Clin Epidemiol. 1993; 46(2):153–62.
18. Martin KA, Rejeski WJ, Miller ME, James MK, Ettinger Jr. WH, Messier SP. Validation of the PASE in older adults with knee pain and physical disability. Med Sci Sports Exerc 1999;31(5):627–633.
19. Sharma L, Cahue S, Song J, Hayes K, Pai YC, Dunlop D. Physical functioning over three years in knee osteoarthritis: role of psychosocial, local mechanical, and neuromuscular factors. Arthritis Rheum. 2003;48(12):3359–70.
20. Dunlop DD, Song J, Semanik PA, Sharma L, Chang RW. Physical activity levels and functional performance in the osteoarthritis initiative: a graded relationship. Arthritis Rheum. 2011;63(1):127–36.
21. Fransen M, Su S, Harmer A, Blyth FM, Naganathan V, Sambrook P, et al. A longitudinal study of knee pain in older men: concord health and ageing in men project. Age Ageing. 2014;43(2):206–12.
22. Cleveland RJ, Luong M-LN, Knight JB, Schoster B, Renner JB, Jordan JM, et al. Independent associations of socioeconomic factors with disability and pain in adults with knee osteoarthritis. BMC Musculoskelet Disorders. 2013;14:297.
23. Neogi T, Zhang Y. Epidemiology Of OA. Rheum Dis Clin N Am. 2013;39(1):1–19.
24. Office for National Statistics. Standard Occupational Classification 2010 (volume 3).
25. Kroenke K, Spitzer RL, Williams JB. The PHQ-9: validity of a brief depression severity measure. J Gen Intern Med. 2001;16(9):606–13.
26. Spitzer RL, Kroenke K, Williams JBW, Löwe B. A brief measure for assessing generalized anxiety disorder: the GAD-7. Arch Intern Med. 2006;166(10):1092–7.
27. MacFarlane GJ, Croft PR, Schollum J, Silman AJ. Widespread pain: is an improved classification possible? J Rheumatol. 1996;23(9):1628–32.
28. StataCorp. Stata statistical software: release 13. College Station, TX: StataCorp LP; 2013.
29. Sterne JAC, White IR, Carlin JB, Spratt M, Royston P, Kenward MG, et al. Multiple imputation for missing data in epidemiological and clinical research: potential and pitfalls. Br Med J. 2009;338:b2393.
30. Hay EM, Dziedzic K, Foster NE, Peat G, van der Windt DA, Bartlam B…Croft, P. Clinical osteoarthritis and joint pain in older people: optimal management in primary care. NIHR Programme grant for Applied Research final report, RP-PG-0407-10386. (in press).
31. Tariss TWA. Primer in longitudinal data analysis. London: SAGE Publications; 2000.
32. Knoop J, Steultjens MPM, Roorda LD, Lems WF, van der Esch M, Thorstensson CA, et al. Improvement in upper leg muscle strength underlies beneficial effects of exercise therapy in knee osteoarthritis: secondary analysis from a randomised controlled trial. Physiotherapy. 2014; 101(2):171–7.
33. Hall AM, Ferreira PH, Maher CG, Latimer J, Ferreira ML. The influence of the therapist-patient relationship on treatment outcome in physical rehabilitation: a systematic review. Phys Ther. 2010;90(8):1099–110.
34. Bennell KL, Kyriakides M, Hodges PW, Hinman RS. Effects of two physiotherapy booster sessions on outcomes with home exercise in people with knee osteoarthritis: a randomized controlled trial. Arthritis Care Res. 2014;66(11):1680–7.
35. Terwee CB, Bouwmeester W, van Elsland SL, de Vet HCW, Dekker J. Instruments to assess physical activity in patients with osteoarthritis of the hip or knee: a systematic review of measurement properties. Osteoarthr Cartil. 2011;19(6):620–33.
36. Prince SA, Adamo KB, Hamel ME, Hardt J, Gorber SC, Tremblay MA. Comparison of direct versus self-report measures for assessing physical activity in adults: a systematic review. The International Journal of Behavioral Nutrition and Physical Activity. 2008;5:56.
37. Craig CL, Marshall AL, Sjöström M, Bauman AE, Booth ML, Ainsworth BE, et al. International physical activity questionnaire: 12-country reliability and validity. Med Sci Sports Exerc. 2003;35(8):1381–95.
38. Adams SA, Matthews CE, Ebbeling CB, Moore CG, Cunningham JE, Fulton J, et al. The effect of social desirability and social approval on self-reports of physical activity. Am J Epidemiol. 2005;161(4):389–98.
39. Polit DF, Yang F. Measurement and the measurement of change. London: Wolters Kluwer; 2015.
40. Svege I, Kolle E, Risberg M. Reliability and validity of the physical activity scale for the elderly (PASE) in patients with hip osteoarthritis. BMC Musculoskelet Disord. 2012;13(1):26.
41. Hendrick P, Milosavljevic S, Hale L, Hurley DA, McDonough SM, Herbison P, et al. Does a patient's physical activity predict recovery from an episode of acute low back pain? A prospective cohort study. BMC Musculoskelet Disorders. 2013;14:126.
42. Kaleth AS, Saha CK, Jensen MP, Slaven JE, Ang DC. Effect of moderate to vigorous physical activity on long-term clinical outcomes and pain severity in fibromyalgia. Arthritis Care and Research. 2013;65(8):1211–8.
43. Steiner JL, Bigatti SM, Ang DC. Trajectory of change in pain, depression, and physical functioning after physical activity adoption in fibromyalgia. J Health Psychol. 2015;20(7):931–41.
44. Szklo M, Nieto FJ. Epidemiology: Beyond the Basics. Jones & Bartlett Publishers; 2014.
45. Warburton D, Nicol CW, Bredin SSD. Health benefits of physical activity: the evidence. Can Med Assoc J. 2006;174(6):801–9.
46. Chodzko-Zajko WJ, Proctor DN, Fiatarone Singh MA, Minson CT, Nigg CR, Salem GJ, et al. Exercise and physical activity for older adults. Med Sci Sports Exerc. 2009;41(7):1510–30.
47. Department of Health. Start Active, Stay Active. 2011;1–62.
48. Autenrieth CS, Kirchberger I, Heier M, Zimmermann A-K, Peters A, Döring A, et al. Physical activity is inversely associated with multimorbidity in elderly men: results from the KORA-age Augsburg study. Prev Med. 2013;57(1):17–9.

9

With a biomechanical treatment in knee osteoarthritis, less knee pain did not correlate with synovitis reduction

Vikram Swaminathan[1,2*], Matthew J Parkes[1,2], Michael J Callaghan[1,2,3,4], Terence W O'Neill[1,2,5], Richard Hodgson[6], Andrew D Gait[6] and David T Felson[1,2,7]

Abstract

Background: Braces are used to treat pain in patellofemoral joint osteoarthritis (PFJOA). In a trial, we previously reported pain improvement after 6-weeks brace use. The pain reduction did not correlate with changes in Magnetic Resonance Imaging (MRI) assessed Bone Marrow Lesion volume or static synovial volume. Studies show that changes in the synovium on dynamic contrast enhanced (DCE) MRI are more closely associated with symptom change than static synovial volume changes. We hypothesised change in synovitis assessed using dynamic imaging could explain the reduction in pain.

Method: One hundred twenty-six men and women aged 40–70 years with painful radiographically confirmed PFJOA were randomised to either brace wearing or no brace for 6-weeks. Pain assessment and DCE-MRI were performed at baseline and 6 weeks. DCE data was analysed using Tofts's equation. Pain measures included a VAS of pain on nominated aggravating activity (VAS_{NA}), and the KOOS pain subscale. Paired t-tests were used to determine within person change in outcome measures and Spearman's correlation coefficients were used to determine the correlation between change in pain and change in the DCE parameters.

Results: Mean age of subjects was 55.5 years (SD = 7.5) and 57% were female. There was clear pain improvement in the brace users compared to controls (VAS_{NA} − 16.87 mm, p = <0.001). There was no significant change to the dynamic synovitis parameters among brace users nor was pain change correlated with change in dynamic synovitis parameters.

Conclusion: The reduction in knee pain following brace wearing in patients with PFJOA is not explained by changes in synovitis.

Keywords: Brace, Patellofemoral, Osteoarthritis, Synovitis, Dynamic contrast enhanced, Magnetic resonance imaging

* Correspondence: vikram.swaminathan@manchester.ac.uk
[1]Arthritis Research UK Centre for Epidemiology, Institute of Inflammation and Repair, Faculty of Medical and Human Sciences, Manchester Academic Health Science Centre, University of Manchester, Stopford Building, Oxford Road, Manchester M13 9PT, UK
[2]NIHR Manchester Musculoskeletal Biomedical Research Unit, Central Manchester NHS Foundation Trust, Manchester Academic Health Sciences Centre, Manchester, UK
Full list of author information is available at the end of the article

Background

Patello-femoral Joint Osteoarthritis (PFJOA) is a common cause of knee pain in middle aged adults. In a recent randomised controlled trial of brace therapy in persons with symptomatic PFJOA we showed that a flexible sleeve knee brace resulted in a significant improvement in pain after 6 weeks and a reduction in bone marrow lesion (BML) volume in the PFJ [1]. The two structures in the knee that are both innervated by nociceptive fibers and reported to be causally related to knee pain are bone [2] and synovitis [3, 4]. In the bone, the most prominently assessed abnormality correlated with pain has been bone marrow lesions [5]. While hyaline cartilage pathology is the signature feature of osteoarthritis [6], this cartilage is not innervated, and it is not clear whether it is a source of pain. The change in pain during the trial was not correlated significantly with change in the BML volume, suggesting other mechanisms explain the pain reduction. Synovial tissue volume decrease has been linked with pain in observational studies [3, 4], but synovial volume assessed in the trial using static contrast enhanced magnetic resonance imaging (CE-MRI) did not shrink with the intervention [1].

Static measures of synovial volume may be less sensitive to pain than measures of synovial perfusion, assessed using dynamic contrast enhanced Magnetic Resonance Imaging (DCE-MRI) is a technique that utilises repeated imaging sequences of the joint whilst injecting contrast agent systemically [7]. This allows enhancement rates of tissues to be calculated as they are perfused by contrast agent. The rate of tissue enhancement has been shown to be more closely linked to active joint inflammation in rheumatoid arthritis (RA) than changes to static tissue volume measures alone, and correlates more strongly with change in pain following intra-articular steroid therapy [8]. We have recently shown that in knee OA, intraarticular steroid treatment leads to a major reduction in perfusion of the synovium as shown by DCE-MRI and that this reduction is far better correlated with pain reduction than measures of static synovial volume [9]. Since braces may diminish contact stress across the joint, leading to less microscopic damage and perhaps less need for the synovium to clear this debris, we hypothesised that the reduction in pain observed following brace use in our recent trial might be explained by changes in synovitis as assessed using DCE-MRI parameters. We therefore undertook a secondary analysis of the trial findings to examine this question.

Methods

Design

One hundred twenty-six subjects aged 40–70 years, recruited from primary and secondary care were randomly allocated to receive a patello-femoral sleeve brace immediately for 6 weeks or no brace. DCE-MRI was performed at both baseline (0 weeks) and at 6 weeks for all subjects. The number of subjects was chosen in advance to provide 80% power to detect an effect of the brace on knee pain (alpha = 0.05, two sided). Recruitment took place between August 2009 to September 2012 and the trial's main results have been reported elsewhere [1]. The primary structural outcome of the brace trial was bone marrow lesion (BML) volume but pain improvement was not significantly correlated with change in BML volume. Our discovery after intraarticular steroid injection that dynamic changes in synovium during DCE-MRI correlated with pain change led us to ask the question as to whether these dynamic changes in synovial volume explained the pain change in the knee brace study as a secondary analysis of these trial data.

Inclusion/exclusion criteria

Subjects were included if they had knee radiographs with a Kellgren and Lawrence (KL) score of grade 2 or 3 in the PFJ. This had to be greater than the KL grade for the tibiofemoral joint. Subjects had daily pain for the previous 3 months which was sufficiently severe to score 40 or above on a 0–100 mm for the visual analogue scale of pain on nominated aggravating activity (VAS_{NA}), and have PF symptoms (such as pain with stairs). Other inclusion/exclusion criteria for eligibility have been reported [1]. As contrast enhanced scans were used, subjects with renal dysfunction or undergoing dialysis were excluded.

Intervention

Subjects remained on their usual OA treatment. The intervention consisted of a Bioskin Patellar Tracking Q Brace (Ossur UK, Manchester, England). This is a Lycra flexible knee support with an optional strap that can be pulled over the patella; no difference in efficacy between the strapped and unstrapped configuration has been reported [10]. Simple randomisation was carried out by the study statistician with allocation using opaque envelopes. There is no known minimal required use to obtain the therapeutic effect of a knee brace, and we arbitrarily chose at least 4 h/day, so that if randomised to brace therapy, participants were instructed to wear it for a minimum of 4 h daily.

Assessments

Knee pain

Following subject recruitment and randomisation, both groups completed questionnaires evaluating their PFJ pain and imaging with DCE-MRI. After 6 weeks, pain evaluation and DCE-MRI was repeated for all subjects in both groups. The primary symptom outcome measure was pain on a VAS_{NA} (0 mm = no pain, 100 mm = worst pain) and the Knee Osteoarthritis Outcome Score (KOOS) pain scale was a secondary outcome measure.

Outcome measures: Structural

MRI assessment

DCE-MRI variables were collected for all subjects at baseline and after 6 weeks using the same magnet and scanning protocol. The enrolled knee only was scanned. Using a 1.5 T Philips Gyroscan ACS NT (Philips, Best Netherlands), axial proton density weighted (PDW) fat saturated (FS) repetition time approximately (TR) 5.5 ms, echo time approximately (TE) 1.9 ms, field of view (FOV) 14 cm × 14 cm, 256 × 256 matrix, slice thickness 3 mm sequences were obtained in all subjects, under the guidance of a musculoskeletal radiologist. The contrast agent Dotarem (gadoteric acid) was administered intravenously.

MRI analysis

The synovitis was segmented on the sagittal image, performed blinded, with computer image analysis excluding cartilage within the segmented area and calculating the proportion of synovial tissue within every voxel [11]. The segmentation was transferred onto the dynamic image using image registration techniques. Repeated MRI sequences were performed every 22 s, and contrast was injected following the 3rd sequence. In our analysis the primary outcome measure was change in enhancement rates of synovium between the baseline and 6-week visit. These variables act as a quantitative assessment of the change in severity of knee synovitis.

Three DCE parameters used in this study were calculated from analysis of the synovial enhancement curve (EC) (Fig. 1) and one was calculated from the Standard Tofts's equation [12]. The relative enhancement rate (RER) is a measurement the initial slope of the EC, which is sensitive to synovial vascularity and capillary permeability which reflects inflammatory activity. The maximum relative enhancement (RE_{max}) and late relative enhancement (RE_{late}) were also measured from the EC. K^{trans}, the volume transfer coefficient calculated from Tofts's equation, also depends on synovial vascularity and capillary permeability. It is thought as synovitis severity increases, DCE parameters will increase correspondingly [8, 12].

Statistical analysis

Our analyses included a comparison of the brace and no brace groups from baseline to 6-weeks. Change in pain (VAS_{NA} and KOOS pain subscale) and the four DCE parameters were assessed by paired t-tests. Following this, unpaired t-tests were performed to identify differences in within person change between brace and control groups. Only subjects with complete data sets at each time point were included in analysis. In addition, bivariate Pearson's correlation coefficients were performed to quantify the strength of associations between change in pain and change in the DCE outcomes in the brace group. The statistical analysis was performed using Stata (V.13.1; Stata Corporation, College Station, Texas, USA).

Results

Subjects

One hundred twenty-six subjects were recruited; 63 were randomised to the intervention and 63 the control group (Fig. 2). The mean age of subjects in the intervention group was 54.5 years (SD = 6.7), body mass index (BMI) was 31.4 Kg/m^2 (SD = 6.3) and 63.5% were female. The control group had a mean age of 56.4 years (SD = 8.1), BMI of

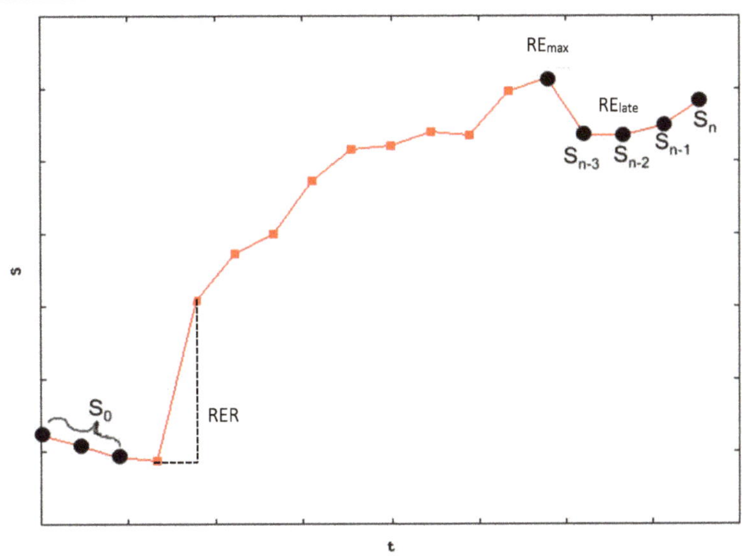

Fig. 1 An example of a typical enhancement curve of a voxel of synovium during and post the administration of contrast agent. Three dynamic enhancement parameters are calculated from analysis of the enhancement curve; these variables (RER, RE_{max} and RE_{late}) are labelled on the curve. The x-axis is time in seconds. There are 22 s between each plotted point on the enhancement curve. The y-axis shows signal intensity, starting at zero

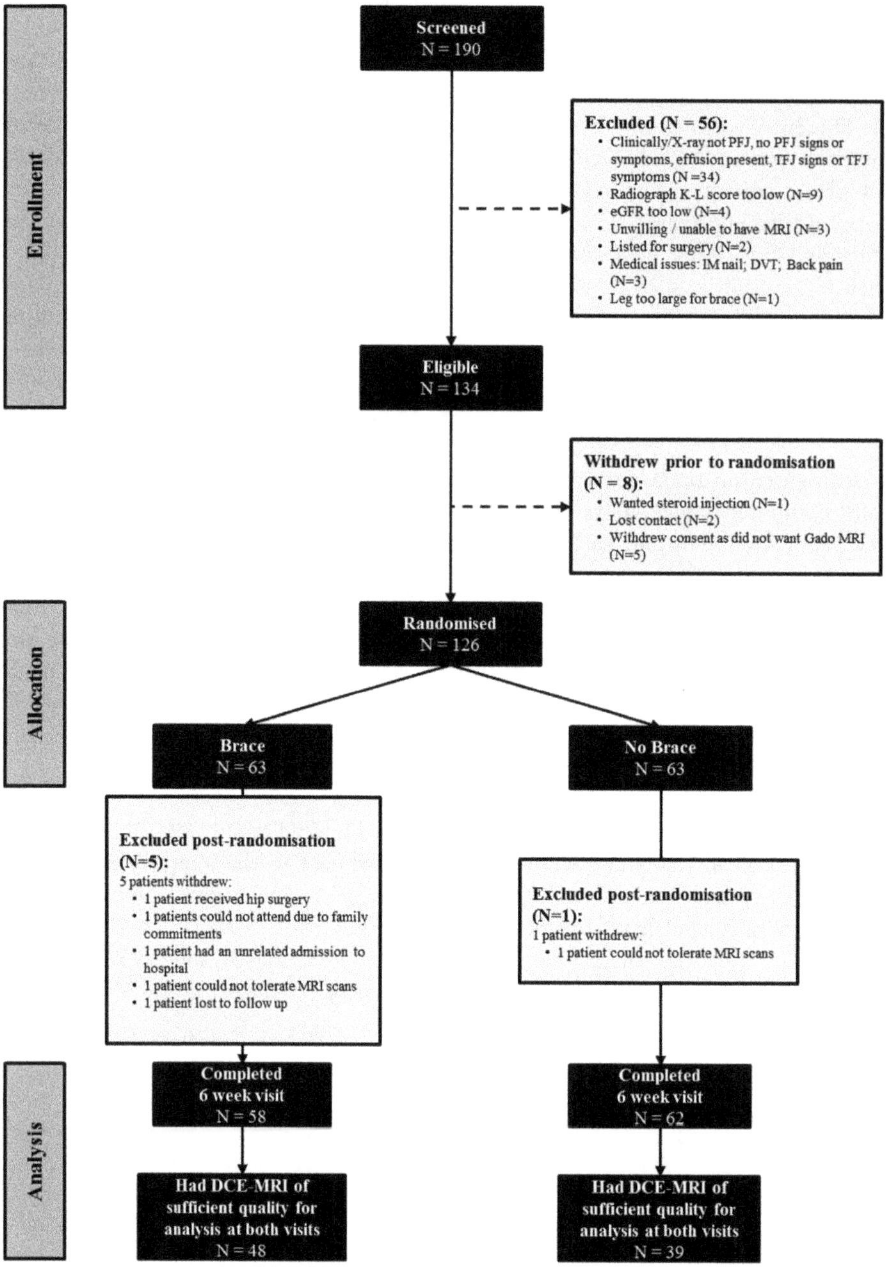

Fig. 2 CONSORT Diagram for the BRACE trial's 6 week period

30.5 Kg/m^2 (SD = 5.1), and 50.8% were female. Baseline pain was similar in both groups (mean VAS_{NA} 6.5). The brace group showed a mean pain reduction of 1.8 on the 10 cm VAS vs. 0 for the no brace group. The mean time the brace was worn was 7.35 h/day (SD = 3.10).

Between group change in pain and synovitis

There was a significantly greater within person reduction in pain in the brace users compared to the controls over the 6-week period (VAS_{NA} $p < 0.001$, KOOS pain $p = 0.01$) (Table 1). In contrast there was no significant difference in within person change in most DCE-MRI parameters between the treated and control group. There was a significant between group difference in the within-group change in RER (RER change 0.008, $p = 0.02$), however, this was primarily due to the significant improvement in the control group (implying reduction in synovitis) rather than a positive change in RER seen in the intervention group (Table 2).

Within group change in pain and DCE parameters

A significant reduction in the VAS_{NA} score (−18.16, $p < 0.001$) and an increase in the KOOS (8.78, $p < 0.001$)

Table 1 Subject baseline characteristics - mean pain scores and DCE parameters of subjects in each group

	Controls (N = 63 randomised, 62 attended 6 week visit)			Brace group (N = 63 randomised, 58 attended 6 week visit)		
Variable	N in analysis	Baseline ean (SD)	6 week visit mean (SD)	N in analysis	Baseline mean (SD)	6 week visit mean (SD)
VAS_{NA}	58[a]	6.17 (2.20)	6.30 (2.14)	56[a]	5.02 (2.55)	6.83 (2.13)
KOOS pain	61[a]	53.03 (18.27)	51.32 (18.30)	57[a]	57.72 (22.93)	48.94 (18.36)
K^{trans}	48	0.016 (0.018)	0.019 (0.018)	39	0.018 (0.018)	0.017 (0.014)
RER	48	0.034 (0.015)	0.039 (0.020)	39	0.038 (0.018)	0.035 (0.010)
RE_{late}	47[b]	2.084 (0.846)	2.186 (0.870)	39	2.128 (0.874)	2.118 (0.634)
RE_{max}	48	2.474 (0.880)	2.635 (0.945)	39	2.569 (0.961)	2.523 (0.639)

[a]Number of observations for KOOS and VAS_{NA} are less than the number attending week 6 visit due to incomplete questionnaires
[b]Dynamic data model error prevented the use of one RE_{late} observation

after 6 weeks brace use, signifying a reduction in pain. However, there were no significant changes to the DCE parameters in this group (Table 2). There was no statistically significant change to pain experienced over 6 weeks in the control group (VAS_{NA} p = 0.61, KOOS pain p = 0.31). There were small but significant changes noted to two of the DCE parameters in the control group; the mean change of K^{trans} was −0.003 (p = 0.05) and RER was −0.005 (p = 0.04), a reduction in enhancement rates of the synovium, suggesting a reduction in synovitis (Table 2).

Pearson's correlations showed weak correlations between change in the dynamic parameters and the two pain measures (r = −0.10 to 0.12).

Discussion

Our result suggest that synovitis, assessed using a sensitive imaging technique, does not improve following sleeve brace wearing. Change in synovitis does not explain the observed improvement in pain. Within the control group there was a small reduction in RER (p = 0.04) and K^{trans} (p = 0.05) variables over the study period suggesting a reduction in synovitis in this group, however, the magnitude of the changes was small and probably not clinically significant.

The DCE technique is a more sensitive method of detecting synovitis than static contrast enhanced imaging. Axelsen et al. demonstrated in 17 RA patients that intra-operative knee synovial biopsies showed histological inflammation which was highly correlated with changes in rates of synovial enhancement on pre-surgical T1 weighted MR images, especially the RER (spearman's correlation coefficient = 0.70, p = 0.001) [8]. A review by Hodgson et al. was consistent with this; the RER was shown in multiple RA studies to correlate with histological, physiological and clinical disease activity changes [13]. Synovitis assessed using DCE-MRI was more strongly associated with change in pain following steroid injection than static MRI imaging [14].

As noted earlier, the two structures consistently linked to pain in knee OA have been bone marrow lesions and synovitis (bone attrition has also been linked to pain but would be unlikely to change in 6 weeks and its change is not readily measurable). The absence of any association with change in synovitis assessed using DCE-MRI suggests that the reduction in pain following brace wearing is not due to change in synovitis and that other mechanisms may be operating. What then is the mechanism for pain reduction? We did find in the trial that the patellar brace caused a reduction in BML volume in the

Table 2 Subject baseline characteristics, mean within-group change following intervention with brace and in controls (without brace), and between-group differences in change (pre- and post-intervention)

	Controls (N = 63 randomised, 62 attended 6 week visit)			Brace group (N = 63 randomised, 58 attended 6 week visit)			Brace group - controls	
Variable	N in analysis	Mean change within group, (95% CI)	P-value	N in analysis	Mean change within group, (95% CI)	P-value	Mean change within group, (95% CI)	P-value
VAS_{NA}	58[a]	−0.13 (−0.64 to 0.38)	0.61	56[a]	−1.82 (−2.39 to −1.24)	<0.001	1.69 (0.93 to 2.44)	<0.001
KOOS pain	61[a]	1.71 (−1.66 to 5.08)	0.31	57[a]	8.78 (4.36 to 13.20)	<0.001	−7.06 (−12.52 to −1.61)	0.01
K^{trans}	48	−0.003 (−0.006 to 0.000)	0.05	39	0.001 (−0.003 to 0.005)	0.63	−0.004 (−0.009 to 0.001)	0.11
RER	48	−0.005 (−0.010 to 0.000)	0.04	39	0.003 (−0.002 to 0.008)	0.19	−0.008 (−0.014 to −0.001)	0.02
RE_{late}	47[b]	−0.102 (−0.280 to 0.076)	0.25	39	0.010 (−0.175 to 0.195)	0.91	−0.112 (−0.367 to 0.142)	0.38
RE_{max}	48	−0.161 (−0.357 to 0.036)	0.11	39	0.045 (−0.166 to 0.256)	0.67	−0.206 (−0.491 to 0.079)	0.15

[a]Number of observations for KOOS and VAS_{NA} are less than the number attending week 6 visit due to incomplete questionnaires. [b]Dynamic data model error prevented the use of one RE_{late} observation
The reduction in RER represents a reduction in the rate of enhancement and was seen significantly more often in the control group, not in the treatment group

patellofemoral compartment but that reduction was not significantly correlated with pain reduction. Although change in BML volume did not explain the pain reduction, it is possible that change in other structural features may have contributed. Ultimately, while pain improved, this was not necessarily accompanied by structural changes (although we may not have had the power to show that the reduction in BML volume was correlated with the pain reduction). The decrease in focal stress across the patellofemoral joint may have decreased nociceptive stimuli without causing a change in imaging parameters, and it is possible that our imaging approaches to pain are still too insensitive to detect the change induced.

This study was a secondary analysis of a trial of 126 patients. The original design did not include a formal sample size calculation for the DCE-MRI analysis. Instead, we made use of all available DCE-MRI scans collected during the course of the trial. Given the observed DCE-MRI trial data, we can calculate an estimated sample size for a future trial of the same design. Using RER as the primary outcome, the observed RER values for the change in the brace (mean change = +0.003; SD = 0.014) and no-brace group (mean change = −0.005; SD = 0.016), alpha of 0.05 and 80% power, a parallel-groups clinical trial testing for differences in the change in RER between the brace and no-brace group after 6 weeks would require 59 patients per group, a similar number to the trial findings presented here. A design using K^{trans} as the primary outcome, using observed values for the brace and no-brace group, would require 137 patients per group. Based on these estimates, it is possible but unlikely that our study was null because of inadequate power. We note that we found significant effects of dynamic measures of synovitis but in the opposite direction expected and that pain reduction effects were highly statistically significant.

The reduction in pain seen in the trial was modest but exceeded the minimum clinically important difference reported by Angst et al. (1.3 on a 10 cm scale) [15].

There are some limitations to be considered. It is possible that the six weeks trial duration may not have been long enough to identify significant physiological changes to synovium in participants who used a brace. This seems unlikely as changes are seen within 2-weeks following an intra-articular steroid injection [11, 16]. DCE-MRI was taken from a fixed region of interest (ROI) in the knee set on computer software. This is due to the standard Tofts's equation requirements and the need to select a fixed area of tissue to make each image comparable between subjects. As each participant did not have the same size knee, the ROI varied between participants. This may have led to the fixed ROI window not capturing all the synovitis in each knee. This discrepancy was not recorded; there may be a difference between the groups with the percentage of total synovitis measured. In addition, sampling was done at intervals longer than might be optimal to detect dynamic change. The low temporal resolution of the DCE-MRI sequence (22 s) limits the accuracy of the model, particularly for estimating K^{trans}. The field of view (FOV) was also limited reflecting the compromise in DCE-MRI between temporal resolution, spatial resolution and FOV in the phase encode directions; these could be improved for measurement of RE_{late} where high temporal resolution is less important. Also, movement between dynamic images may degrade reproducibility of measurements such as RER. This could be reduced by use of image registration (4).

Conclusion

Brace therapy in symptomatic knee PFJOA is linked in the short term with a reduction in knee pain. There was no corresponding reduction in the observed DCE-MRI parameters of knee synovitis.

Abbreviations

BML: Bone marrow lesion; CE-MRI: Contrast enhanced magnetic resonance imaging; DCE-MRI: Dynamic contrast enhanced Magnetic Resonance Imaging; FOV: Field of view; KL: Kellgren and Lawrence; KOOS: Knee osteoarthritis outcome score; K^{trans}: Volume transfer coefficient calculated from Tofts's equation; MRI: Magnetic resonance imaging; PFJOA: Patellofemoral joint osteoarthritis; RA: Rheumatoid arthritis; RE_{late}: Late relative enhancement; RE_{max}: Maximum relative enhancement; ROI: Region of interest; VAS_{NA}: Visual Analog Scale of pain on nominated aggravating activity

Acknowledgements

The authors appreciate the assistance of Helen Williams, Laura Heathers, Laura Forsythe and Rosie Perry for their support with the research study.

Funding

This research was funded by Arthritis Research UK grant 20,380, and special strategic award grant 18,676. This report includes independent research supported by (or funded by) the National Institute for Health Research Biomedical Research Unit Funding Scheme. The views expressed in this publication are those of the author(s) and not necessarily those of the NHS, the National Institute for Health Research or the Department of Health. The Research in Osteoarthritis Manchester (ROAM) group is supported by the Manchester Academic Health Sciences Centre (MAHSC). DTF is supported by NIH AR4778.

Author contributions

VS developed the idea and wrote the paper; MJP analysed the data and helped write the paper; MJC Evaluated study participants and helped write the paper; TWO developed the idea and helped write the paper; RH oversaw the protocol to analyse the MRI images and interpreted the dynamic MRI data; helped write the paper; ADG carried out the analysis of images and helped write the paper; DTF funded the study, developed the idea for the paper and helped write it. All authors read and approved the final manuscript.

Consent for publication

Not applicable.

Competing interests

The authors declare that they have no competing interests.

Author details

[1]Arthritis Research UK Centre for Epidemiology, Institute of Inflammation and Repair, Faculty of Medical and Human Sciences, Manchester Academic Health Science Centre, University of Manchester, Stopford Building, Oxford Road, Manchester M13 9PT, UK. [2]NIHR Manchester Musculoskeletal Biomedical Research Unit, Central Manchester NHS Foundation Trust, Manchester Academic Health Sciences Centre, Manchester, UK. [3]Faculty of Health, Psychology, and Social Care, Department of Health Professions, Manchester Metropolitan University, Manchester, UK. [4]Central Manchester University Hospitals NHS Foundation Trust, Manchester, UK. [5]Department of Rheumatology, Salford Royal NHS Foundation Trust, Salford, UK. [6]Centre of Imaging Sciences, Institute of Population Health, University of Manchester, Manchester, UK. [7]Clinical Epidemiology Unit, Boston University School of Medicine, Boston, MA, USA.

References

1. Callaghan MJ, Parkes MJ, Hutchinson CE, Gait AD, Forsythe LM, Marjanovic EJ, et al. A randomised trial of a brace for patellofemoral osteoarthritis targeting knee pain and bone marrow lesions. Ann Rheum Dis. 2015;74: 1164–1170. doi:10.1136/annrheumdis-2014-206376.
2. Felson DT. Imaging abnormalities that correlate with joint pain. Brit J Sport Med. 2011;45(4):289–91.
3. Baker K, Grainger A, Niu J, Clancy M, Guermazi A, Crema M, et al. Relation of synovitis to knee pain using contrast-enhanced MRIs. Ann Rheum Dis. 2010;69(10):1779–83.
4. Hill A, Mehnert A, Crozier S, Leung C, Wilson S, McMahon K, et al. Dynamic breast MRI: image registration and its impact on enhancement curve estimation. Conf Proc IEEE Eng Med Biol Soc. 2006;1:3049–52.
5. Yusuf E, Kortekaas MC, Watt I, Huizinga TW, Kloppenburg M. Do knee abnormalities visualised on MRI explain knee pain in knee osteoarthritis? A systematic review. Ann Rheum Dis. 2011;70(1):60–7.
6. Musumeci G, Aiello FC, Szychlinska MA, Di Rosa M, Castrogiovanni P, Mobasheri A. Osteoarthritis in the XXIst century: risk factors and Behaviours that influence disease onset and progression. Int J Mol Sci. 2015;16(3):6093–112.
7. Gait AD, Hodgson R, Parkes MJ, Hutchinson CE, O'Neill TW, Maricar N, et al. Synovial volume vs synovial measurements from dynamic contrast enhanced MRI as measures of response in osteoarthritis. Osteoarthr Cartilage. 2016;24(8):1392–8.
8. Axelsen MB, Stoltenberg M, Poggenborg RP, Kubassova O, Boesen M, Bliddal H, et al. Dynamic gadolinium-enhanced magnetic resonance imaging allows accurate assessment of the synovial inflammatory activity in rheumatoid arthritis knee joints: a comparison with synovial histology. Scand J Rheumatol. 2012;41(2):89–94.
9. Gait A, Hodgson R, Parkes M, Hutchinson C, O'Neill T, Maricar N, et al. Synovial volume vs. enhancement of synovium as measures of response in osteoarthritis. Osteoarthritis & Cartilage. 2016;submitted: OAC2920; in revision.
10. Hunter DJ, Harvey W, Gross KD, Felson D, McCree P, Li L, et al. A randomized trial of patellofemoral bracing for treatment of patellofemoral osteoarthritis. Osteoarthr Cartil. 2011;19(7):792–800.
11. O'Neill TW, Parkes MJ, Maricar N, Marjanovic EJ, Hodgson R, Gait AD, et al. Synovial tissue volume: a treatment target in knee osteoarthritis (OA). Ann Rheum Dis. 2015;
12. Tofts PS. T1-weighed DCE Imaging Concepts: Modelling, Acquisition and Analysis. Magnetom Flash 2010 [cited 2015 20/05/2015]; Available from: http://usa.healthcare.siemens.com/siemens_hwem-hwem_ssxa_websites-context-root/wcm/idc/siemens_hwem-hwem_ssxa_websites-context-root/wcm/idc/groups/public/@global/@imaging/@mri/documents/download/mdaw/mde0/~edisp/t1-weighted_dce_imaging_concepts-00014355.pdf.
13. Hodgson RJ, O'Connor P, Moots R. MRI of rheumatoid arthritis image quantitation for the assessment of disease activity, progression and response to therapy. Rheumatology (Oxford). 2008;47(1):13–21.
14. Wenham CY, Balamoody S, Grainger AJ, Hensor EM, Draycott S, Hodgson R, et al. The responsiveness of novel, dynamic, contrast-enhanced magnetic resonance measures of total knee synovitis after intra-articular corticosteroid for painful osteoarthritis. Osteoarthr Cartil. 2014;22(10):1614–8.
15. Angst F, Aeschlimann A, Michel BA, Stucki G. Minimal clinically important rehabilitation effects in patients with osteoarthritis of the lower extremities. J Rheumatol. 2002;29(1):131–8.
16. O'Neill TW, Parkes MJ, Maricar N, Marjanovic EJ, Hodgson R, Gait AD, et al. Response to: 'Synovial tissue volume and reduction in pain following intra-articular steroid therapy' by Wei et al. Ann Rheum Dis. 2015;

10

Cross-cultural adaptation and psychometric analysis of the Arabic version of the oxford knee score in adult male with knee osteoarthritis

Ahmad H. Alghadir[1], Einas S. Al-Eisa[1] and Shahnawaz Anwer[1,2*]

Abstract

Background: There are varieties of self-assessment questionnaire used for the evaluation of pain, functional disability, and health related quality of life in individuals with knee osteoarthritis (OA). The present study intended to adapt and translate the oxford knee score into the Arabic and investigated its psychometric properties in adult male with knee OA.

Methods: Ninety-seven adult male (mean age 57.55 ± 11.49 years) with knee OA participated. Patients were requested to complete the adapted Arabic version of the Oxford knee score (OKS-Ar), reduced "Western Ontario and McMaster Universities Index (WOMAC)", and the Visual analogue scale (VAS). Patients were requested to complete 2nd form of OKS-Ar at least 1 week apart to assess the reproducibility of the score. The OKS was adapted and translated into Arabic by two independent Arabic native speakers (one rehabilitation professional having experience of knee OA patients and another one a trained translator) according to the international guidelines.

Results: All the participants completed the 2nd form of OKS-Ar (Response rate 100%). Reliability and internal consistency was high with an ICC of 0.97, and the Cronbach's alpha coefficient of 0.987, respectively. A significant relationship between the OKS-Ar and the WOMAC and VAS scores confirmed the construct validity ($p < 0.001$). The standard error of measurement (SEM) and the minimum detectable change (MDC) were 2.2 and 6.2, respectively.

Conclusions: The adapted Arabic version of the OKS demonstrated acceptable psychometric properties, including reliability, internal consistency, and the validity. The present study indicates that the OKS-Ar is a suitable questionnaire to measure pain and physical function in the Arabic speaking adult male patients with knee OA.

Keywords: Arabic, Osteoarthritis, Knee, Oxford knee score, Validity, Reliability

Background

Knee osteoarthritis (OA) is the commonest degenerative joint disease affecting both men and women, and is represented by pain and impaired physical function that can significantly influence the health related quality of life [1–3]. Previous study reported that approximately 60.9% female and 53.3% male adults aged 30–93 years had shown radiographic evidence of knee OA in the Middle East [4]. Another study reported the prevalence of knee OA in the Saudi Arabia was around 30.8% in the adult aged 46–55 years and 60.6% in the adult aged 66–75 years [5]. The world-wide prevalence of the symptomatic knee OA with the radiographic evidence was about 3.8% in the year 2010 [6]. The prevalence of knee OA was higher in females than males (4.8% vs 2.8%) [6]. In the year 2010, the Asia Pacific high-income nations had highest prevalence of Knee OA, followed by Middle East North Africa (MENA) region [6]. In the year 2010, hip and knee OA was reported to be 11th highest contributor causing global disability world-wide [6].

Patients-rated self-assessment questionnaire are widely used to evaluate the outcomes of various interventions [7–10]. These questionnaires often assess pain, disability, and the quality of life. There are varieties of self-assessment

* Correspondence: anwer_shahnawazphysio@rediffmail.com
[1]Rehabilitation Research Chair, College of Applied Medical Sciences, King Saud University, P.O.Box-10219, Riyadh 11433, Saudi Arabia
[2]Dr. D. Y. Patil College of Physiotherapy, Dr. D. Y. Patil Vidyapeeth, Pune, India

questionnaire used for the evaluation of pain, disability, and quality of life in individuals with knee OA [11–16]. Out of these scales, the Oxford Knee Score (OKS) is a 12 item short self-reported scale designed to evaluate pain and function in individuals undergoing total knee arthroplasty (TKA) [12]. It was reported to be amongst the most sensitive, responsive, reliable, and valid patients-reported knee-specific questionnaire [17]. This questionnaire has been validated into various languages, including Italian [18], Chinese [19], Korean [20], Japanese [21], Swedish [22], Thai [23], Persian [24], Dutch [25], Portuguese [26], German [27], Turkish [28], and French [29].

The original English version and the subsequent adapted and translated versions of the OKS have been validated in individuals with knee OA who were either waiting for or undergoing knee replacement surgery [12, 18–20, 22, 23, 25–27, 29]. A few studies have validated the OKS in patient with knee OA [21, 24, 28, 30]. In addition, there was no validation of OKS in Arabic speaking population, therefore, in order to utilize this scale in Arab nation, a validation of the Arabic version OKS was required. The present study intended to adapt and translate the OKS for the Arabic speaking population and investigated its psychometric properties in adult male with knee OA.

Methods

Participants and criteria

Ninety-seven adult male diagnosed with knee OA as indicated by the criteria given by the "American

Table 1 Backward English translation of Arabic Version of the Oxford Knee Score (OKS-Ar)

PROBLEMS IN YOUR KNEE (put a tick mark only one box of each question)

1. During the past four weeks ...... How will you describe the pain your knee often have?
   □ None
   □ Very little
   □ Little
   □ Moderate
   □ Severe
2. During the past four weeks ..... Do you have any problems in washing or drying your entire body because of your knee pain?
   □ None at all
   □ Very little difficulty
   □ Moderate difficulty
   □ Severe difficulty
   □ Hard to do this
3. During the past four weeks .... Do you have any problems in the entry and exit of your car or when using public transport because of your knee ?(Whichever is used)
   □ None at all
   □ Very little difficulty
   □ Moderate difficulty
   □ Severe difficulty
   □ Hard to do this
4. During the past four weeks ... How long you can be able to walk before it becomes severe knee pain? (With or without a stick)
   □ No pain (For more than 30 min)
   □ No pain (for 16–30 min)
   □ No pain (for 5–15 min)
   □ No pain (Just around house only)
   □ There is no time at all without pain/severe pain when walking
5. During the past four weeks ... After sitting on the table to eat, how much was the pain that you feel when getting up from the chair because of your knee?
   □ There is no pain at all
   □ Little Pain
   □ Moderate Pain
   □ Severe Pain
   □ Worst pain
6. During the past four weeks ... Do you feel stumbling when walking because of your knee?
   □ Rarely/Never
   □ Sometimes, or just at the beginning
   □ Often, not only at the beginning
   □ Most of the time
   □ All times
7. During the past four weeks ... Are you able to kneel down and after that getup from the kneel down position?
   □ Yes, easily
   □ Little difficulty
   □ Moderate difficulty
   □ Severe difficulty
   □ No, it is impossible to do so
8. During the past four weeks ... Do you suffer from pain in your knee in bed during the night?
   □ No nights
   □ A night or two nights only
   □ Some nights
   □ Most nights
   □ Every night
9. During the past four weeks ... How much was the amount of the impact of knee pain on your usual work (including housework)?
   □ No impact
   □ Little impact
   □ Moderate impact
   □ Considerable impact
   □ Total impact
10. During the past four weeks ... Have you ever felt that perhaps your knees are unstable or may make you fall?
   □ Rarely/Never
   □ Sometimes, or just at the beginning
   □ Often, not only at the beginning
   □ Most of the time
   □ All times
11. During the past four weeks... Is it possible for you to do shopping for yourself?
   □ Yes, easily
   □ Little difficulty
   □ Difficulty Medium
   □ With great difficulty
   □ No, it is impossible to do so
12. During the past four weeks ... Is it possible for you to descend the one step of stairs?
   □ Yes, easily
   □ Little difficulty
   □ Moderate Difficulty
   □ Severe Difficulty
   □ No, it is impossible to do so

Finally, please check that you have answered all the questions. Thank you so much

College of Rheumatology (ACR)" participated in this study [31]. Severity of knee was measured using the "Kellgren and Lawrence scale" [32]. Due to the lack of access to the female patients, only male patients were recruited. Patients aged 40–80 years and who can read and understand Arabic language was participated. Patients were excluded if they had secondary OA, inflammatory joint disease, and trauma to knee joint. Patients with peripheral vascular diseases or cardiac diseases were also excluded. Rehabilitation Research Chair, King Saud University, Riyadh, Saudi Arabia, approved this study. Each patient provided an informed consent before the participation.

Table 2 Participants' characteristics and the baseline scores

	$N = 97$
Age, years	
Mean (SD)	57.55 (11.49)
Range	40–80
Height, m	
Mean (SD)	1.69 (0.04)
Range	1.58–1.80
Weight, kg.	
Mean (SD)	77.81 (10.91)
Range	55–110
BMI, kg/m^2	
Mean (SD)	27.12 (3.70)
Range	18.8–38.5
OKS-Ar, 1st test	
Mean (SD)	28.28 (12.80)
Range	12–58
OKS-Ar, Re-test	
Mean (SD)	28.47 (13.06)
Range	12–59
VAS	
Mean (SD)	4.61 (3.01)
Range	0–10
WOMAC, pain scale	
Mean (SD)	7.41 (4.19)
Range	0–17
WOMAC, function scale	
Mean (SD)	11.38 (6.62)
Range	0–27
WOMAC, total scale	
Mean (SD)	18.79 (10.64)
Range	0–41

SD Standard deviation, *BMI* Body mass index, *OKS-Ar* Arabic version of the oxford knee score, *VAS* Visual analogue scale, *WOMAC* Western Ontario and McMaster Universities Index

Translation and cross-cultural adaptation

The OKS was adapted and translated into Arabic according to the international guidelines [33–36], as per the license of the OKS copyright holder (©Isis Innovation Limited, 1998. All rights reserved. www.isis-innovation.com). The English OKS [12] was translated into Arabic language by two independent Arabic native speakers (one rehabilitation professional having experience of knee OA patients and another one a trained translator). The first draft of the preliminary version was developed after the discussion of the obtained translations in a first consensus panel. The Arabic adapted version was translated back to English by two independent translators, who were unaware with the original variant (Table 1). The second draft of the preliminary version was developed after the discussion of the forward and backward translations in a second consensus panel. This pre-final version was tested by knee OA ($n = 10$) to identify whether all the items of the questionnaire were easy to understand. They were requested to suggest the word or sentences to replace existing word or sentences, if they find any difficulty to understand any word or sentences. This stage confirmed that the questionnaire was easy to understand and no further changes in the questionnaire were required. Finally, a third consensus panel discussed and developed the final Arabic version of OKS-Ar.

Psychometric measurements

Patients were asked to complete all the outcome scores including, OKS-Ar, the reduced "Western Ontario and McMaster Universities Osteoarthritis index (WOMAC)" [16, 37], and the visual analogue scale (VAS) [38, 39] at first sessions. A second form of the OKS-Ar was

Table 3 Internal consistency of the Arabic version of the Oxford Knee Score (OKS-Ar)

Items	Mean score ± SD	Corrected item-total correlation	Alpha if item deleted
1	3.18 ± 1.16	.83	.98
2	2.13 ± 1.06	.92	.97
3	2.21 ± 1.04	.93	.97
4	2.06 ± 1.11	.89	.98
5	2.46 ± 1.08	.88	.98
6	2.54 ± 1.37	.88	.98
7	2.57 ± 1.18	.90	.97
8	2.31 ± 1.21	.91	.97
9	2.22 ± 1.12	.90	.97
10	2.24 ± 1.17	.90	.97
11	2.10 ± 1.22	.86	.98
12	2.25 ± 1.23	.91	.97

SD Standard deviation

Table 4 Reliability of test-retest scores of the Arabic version Oxford knee score (OKS-Ar)

Items	1st Test (Mean ± SD)	Re-test (Mean ± SD)	ICC (95% CI)	[a]P-value
Total	28.28 ± 12.80	28.47 ± 13.06	.97 (.96–.98)	.84
1	3.18 ± 1.16	3.23 ± 1.168	.85 (.79–.90)	.39
2	2.13 ± 1.06	2.14 ± 1.051	.94 (.91–.95)	.78
3	2.21 ± 1.04	2.19 ± 1.024	.90 (.85–.93)	.65
4	2.06 ± 1.11	2.12 ± 1.120	.91 (.86–.93)	.20
5	2.46 ± 1.08	2.48 ± 1.174	.86 (.81–.91)	.72
6	2.54 ± 1.37	2.51 ± 1.363	.92 (.89–.94)	.56
7	2.57 ± 1.18	2.62 ± 1.220	.91 (.87–.94)	.31
8	2.31 ± 1.21	2.31 ± 1.228	.90 (.85–.93)	.98
9	2.22 ± 1.12	2.30 ± 1.165	.88 (.83–.92)	.16
10	2.24 ± 1.17	2.30 ± 1.243	.90 (.86–.93)	.24
11	2.10 ± 1.22	2.12 ± 1.210	.88 (.82–.91)	.74
12	2.25 ± 1.23	2.23 ± 1.254	.91 (.88–.94)	.68

SD Standard deviation
[a]Wilcoxon sign ranked test

completed at least 1 week apart to evaluate the reproducibility of the score. The construct validity of the OKS-Ar was investigated by testing the hypothesis that the scores of OKS-Ar should correlate with the WOMAC and VAS score.

Statistical analyses

Descriptive data were recorded as mean (standard deviation) and the range (minimum – maximum). Intraclass correlation coefficients ($ICC_{2,1}$) was applied to determine the reliability. Wilcoxon sign ranked test was used to investigate any systematic differences between two test scores of OKS-Ar. Cronbach's α coefficient was applied to determine the internal consistency. Absolute reliability was investigated by Bland-Altman plot method [37, 40]. The absolute measurement error was calculated using the standard error of measurement (SEM) and the minimal detectable change (MDC) ($MDC = 1.96 \times \sqrt{2} \times SEM$) [41, 42]. Spearman's correlation coefficient between the OKS-Ar, WOMAC, and the VAS scores was used to assess the construct validity. In all the tests, the $p < 0.05$ was considered as level of significance. All the statistical analysis was done using the statistical package for the social sciences for Windows version 22 (IBM Inc., Chicago, Illinois, USA).

Results

All the participants were male [$n = 97$; mean age (standard deviation), 57.55 (11.49) years]. Table 2 presented the participants characteristics and baseline scores of OKS-Ar (test and retest), VAS, WOMAC pain score, WOMAC function score, and the WOMAC total score. All the participants completed the 2nd form of OKS-Ar (Response rate 100%). The results of the OKS-Ar total score indicate no floor (2.1%) or ceiling effect (1%).

Internal consistency

Table 3 presented the results of internal consistency. The internal consistency of OKS-Ar was excellent with the Cronbach's alpha (CA) values of 0.98 for total scores. Similarly, the corrected item-total correlations

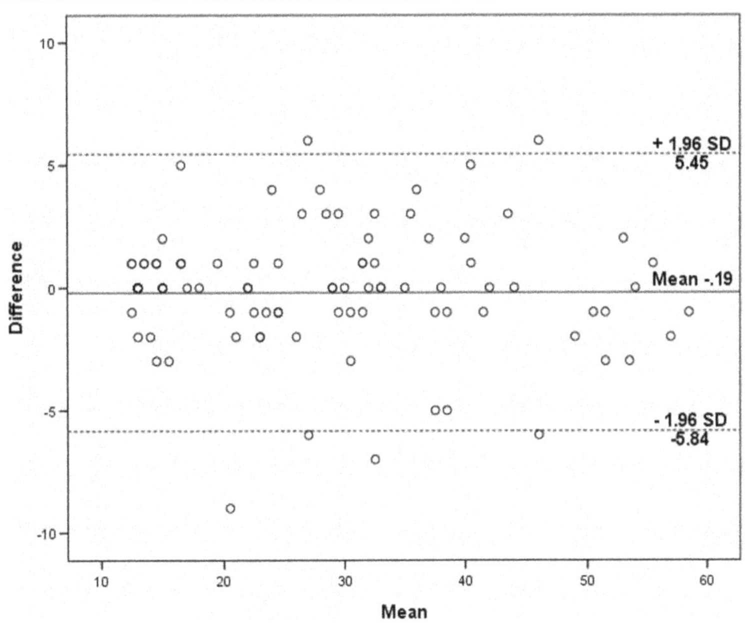

Fig. 1 Bland-Altman plot showing reliability of the Oxford Knee Score (OKS-Ar)

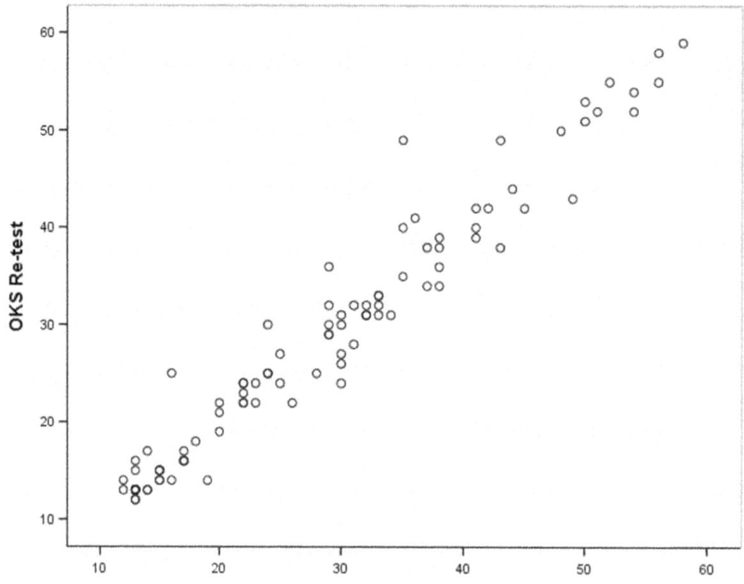

Fig. 2 Scatter diagram showing the correlation between first test and re-test of OKS-Ar

for all the items were high (range, 0.83–0.93]). The CA values did not improve higher than 0.98, if one item deleted.

Reliability

Table 4 presented the reliability of test-retest scores of OKS-Ar. Mean scores of test and retest assessment of OKS-Ar were 28.28 ± 12.8 and 28.47 ± 13.06, respectively. The ICCs for total score and each item were very high (range, .85–.97). In addition, there were no significant difference between test and retest scores of each item as well as total scores ($p > 0.05$). Figure 1 showed the Bland – Altman plot indicating most of the scores were within the limits of agreement. The Spearman's correlation coefficient between the test and retest of OKS-Ar was high ($r = 0.973$, $p < 0.001$) (Fig. 2) (Table 5). The calculated SEM and MDC were 2.2 and 6.2, respectively.

Table 5 Correlations between the Oxford knee score (OKS-Ar) and visual analogue scale (VAS) and the Western Ontario and McMaster Universities Osteoarthritis Index (WOMAC)

Scales	OKS-Ar
OKS-Ar (re-test)	.973[a]
WOMAC, pain subscale	.885[a]
WOMAC, function subscale	.883[a]
WOMAC, total scale	.895[a]
VAS	.841[a]

[a]Correlations $p \leq 0.001$

Validity

Table 5 presented the correlations between OKS-Ar and the WOMAC and VAS score. OKS-Ar was significantly associated with the VAS, WOMAC pain score, WOMAC function score, and the WOMAC total score ($p < 0.001$). The best degree of association was found between the OKS-Ar and the WOMAC total score ($r = 0.895$) (Fig. 3).

Discussion

In the present study, the stage of translation and cross-cultural adaptation of the OKS to the Arabic language was described and the psychometric properties including internal consistency, reliability, and validity in adult male patients with knee OA were presented. In the present study, the Arabic version of the OKS demonstrated good psychometric properties including reliability, internal consistency, and validity in a sample of adult male with knee OA. As per literature review, this is the first study validating Arabic version of the OKS in Saudi Arabia.

The original English variant of OKS was designed to evaluate pain and physical function in individuals undergoing TKA [12]. Similarly, the questionnaire has been validated in a various languages and used in knee OA patients who were either waiting for or undergoing knee replacement surgery [18–20, 22, 23, 25–27, 29]. Till date, a few studies have validated the OKS in individuals with knee OA [21, 24, 28, 30]. In the present study, the reliability and the internal consistency of the Arabic version of the OKS were high (ICC 0.97 and CA 0.98). Similarly, previous studies reported high values of reliability (ICC 0.85 to 0.99) and internal consistency (CA 0.90 to 0.95) for

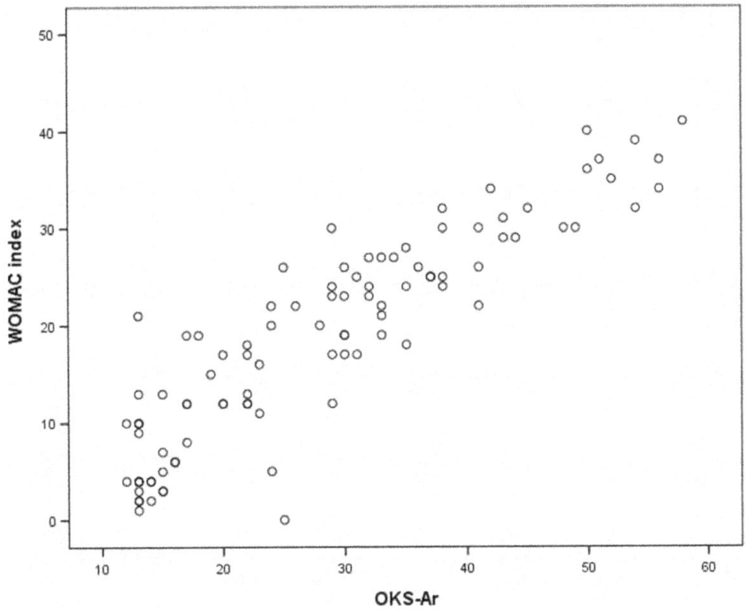

Fig. 3 Scatter diagram showing the correlation between the OKS-Ar and the WOMAC index

different languages of the OKS in patients with knee OA [21, 24, 28]. In contrast, other studies reported a little lower internal consistency (CA 0.80 to 0.87) for different languages of the OKS as well as the original English version [12, 19, 23, 26, 27]. However, in the validation of the OKS, these studies involved knee OA patients who were either waiting for or undergoing knee replacement surgery. While, in the present study, only patients with knee OA with no any surgical intervention participated.

A good correlation between the OKS-Ar and the WOMAC and VAS scores confirmed the construct validity. Similarly, Turkish and Japanese version of the OKS demonstrated a good correlation between the OKS and the WOMAC index [21, 28]. In addition, original English version and the Korean version of the OKS demonstrated a moderate relationship between the OKS and the VAS score [12, 20]. Furthermore, Portuguese version of the OKS demonstrated a weak correlation between the OKS and the VAS score [26].

In addition, the SEM and MDC were calculated for the OKS-Ar in people with knee OA. As per literature review, neither original English version nor the subsequent adapted versions of the OKS have reported the SEM and MDC. Previous studies encouraged using SEM to determine the statistically meaningful change of a health outcome questionnaire [41, 42].

The present study acknowledged some potential limitations. The present study is limited to adult male patients with knee osteoarthritis. Due to the lack of access to the female patients, only male patients were recruited. Further validation with the female patients is recommended. In addition, sample size of the present study was fairly small. Furthermore, the present study did not assess the responsiveness of the Arabic version of the OKS. Further testing with the larger sample is required to complete the evaluation of this important psychometric property.

Conclusions

The adapted Arabic version of the OKS demonstrated acceptable psychometric properties, including reliability, internal consistency, and the validity. The present study indicates that the OKS-Ar is a suitable questionnaire to measure pain and function in the Arabic speaking adult male with knee osteoarthritis.

Abbreviations

MDC: Minimum detectable change; OA: Osteoarthritis; OKS: Oxford Knee Score; SEM: Standard error of measurement; VAS: Visual analogue scale; WOMAC: Western Ontario and McMaster Universities Index.

Acknowledgements

The authors are grateful to the Deanship of Scientific Research, King Saud University for funding through Vice Deanship of Scientific Research Chairs.

Funding

This project was funded by the Deanship of Scientific Research, King Saud University through Vice Deanship of Scientific Research Chairs. The funding body played no role on study design, the writing of the manuscript or the decision to submit the manuscript for publication.

Authors' contributions

SA: Corresponding author, participated in the design of the study, participated in the data collection, drafted the manuscript and finished the manuscript. AA: participated in the design of the study, helped in ethics applications and revised the manuscript critically. EA: participated in the design of the study and revised the manuscript critically. All authors read and approved the final manuscript.

Competing interests
The authors declare that they have no competing interests.

Consent for publication
Not applicable.

References

1. Cho HJ, Chang CB, Kim KW, Park JH, Yoo JH, Koh IJ, et al. Gender and prevalence of knee osteoarthritis types in elderly Koreans. J Arthroplasty. 2011;26(7):994–9.
2. Hochberg MC, Altman RD, Brandt KD, Clark BM, Dieppe PA, Griffin MR, et al. Guidelines for the medical management of osteoarthritis. Part I. Osteoarthritis of the hip. American College of Rheumatology. Arthritis Rheum. 1995;38(11): 1535–40.
3. Hochberg MC, Altman RD, Brandt KD, Clark BM, Dieppe PA, Griffin MR, et al. Guidelines for the medical management of osteoarthritis. Part II. Osteoarthritis of the knee. American College of Rheumatology. Arthritis Rheum. 1995;38(11): 1541–6.
4. Al-Arfaj A, Al-Boukai AA. Prevalence of radiographic knee osteoarthritis in Saudi Arabia. Clin Rheumatol. 2002;21(2):142–5.
5. Al-Arfaj AS, Alballa SR, Al-Saleh SS, Al-Dalaan AM, Bahabry SA, Mousa MA, et al. Knee osteoarthritis in Al-Qaseem, Saudi Arabia. Saudi Med J. 2003; 24(3):291–3.
6. Cross M, Smith E, Hoy D, Nolte S, Ackerman I, Fransen M, et al. The global burden of hip and knee osteoarthritis: estimates from the global burden of disease 2010 study. Ann Rheum Dis. 2014;73(7):1323–30.
7. Beaton DE, Schemitsch E. Measures of health-related quality of life and physical function. Clin Orthop Relat Res. 2003;413:90–105.
8. Fitzpatrick R, Davey C, Buxton MJ, Jones DR. Evaluating patient-based outcome measures for use in clinical trials. Health Technol Assess. 1998; 2(14):i–iv. 1–74.
9. Whitehouse SL, Blom AW, Taylor AH, Pattison GT, Bannister GC. The Oxford Knee Score; problems and pitfalls. Knee. 2005;12(4):287–91.
10. Marx RG. Knee rating scales. Arthroscopy. 2003;19(10):1103–8.
11. Bellamy N, Buchanan WW, Goldsmith CH, Campbell J, Stitt LW. Validation study of WOMAC: a health status instrument for measuring clinically important patient relevant outcomes to antirheumatic drug therapy in patients with osteoarthritis of the hip or knee. J Rheumatol. 1988;15(12):1833–40.
12. Dawson J, Fitzpatrick R, Murray D, Carr A. Questionnaire on the perceptions of patients about total knee replacement. J Bone Joint Surg (Br). 1998;80(1):63–9.
13. Lysholm J, Tegner Y. Knee injury rating scales. Acta Orthop. 2007;78(4):445–53.
14. Mahler E, Cuperus N, Bijlsma J, Vliet Vlieland T, van den Hoogen F, den Broeder AA, et al. Responsiveness of four patient-reported outcome measures to assess physical function in patients with knee osteoarthritis. Scand J Rheumatol. 2016;45(6):518–27.
15. Roos EM, Roos HP, Lohmander LS, Ekdahl C, Beynnon BD. Knee Injury and Osteoarthritis Outcome Score (KOOS) – development of a self-administered outcome measure. J Orthop Sports Phys Ther. 1998;28(2):88–96.
16. Whitehouse SL, Lingard EA, Katz JN, Learmonth ID. Development and testing of a reduced WOMAC function scale. J Bone Joint Surg (Br). 2003;85(5):706–11.
17. Garratt AM, Brealey S, Gillespie WJ, Team DT. Patient-assessed health instruments for the knee: a structured review. Rheumatology (Oxford). 2004;43(11):1414–23.
18. Padua R, Zanoli G, Ceccarelli E, Romanini E, Bondi R, Campi A. The Italian version of the Oxford 12-item Knee Questionnaire-cross-cultural adaptation and validation. Int Orthop. 2003;27(4):214–6.
19. Xie F, Li SC, Lo NN, Yeo SJ, Yang KY, Yeo W, et al. Cross-cultural adaptation and validation of Singapore English and Chinese Versions of the Oxford Knee Score (OKS) in knee osteoarthritis patients undergoing total knee replacement. Osteoarthritis Cartilage. 2007;15(9):1019–24.
20. Eun IS, Kim OG, Kim CK, Lee HS, Lee JS. Validation of the Korean version of the Oxford Knee Score in patients undergoing total knee arthroplasty. Clin Orthop Relat Res. 2013;471(2):600–5.
21. Takeuchi R, Sawaguchi T, Nakamura N, Ishikawa H, Saito T, Goldhahn S. Cross-cultural adaptation and validation of the Oxford 12-item knee score in Japanese. Arch Orthop Trauma Surg. 2011;131(2):247–54.
22. Dunbar MJ, Robertsson O, Ryd L, Lidgren L. Translation and validation of the Oxford-12 item knee score for use in Sweden. Acta Orthop Scand. 2000; 71(3):268–74.
23. Charoencholvanich K, Pongcharoen B. Oxford knee score and SF-36: translation & reliability for use with total knee arthroscopy patients in Thailand. J Med Assoc Thai. 2005;88(9):1194–202.
24. Ebrahimzadeh MH, Makhmalbaf H, Birjandinejad A, Soltani-Moghaddas SH. Cross-cultural adaptation and validation of the persian version of the oxford knee score in patients with knee osteoarthritis. Iran J Med Sci. 2014;39(6): 529–35.
25. Haverkamp D, Breugem SJ, Sierevelt IN, Blankevoort L, van Dijk CN. Translation and validation of the Dutch version of the Oxford 12-item knee questionnaire for knee arthroplasty. Acta Orthop. 2005;76(3):347–52.
26. Goncalves RS, Tomas AM, Martins DI. Cross-cultural adaptation and validation of the Portuguese version of the Oxford Knee Score (OKS). Knee. 2012;19(4):344–7.
27. Naal FD, Impellizzeri FM, Sieverding M, Loibl M, von Knoch F, Mannion AF, et al. The 12-item Oxford Knee Score: cross-cultural adaptation into German and assessment of its psychometric properties in patients with osteoarthritis of the knee. Osteoarthritis Cartilage. 2009;17(1):49–52.
28. Tugay BU, Tugay N, Guney H, Kinikli GI, Yuksel I, Atilla B. Oxford Knee Score: cross-cultural adaptation and validation of the Turkish version in patients with osteoarthritis of the knee. Acta Orthop Traumatol Turc. 2016;50(2):198–206.
29. Jenny JY, Diesinger Y. Validation of a French version of the Oxford knee questionnaire. Orthop Traumatol Surg Res. 2011;97(3):267–71.
30. Xie F, Ye H, Zhang Y, Liu X, Lei T, Li SC. Extension from inpatients to outpatients: validity and reliability of the Oxford Knee Score in measuring health outcomes in patients with knee osteoarthritis. Int J Rheum Dis. 2011;14(2):206–10.
31. Altman R, Asch E, Bloch D, Bole G, Borenstein D, Brandt K, et al. Development of criteria for the classification and reporting of osteoarthritis. Classification of osteoarthritis of the knee. Diagnostic and Therapeutic Criteria Committee of the American Rheumatism Association. Arthritis Rheum. 1986;29(8):1039–49.
32. Kellgren JH, Lawrence JS. Radiological assessment of osteo-arthrosis. Ann Rheum Dis. 1957;16(4):494–502.
33. Wild D, Grove A, Martin M, Eremenco S, McElroy S, Verjee-Lorenz A, et al. Principles of Good Practice for the Translation and Cultural Adaptation Process for Patient-Reported Outcomes (PRO) Measures: report of the ISPOR Task Force for Translation and Cultural Adaptation. Value Health. 2005;8(2):94–104.
34. Acquadro C, Conway K, Hareendran A, Aaronson N, Quality ERI. Literature review of methods to translate health-related quality of life questionnaires for use in multinational clinical trials. Value Health. 2008;11(3):509–21.
35. Beaton DE, Bombardier C, Guillemin F, Ferraz MB. Guidelines for the process of cross-cultural adaptation of self-report measures. Spine. 2000;25(24):3186–91.
36. Guillemin F, Bombardier C, Beaton D. Cross-Cultural Adaptation of Health-Related Quality-of-Life Measures - Literature-Review and Proposed Guidelines. J Clin Epidemiol. 1993;46(12):1417–32.
37. Alghadir A, Anwer S, Iqbal ZA, Alsanawi HA. Cross-cultural adaptation, reliability and validity of the Arabic version of the reduced Western Ontario and McMaster Universities Osteoarthritis index in patients with knee osteoarthritis. Disabil Rehabil. 2016;38(7):689–94.
38. Hjermstad MJ, Fayers PM, Haugen DF, Caraceni A, Hanks GW, Loge JH, et al. Studies comparing Numerical Rating Scales, Verbal Rating Scales, and Visual Analogue Scales for assessment of pain intensity in adults: a systematic literature review. J Pain Symptom Manage. 2011;41(6):1073–93.
39. Gallasch CH, Alexandre NM. The measurement of musculoskeletal pain intensity: a comparison of four methods. Rev Gaucha Enferm. 2007;28(2):260–5.
40. Alsanawi HA, Alghadir A, Anwer S, Roach KE, Alawaji A. Cross-cultural adaptation and psychometric properties of an Arabic version of the Shoulder Pain and Disability Index. Int J Rehabil Res. 2015;38(3):270–5.
41. Lydick E, Epstein RS. Interpretation of quality of life changes. Qual Life Res. 1993;2(3):221–6.
42. Wyrwich KW, Wolinsky FD. Identifying meaningful intra-individual change standards for health-related quality of life measures. J Eval Clin Pract. 2000; 6(1):39–49.

11

Identification of pain categories associated with change in pain in patients receiving placebo: data from two phase 3 randomized clinical trials in symptomatic knee osteoarthritis

Asger Reinstrup Bihlet[1*], Inger Byrjalsen, Anne-Christine Bay-Jensen[1], Jeppe Ragnar Andersen[1], Claus Christiansen[1], Bente Juel Riis[1], Ivo Valter[2], Morten A. Karsdal[1] and Marc C. Hochberg[3]

Abstract

Background: Pain is the principal clinical symptom of osteoarthritis (OA), and development of safe and effective analgesics for OA pain is needed. Drug development of new analgesics for OA pain is impaired by substantial change in pain in patients receiving placebo, and more data describing clinical characteristics and pain categories particularly associated with this phenomenon is needed.
The purpose of this post-hoc analysis was to investigate clinical characteristics and pain categories and their association with radiographic progression and placebo pain reduction (PPR) in OA patients as measured the Western Ontario and McMasters Arthritis (WOMAC).

Methods: Pooled data from the placebo groups of two phase III randomized clinical trials in patients with knee OA followed for 2 years were analyzed. Differences between individual sub-scores and pain categories of weight-bearing and non-weight bearing pain over time were assessed. Selected patient baseline characteristics were assessed for association with PPR. Association between pain categories and radiographic progression was analyzed.

Results: The reduction of pain in placebo-treated patients was significantly higher in the composite of questions related to weight-bearing pain compared to non-weight-bearing pain of the target knee. Baseline BMI, age and JSW were not associated with pain change. Pain reduction was higher in the Target knee, compared to the Non-Target knee at all corresponding time-points. A very weak correlation was found between weight-bearing pain and progression in the non-target knee.

Conclusions: These results indicate that the reduction in pain in patients treated with placebo is significantly different between pain categories, as weight-bearing pain was significantly more reduced compared to non-weight-bearing pain. Further research in pain categories in OA is warranted.

Keywords: Pain categories, Placebo-response, Radiographic progression

* Correspondence: abi@nordicbioscience.com
[1]Nordic Bioscience, Herlev Hovedgade 207, DK2730 Herlev, Denmark
Full list of author information is available at the end of the article

Background

Osteoarthritis (OA) is the most common arthritic disease, affecting more than 250 million people in the world [1]. Pain is the principal clinical symptom of osteoarthritis (OA), and while several approved medical treatments for OA pain exist, new safe and effective analgesics are still needed [2]. OA pain itself is considered to be the result of several pathological conditions, manifested as allodynia, hyperalgesia and central sensitization, to varying degrees [3–5]. This diffuse construct of features combined with elements of psychosocial factors has proven particularly difficult to treat [6, 7]. Whether and how knee pain is linked to increased risk of radiographic progression is controversial [8–10]. Indeed OA pain is considered to be multifactorial [3, 4], and there is no clear-cut association of single-factors with disease activity and structural degradation. Clinical research evaluating new efficacious analgesic treatments in OA is also impaired by a substantial placebo-response, requiring large sample sizes, complex study designs or cumbersome methods of study participant selection to facilitate demonstration of statistically significant improvement in reported pain levels [11]. Several mechanisms are thought to be involved in placebo-response [12–14], but data describing if different categories of pain are similarly affected by placebo-response are lacking, and links between pain categories and disease activity remains unclear.

Specialized and validated methods of subtyping pain into elements of central sensitization [15], neuropathic pain [16], among others, exist. The use of more crude, exploratory methods include the subscores of the well-recognized Western Ontario and McMaster Universities Osteoarthritis Index (WOMAC) [17] as a potential indicator of differences in pain categories. In a report by Lo et al. from 2009, the authors found that WOMAC pain while the joint is load-bearing is likely to be linked to bone marrow lesions and effusion assessed using magnetic resonance imaging (MRI), but pain while idle is not, indicating that pain is multifactorial [18]. Further in support of differences behind weight-bearing and non-weight-bearing pain is a report by Hensor et al. analyzing periodic individual WOMAC questions from the OsteoArthritis Initiative (OAI) of people at high risk of developing OA over a period of 7 years, showed that pain while walking up or down stairs was the first to manifest as a symptom of OA, and pain while in bed at night was registered as the last [19].

A report by Stratford et al. further concluded that these two pain categories, pain while weight-bearing vs. non-weight-bearing pain, reflect different pain constructs [20]. Thus, attempts to quantify pain using the total WOMAC pain composite may not be ideal, and additional, exploratory information which may point to differences in pain etiology may be derived from analyzing the two pain constructs separately.

In the absence of existing research describing the origin of pain categories and their association with placebo pain reduction (PPR), this report will assess associations between age, clinical and radiographic features and pain categories with reduction in pain as reported by patients receiving placebo as well as associations between pain categories and risk of radiographic progression in two pooled randomized controlled trials.

Methods

Study population

This is a post-hoc analysis of the placebo groups in two, double-blinded, randomized, placebo-controlled and multicenter phase III clinical trials assessing the efficacy and safety of an oral formulation of 0.8 mg salmon calcitonin in patients with painful knee OA (NCT00486434 (trial 1) and NCT00704847 (trial 2)). Each independent trial recruited patients aged 51–80 years with painful OA in the target knee, defined as a Visual Analogue Score of ≥150 mm on the WOMAC pain subscale (500 mm being the maximum score). In study 2, patients scoring ≤150 mm on the pain sub-score were allowed to participate if they also scored ≥510 mm on the WOMAC function sub-scale (1700 mm being the maximum score). The radiographic inclusion criteria for target knees included Kellgren-Lawrence (KL) grades 2 or 3, and a Joint Space Width (JSW) of ≥2.0 mm. A total of 2206 patients were recruited at 19 sites in 11 countries. Details regarding trial design and results are published elsewhere [21]. The present analysis includes the 771 placebo-treated subjects in the per-protocol population with no missing values during the trial. The Per-Protocol Population was chosen as it constitutes the most protocol compliant dataset, including treatment/placebo compliance, completion of planned visits including pain questionnaires and scheduled X-rays, and absence of protocol deviations such as use of analgesic treatment or surgical procedures which may interfere with pain questionnaires. A single target knee was selected for each patient, and the patient was made aware of which knee was the target knee. Target knee designation was made based on eligibility criteria as described above. If both knees were deemed eligible, the knee with the lowest eligible KL-score was selected (KL 2), and if both knees were KL 2, the knee with the highest pain score was selected as the target knee. In Study 2, data on pain in the non-target knee was only collected at baseline. For analysis of pain change of the non-target knee in subjects receiving placebo, a sub-group consisting of non-target knees matching the pain inclusion criteria as mentioned above, were selected, to improve comparability between the two groups of knees and reduce noise originating from small numerical changes in knees with very little baseline pain leading to large proportional (percentage) change. In addition, only non-target knees with no missing pain data throughout the trial were selected. Thus, 771 target knees and 256 non-target knees are analyzed.

For the analysis of baseline pain categories and risk of Joint-Space Narrowing (JSN), data of all baseline 771 target knees and contralateral 733 non-target knees with both baseline and Year 2 radiographic assessments were analyzed, regardless of baseline pain level. The studies were conducted in full compliance with the Helsinki Declaration, and were approved by all applicable Instiutional Review Boards, Ethical Committees and Competent Authorities in the countries in which they were conducted.

Radiographic evaluation

X-ray images of both knees using fixed-flexion were obtained at the screening to assess the eligibility for study participation and to select the target knee. Each X-ray image was read by one expert radiologist for absolute JSW and KL-grade. Additional X-ray images were obtained at months 12 and 24 to, upon final data analysis, assess JSN defined as absolute change in JSW in millimeters during the 24 month period.

Pain assessment

Pain, stiffness and function of both the target- and non-target knees were assessed by the WOMAC version VA3.1 questionnaire. In Study 2, pain in the non-target knee was only assessed at baseline. For the present analysis, only the pain sub-scale is used. The subjects were instructed to read each question carefully and mark an X on a 100 mm line, on which 0 mm equaled "No Pain" and 100 equaled "Worst Pain Imaginable".

The pain sub-scale records patient assessments in the following five situations: 1; during walking on a flat surface, 2; using stairs (up or down), 3; at night while in bed, 4; sitting or lying, and 5; while standing. Composites of the WOMAC pain subscale were constructed to detect associations with radiographic progression: A) pain experienced while the joint was under load, and/or the patient was active (questions 1, 2, and 5) or B) pain experienced while idle and while the joint was free of mechanical load (questions 3 and 4).

Statistical analyses

The baseline total WOMAC pain score and each pain sub-scale score was normalized to a percentage of the maximum possible score and mean levels were compared in a mixed model with pain level as the dependent variable, the question as a fixed effect, and the patient as a random effect.

The change in pain level from baseline of each patient at a given time point was calculated as a proportionate change in percent, e.g. a change from 40 mm to 20 mm equals a 50% reduction, and the mean change in percent for each variable was used. Changes in percent from baseline pain were calculated at months 1, 6, 12 and 24, and differences between individual questions were assessed using a repeated measures ANOVA. Pain values below 10 of 100 were set arbitrarily at 10 to normalize output and reduce noise. Pain by category ("weight-bearing"; WOMAC questions 1, 2 and 5 and "non-weight-bearing"; WOMAC questions 3 and 4) was similarly analyzed for change over time, and compared in a repeated measures ANOVA. Similar to the individual WOMAC scores, if at any timepoint the score of a category was below 10, the value was set at 10 to normalize output and reduce noise. Selected patient baseline characteristics; pain by WOMAC question, Joint-space width, age, sex, and body mass index (BMI) were assessed for association with PPR defined as change in percent from baseline to year two using Spearman's correlation.

Spearman's correlation analysis was used to assess the relationship between baseline WOMAC pain levels (levels of WOMAC pain score, each pain sub--scale question, and composite pain questions) and the radiographic progression measured as change from baseline in JSW at year two, i.e. Joint Space Narrowing (JSN), for both target- and non-target knees. Data were calculated both unadjusted and adjusted for BMI and KL-grade as predictors. These parameters have previously been shown to be associated with progression in the study population used for this analysis [22]. Results of the spearman's correlation analyses were considered exploratory, and were not adjusted for multiplicity. To graphically depict associations between baseline WOMAC pain level and radiographic progression, all available Target ($N = 771$) and Non-Target knees ($N = 733$) of the Per Protocol population were divided by pain quintiles (A-E) for each WOMAC question (Q1–5), and plotted against JSN at year two.

Regression to the mean

As described by Barnett and colleagues [23] the impact of regression to the mean (RTM) in the current report was estimated using a SAS-script as supplied by Barnett incorporating within- and between-patient variance in pain reporting. The estimated RTM was calculated as change in pain from baseline to year two, and then subtracted from the observed change in pain from baseline for each pain category to estimate the change in pain excluding the influence of RTM.

Results

The baseline characteristics and mean pain levels are shown in Table 1.

Pain categories and pain placebo reduction

A reduction in pain in patients receiving placebo was evident from month 1, at which point the mean reduction in pain from baseline was 8.1%.

WOMAC Q2 was associated with the highest reduction in pain for both Target (T), and NT (Non-Target) knees (36.8% ±52.4 (SD) and 28.0% ±44.4,

Table 1 Demographic characteristics by study and overall per protocol population

Demographic characteristics placebo group, per protocol population				
Parameter	Target knee *N* = 771		Non-target knee *N* = 256	
Sex - *n* (%)				
Male	280 (36.3)		82 (32.0)	
Female	491 (63.7)		174 (68.0)	
Age (years)				
Mean (SD)	64.5 (6.5)		64.70 (6.3)	
Median (min, max)	64.1 (50, 81)		64.5 (50.4, 79.5)	
Age group (years) – *n* (%)				
< 65	456 (59.1)		137 (53.5)	
≥ 65	315 (40.9)		119 (46.5)	
Race – *n* (%)				
Caucasian	666 (86.4)		228 (89.1)	
Asian	103 (13.4)		27 (10.5)	
Other	2 (0.3)		1 (0.4)	
BMI (kg/m^2)				
Mean (SD)	28.6 (4.7)		28.6 (4.4)	
Median (min, max)	27.9 (17.3, 45.9)		28.1 (19.6, 43.3)	
KL Score - *n* (%)				
KL 0	N/A		5 (2)	
KL 1	N/A		37 (14.5)	
KL 2	641 (83.1)		130 (50.8)	
KL 3	130 (16.9)		73 (28.5)	
KL4	N/A		10 (3.9)	
JSW (mm)				
Mean (SD)	3.43 (0.99)		3.15 (1.56)	
Median (min, max)	3.4 (1.8, 6.7)		3.39 (0.0, 7.3)	
WOMAC pain score (normalized 0–100)	Mean (SD)	Median (min, max)	Mean (SD)	Median (min, max)
Total pain (Q1–5)	49 (15)	47 (10, 100)	50 (16)	47 (30, 96)
Walking on flat surface (Q1)	47 (20)	47 (2, 100)	47 (21)	46 (2, 99)
Stairs (up or down) (Q2)	65 (18)	65 (2, 100)	65 (19)	63 (13, 100)
In bed at night (Q3)	42 (26)	41 (0, 100)	44 (24)	44 (0, 98)
Sitting or lying (Q4)	42 (22)	40 (0, 100)	43 (22)	43 (0, 100)
Standing(Q5)	49 (21)	49 (0, 100)	49 (20)	48 (3, 100)
Weight-bearing Composite (Q1, 2, 5)	53 (15)	52 (2, 100)	53 (17)	51 (18, 96)
Non-weight-bearing Composite (Q3, Q4)	42 (21)	40 (0, 100)	44 (21)	41 (0–96)

Trial 1: NCT00486434. Trial 2: NCT00704847. Non-target knees is a sub-group matching the pain inclusion criteria of the target knee within the per-protocol population. Both trials 1 and 2 were phase three randomized trials with a duration of 2 years, evaluating the effect of oral salmon calcitonin in symptomatic knee osteoarthritis on radiographic progression and symptoms. *BMI* Body Mass Index, *KL-score* Kellgren-Lawrence, *JSW* Joint Space Width, *WOMAC* Western Ontario and McMaster Universities Arthritis Index

respectively) at year two. Notably the observed pain reduction was higher in the T knee, compared to the NT knee at all corresponding time-points.

The level of placebo pain reduction was significantly higher in questions related to weight-bearing pain compared to non-weight-bearing pain. This was statistically significant in the T knee ($p < 0.005$) at month 1 and onwards, but did not reach statistical significance for the NT knee (Fig. 1). No differences were observed between questions within the two categories (weight-bearing and non-weight-bearing) at any time-points. Notably the main divergence between the two categories occurred during the first month, at which point the difference in change from baseline between the two categories is 10%; a difference which remains largely unchanged through the remainder of the trial.

Regression to the mean as a result of chance should be considered as a confounder in all assessments of change in pain over time [24]. The assessment of RTM in the current dataset (Table 2) indicates that data of pain change during the trial of the target knee may have affected by RTM for both composites and individual questions of weight-bearing and non-weight-bearing pain. When adjusting the observed pain change during the trial for the RTM estimate, the non-weight-bearing pain composite appears to change much less from baseline levels during the trial, while a modest decline in weight-bearing pain is observed (Fig. 1c).

Baseline clinical and radiographic features and pain change in patients receiving placebo

Baseline BMI, age, sex and JSW were not associated with pain change in the placebo-treated patients at year two.

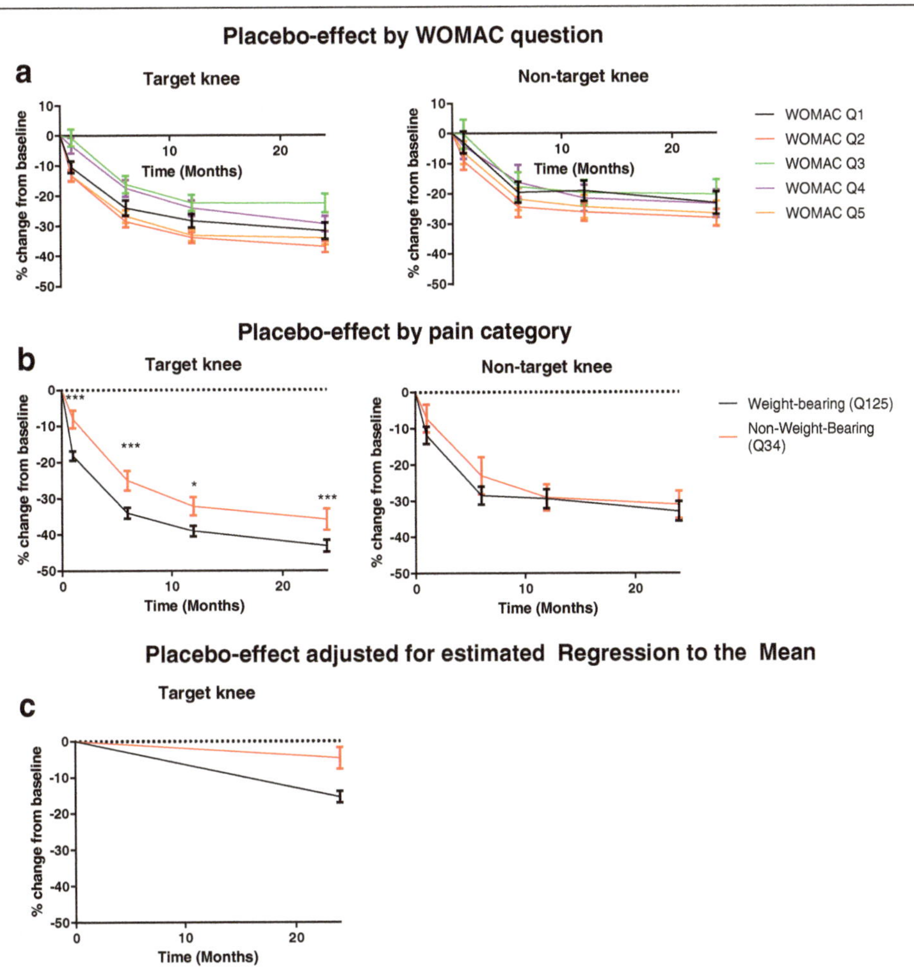

Fig. 1 Target knee ($n = 771$) and Non-target knee ($n = 256$) mean pain change from baseline in % over 24 months, normalized (0–100), by pain question (**a**) and category; Weight-bearing pain (WOMAC questions 1, 2 and 5), and non-weight-bearing pain (WOMAC questions 3 and 4) (**b**). Baseline values below 10 are set to 10 to reduce noise. Non-target knees were selected to include only those meeting the pain inclusion criteria of the target knee for comparability. **c** depicts mean change from baseline in %, adjusted for the estimated regression to the mean as listed in Table 2. Error bars are SEM. *: $p < 0.05$ ***: $p < 0.001$

Table 2 Estimated Regression-to-the-mean

WOMAC sub-score	SD	σ_b^2	σ_w^2	Estimated RTM effect from BL to Y2 (%)	Pain change from BL to Y2 adjusted for estimated RTM effect (%)
Question 1: Walking on flat surface	56	1602.5	1533.5	32.6	0.9
Question 2: On stairs	38	735.0	709.0	26.0	−10.9
Question 3: Lying in bed	80	3872.0	2528.0	33.7	11.2
Question 4: Sitting or lying	69	2551.9	2209.1	35.6	6.3
Question 5: Standing	57	1614.8	1634.3	33.9	−0.1
Questions 1, 2, and 5: Weight-bearing	39	734.6	786.4	27.8	−15,4
Questions 3 and 4: Non-weight-bearing	65	2433.6	1791.4	31.2	−4.6

The percentage of RTM of the Target knee as estimated using the method of Barnett et al. [24]. Calculation of σ_w^2 was based on within patient data from screening visit and subsequent baseline visit, between 1 and 3 weeks apart. σ_b^2: Between patient-variance. σ_w^2: Within patient-variance. *BL* Baseline. *Y2* Year 2, *RTM* Regression to the mean

Associations of baseline pain and radiographic joint-space narrowing

Target knee

In target knees, Spearman's correlation of individual WOMAC pain questions showed very weak correlations between baseline pain score and change in JSW at year 2. WOMAC question 2 (pain while walking on stairs) was found to be negatively correlated with change in JSW (rho = – 0.079, $p = 0.028$). Consequently neither of the composite scores of pain while under load (Q1, Q2 and Q5) or pain while idle (Q3 and Q4) were significantly correlated with change in JSW at year 2. Adjustments for KL-score and BMI did not lead to significant changes in correlations between pain severity and radiographic progression.

The average JSN in target knees at year 2 ranged from 0.34 mm to 0.49 mm with little apparent influence of degree or, type of baseline pain (Fig. 2).

Non-target knee

As shown in Table 3, all WOMAC questions apart from Q3 (pain at night while in bed) were very weakly, positively associated with a change in JSW at year 2, indicating that a higher baseline pain score may contribute, albeit very modestly to a higher risk of progression in the NT knee. WOMAC question 5 (pain while standing), appeared most associated with progression (rho = 0.10, $p = 0.007$). The correlation coefficients of the composite score of weight-bearing pain (Q1, Q2 and Q5) to JSN were rho = 0.10, $p = 0.007$, while non-weight-bearing pain (Q3 and Q4) was weaker, with a rho = 0.05, $p = 0.14$.

After adjustment for KL-score and BMI, WOMAC Q5 and the composite score of weight-bearing pain were rho = 0.08, $p = 0.02$ and rho = 0.08, $p = 0.03$, respectively).

JSN in the non-target knees varied from very low to moderate, as progression rates ranged from 0.13 mm to 0.32 mm during the two-year study period. Visual inspection of Fig. 2 indicates a dose-dependent association between weight-bearing pain components, particularly pain while walking on stairs and JSN, but not non-weight-bearing pain.

Discussion

Placebo-response

This report is the first to describe differences in pain reduction between separate pain categories in in patients receiving placebo in OA trials. Several reports have investigated biochemical, psychological and psycho-social determinants of analgesic placebo-response, but to the knowledge of the authors, no investigations regarding disease-specific categories have been performed, identifying differences in susceptibility to placebo pain reduction.

The common change in pain observed in the placebo-groups of OA clinical trials can be regarded as the sum of three distinct elements; natural OA pain progression (discussed below), regression to the mean, and the true placebo response. Using a crude estimate of RTM, we report that regression to the mean may account for a part of the observed change in particularly non-weight-bearing pain, indicating a less pronounced true placebo-response on this parameter, as opposed to weight-bearing pain. The results indicate that the impact of RTM may have been overlooked as a significant driver of change in pain over time in clinical trials, but further research is needed to draw conclusions on this issue.

The findings that measures of weight-bearing pain appear more susceptible to change in patients receiving placebo than measures of non-weight bearing pain can be interpreted in several ways: 1): These measures are simply more susceptible to placebo-response, and should therefore be limited as a means of quantifying pain response in clinical trials. 2): The weight-bearing pain-measures are more sensitive to change, and therefore also more sensitive to neurobiological changes caused psychological factors such as expectations to treatment efficacy etc., but perhaps also more sensitive to change using an efficacious treatment. 3): The non-weight-bearing pain measures may be driven by a distinct pain mechanism, perhaps central sensitization, which may be less sensitive to change in patients receiving placebo, but perhaps also less sensitive to otherwise efficacious, non-neurologically-targeted analgesic treatments. As discussed below, the current report lacks suitable controls to adequately address these questions, which will need

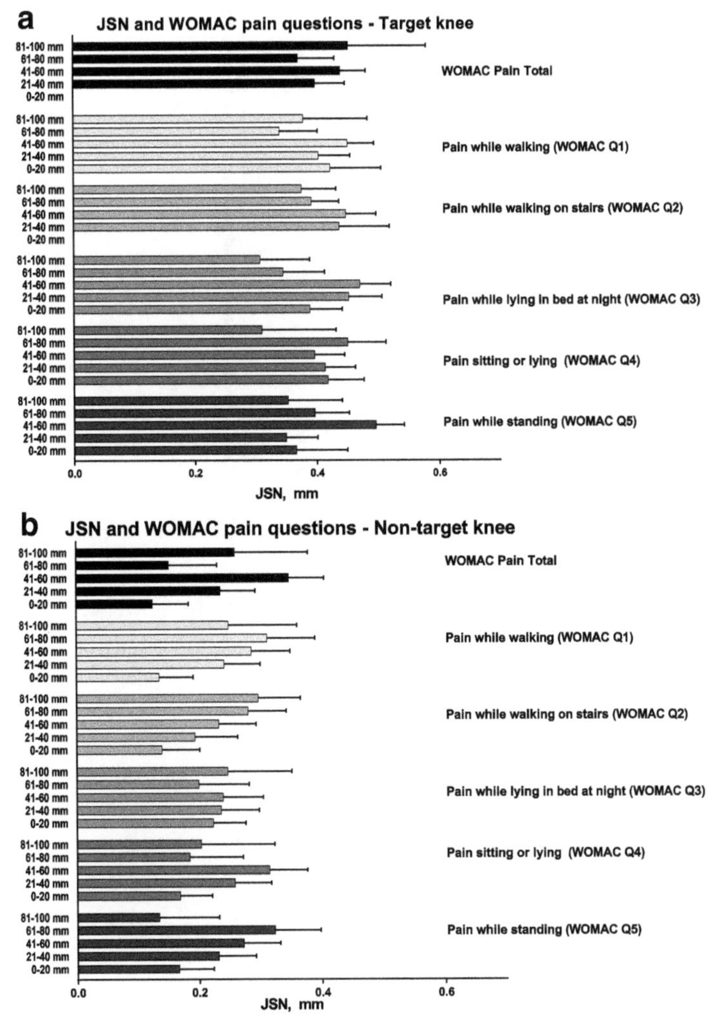

	WOMAC pain total		WOMAC Q1 Walking		WOMAC Q2 Stairs		WOMAC Q3 In bed		WOMAC Q4 Sitting/lying		WOMAC Q5 Standing	
	T	NT	T	NT	T	NT	T	NT	T	NT	T	NT
0-20 mm	7*	193	71	262	7*	162	190	323	147	295	69	236
21-40 mm	247	238	218	196	72	118	189	165	243	195	205	184
41-60 mm	352	199	313	161	230	180	216	134	223	151	278	180
61-80 mm	138	74	128	80	297	158	106	72	127	63	163	88
81-100 mm	27	29	41	34	165	115	70	39	31	29	56	45

Fig. 2 Joint-space narrowing (JSN) at year 2 by baseline pain severity level of individual and total WOMAC pain scores of target (**a**)- and non-target (**b**) knees. Data on JSN are mixed-model least-square means (standard error) adjusted for KL-score, BMI, study code, and sex. Pain severity is divided into quintile subgroups of normalized maximum possible score ranging from 0 mm (least possible pain) to 100 mm (worst imaginable pain for each WOMAC pain category. The number of observations (knees) in each category are shown in the table below the figures. Sub-groups with less than 10 observations, marked with * in the table, are excluded from the figure. Target knee. NT: Non-target knee. WOMAC: Western Ontario and McMaster's Universities Arthritis Index. Error bars are SEM

to be addressed in experiments designed fully or in part with that purpose.

The results are interesting since they could indicate distinct differences in etiology of each pain category, as mentioned above. As can be imagined, pain experienced while the joint is free of mechanical load, such as lying in bed at night (WOMAC pain question 3), is likely to have a significantly different etiology compared to pain evoked by mechanical loading and movement. The work of Arendt-Nielsen and colleagues describes that chronic, nociceptive pain can lead to lowered pain thresholds in parts of the body remote from that of the diseased joint [5, 25]. With reference to the findings of Hensor et al., documenting the sequential emergence of first weight-bearing pain symptoms, and finally non-weight-bearing symptoms in the gradual development of OA [19], it is plausible that non-weight bearing pain itself may partly be a product of continuous, constant nociceptive pain

Table 3 Correlations between baseline WOMAC scores, composite WOMAC scores and change in joint-space width (JSW) at year two

Variables		WOMAC Q1		WOMAC Q2		WOMAC Q3		WOMAC Q4		WOMAC Q5		WOMAC Weight-bearing		WOMAC idle		Total WOMAC pain score	
		adj	unadj	adj	unadj	adj	unadj	adj	unadj	adj	unadj	adj	unadj	adj	unadj	adj	unadj
Target chg in JSW yr. 2	Spearman	−0.03	− 0.01	**− 0.10**	**−0.08**	− 0.05	−0.03	0.00	0.00	0.04	0.05	−0.04	−0.02	− 0.02	−0.02	− 0.04	−0.02
	P	0.40	0.70	**0.006**	**0.03**	0.27	0.36	0.98	0.90	0.29	0.15	0.31	0.59	0.54	0.62	0.33	0.60
	N	771	771	**771**	**771**	771	771	771	771	771	771	771	771	771	771	771	771
Non Target chg in JSW yr. 2	Spearman	0.07	**0.09**	0.06	**0.09**	0.01	0.03	0.06	**0.07**	**0.08**	**0.10**	**0.08**	**0.10**	0.04	0.05	**0.07**	**0.09**
	P	0.07	**0.02**	0.09	**0.02**	0.71	0.40	0.10	**0.05**	**0.02**	**0.007**	**0.03**	**0.007**	0.27	0.14	**0.05**	**0.01**
	N	733	**733**	733	**733**	733	733	733	**742**	**733**	**742**	**733**	**739**	733	733	**733**	**733**

"Unadj" refers to unadjusted data. "Adj" is adjusted for Kellgren-Lawrence grade and Body Mass Index. Correlations with a *p*-value < 0.05 are highlighted in bold. *WOMAC* Western Ontario and McMaster's Universities Arthritis Index

signaling leading to central allodynia and hyperalgesia, but in itself be a poorer reflection of disease activity than weight-bearing pain. This may also help to explain some weak associations between radiographic progression of disease and pain as described in the literature [8, 26, 27].

The trajectories of pain change during the trial of both the target and the non-target knees were similar. While the differences between weight-bearing and non-weight-bearing pain was not found to be significantly different for the non-target knee, the analysis of each individual pain question revealed the same hierarchy for both knees. The overall level of change was notably higher in the target knees compared to the non-target knees, which could indicate a contribution to the placebo-effect derived from increased patient focus on the knee under study.

Intuitively, removal of the source of pain should lead to elimination of pain, but studies of total joint replacements, which indeed removes the primary source of pain, are discrepant. In trials evaluating the outcome of total knee arthroplasty, particularly on pain, results show either complete elimination of pain [28] or that while a majority of patients experience a significant reduction in pain, pain does not seem to be completely abolished [25, 29], and it has been reported that approximately 15% of patients continue to experience severe pain even after joint replacement surgery [30]. The lack of complete pain resolution might indicate a residual, non-joint specific pain mechanism, such as a state of central sensitization persisting even after surgical removal of the stimuli initiating this condition, which could render the patient less likely to respond to any analgesic treatment without undergoing arthroplastic surgery. The relevance of this observation is the presence of a possibly less dynamic pain category, which is harder to manipulate and may have a central origin rather than a peripheral. As the current results indicate that the elements of non-weight-bearing pain are less likely to change by placebo-treatment, this could be in support on this hypothesis, yet more research is needed.

The main limitations of this report is the lack of an untreated OA control, as well as a positive control. Inclusion of an untreated OA control would facilitate comparisons to a natural development of OA pain over time to determine the true placebo-response. In an analysis of pain trajectories in patients with established OA from the Cohort Hip and Cohort Knee study (CHECK), it was found that only 3% of the sample size experienced a major regression in pain, while 67.7% of subjects experienced constant or worsening pain during the 5 year follow up [31]. While it is common that OA placebo-treatments lead to placebo-response [12], the majority of OA patients participating in trials as untreated controls are not expected to achieve a notable regression of pain, nor a significant increase in pain over time [32–34]. It is therefore regarded as plausible that the observed reduction in pain in the current analysis is to a large extent attributable to a true placebo-response and potential effect of RTM rather than a result of natural history. The inclusion of an untreated control group would facilitate analyses of sensitivity to change in each pain category, as well as an estimate of the impact of the patient-practitioner interaction without medical treatment per se. This limitation is important, as the implications of the findings are not necessarily to exclude patients with a high level of weight-bearing pain, but perhaps rather to expand the view on OA pain: From one single concept to at least two possibly distinct elements of disease, which may require hitting multiple targets to be affected.

The use of subscore and individual WOMAC items to category pain may appear crude in relation to speculation regarding associations with the potential underlying mechanism of pain; neuropathic, central sensitization etcetera, particularly in the presence of other, specialized psychometric tools and devices developed to assess these particular pain elements [15, 16]. But in the absence of more or less cumbersome and experimental methods of quantifying separate pain features, as the most widely used, and simple method of assessing OA pain, the WOMAC questionnaire may provide a suitable basis for hypothesis generation to be further evaluated using more specialized tools in adequately designed trials.

Pain categories and risk of radiographic progression

The weak correlations between different categories of pain and progression are in line with previous findings that pain is not clearly associated with radiographic progression [8, 35]. This supports the current belief that progression is likely associated with several factors affecting JSN, of which pain is only one. The lack of clarity between findings of the NT and the T knee, and the very weak correlations limits the options for clinical translation of the results. As a number of different readers were engaged in the radiographic readings and there was no assessment of inter-reader reliability, the resulting measurement error may contribute to the low correlations reported in Table 3. The results do indicate differences, although of unknown clinical significance, between elements of weight-bearing, and non-weight-bearing pain, most clearly shown for questions of weight-bearing pain (WOMAC questions 1,2 and 5) in the NT knee in Fig. 2. These findings warrant further research. The reasons for the discrepancies between the observations of pain and progression in the T- and NT knees are unknown. As described by Felson and colleagues, OA disease progression is likely to be

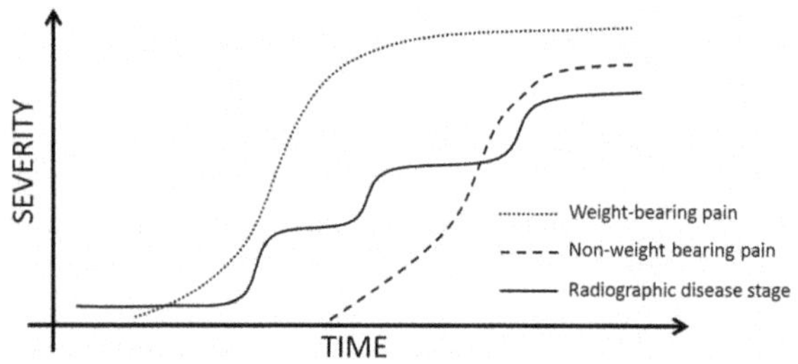

Fig. 3 Hypothetical depiction of pain category severity and progressive disease stage over time. While disease progression is likely occurring in limited periods follow by periods of inertia [35], pain trajectories appear to be progressing more steadily, although slowly [19, 32, 33]. Weight-bearing pain is the first pain category to present, followed by non-weight-bearing pain [19]. Variable radiographic disease progression rates may blur the otherwise expected hypothetical association between pain severity and risk of progression at one or very few given time points

characterized as a state of inertia, followed by periods of progression [36], while Hensor as well as the data in this report indicates that pain progression may evolve at a more constant rate, although weight-bearing pain surfacing before non-weight-bearing pain [19]. This discrepancy in progression rate between objectively measurable disease parameters and pain may limit the possibilities of assessing any association between pain severity and the risk of radiographic progression at one or few given point(s) in time, while an association may be found at other times, as illustrated in Fig. 3.

Due to inclusion criteria, the distribution of pain in the target knees is concentrated in the range of moderate pain. This is likely to have affected the correlation between pain and progression of the target knee, which may introduce a bias towards a lower correlation coefficient as low pain values with low progression rates are not present or very scarce.

Conclusions

These results indicate that the reduction in pain in patients treated with placebo is different between pain categories, as weight-bearing pain was significantly more reduced compared to non-weight-bearing pain. Further research in pain categories in OA is warranted.

Abbreviations

ANOVA: Analysis of Variance; BMI: Body Mass Index; CHECK: Cohort Hip and Cohort Knee; JSN: Joint Space Narrowing; JSW: Joint Space Width; KL: Kellgren-Lawrence; NT: Non-target; OA: Osteoarthritis; OAI: Osteoarthritis Initiative; PPR: Placebo pain reduction; RTM: Regression to the mean; T: Target; WOMAC: Western Ontario and McMasters Osteoarthritis Index

Acknowledgments

We wish to sincerely thank all the participants and investigators Peter Alexandersen, Merete Holm-Bentzen, Hans Christian Hoeck, Edith Lau, Tomas Hala, Ivo Valter, Florin Radulescu, Beata Jendrych and Janusz Badurski of the CSMC021C2301 and the participants and investigators Peter Alexandersen, Merete Holm-Bentzen, Sonja Snel, Edith Lau, Beata Jendrych, Tomas Hala, Tom Maxwell, Andre Beaulieu, Florin Radulescu, James Farrel, Jean-Pierre Devogelaer, Thomas Schnitzer, Nancy Lane, Roland Moskowitz, Emilio Martin-Mola, Janusz Badurski, Craig Buettner and Beth Jonas of the CSMC021C2302 study, as well as the IDMC board: Marc Hochberg, Nigel Stallard, Robert Wallace, Dieter Felsenberg and Michael Farkouh.

Funding

Novartis and Nordic Bioscience co-sponsored the trials. Novartis provided the medications for the study.

Authors' contributions

ARB and MAK drafted the first manuscript. ARB, IB, CC, BJR, MAK, ACBJ, and JRA participated in trial design, data acquisition, analysis and interpretation of data, critical review and final approval. IV contributed with clinical expertise, conduct of patient visit procedures, data collection, data interpretation and final approval of the manuscript. IB performed all statistical analyses. MH contributed with data analysis and interpretation, critical review, and final approval of the manuscript.

Competing interests

ARB, IB, ACBJ, CC, BJR, JRA, and MAK are full-time employees in Nordic Bioscience, a company engaged in biomarker research and development of treatments for OA. ARB, ACBJ, CC, BJR, JRA and MK are shareholders of Nordic Bioscience. BJR and CC are major shareholders and board members of Nordic Bioscience. IV is a full-time employee of BioClinica. MH does not have any conflicts of interest to declare.

Author details

[1]Nordic Bioscience, Herlev Hovedgade 207, DK2730 Herlev, Denmark. [2]Bioclinica, Tallinn, Estonia. [3]University of Maryland School of Medicine, Baltimore, USA.

References

1. Vos T, Flaxman AD, Naghavi M, Lozano R, Michaud C, Ezzati M, et al. Years lived with disability (YLDs) for 1160 sequelae of 289 diseases and injuries 1990-2010: a systematic analysis for the global burden of disease study 2010. Lancet. 2012;380:2163–96.
2. TE MA, Bannuru RR, Sullivan MC, Arden NK, Berenbaum F, Bierma-Zeinstra SM, et al. OARSI guidelines for the non-surgical management of knee osteoarthritis. Osteoarthritis. Cartilage. 2014;22:363–88.
3. Kavchak AJ, Fernandez-de-las-Penas C, Rubin LH, rendt-Nielsen L, Chmell SJ, Durr RK, et al. Association between altered somatosensation, pain, and knee stability in patients with severe knee osteoarthrosis. Clin J Pain. 2012;28:589–94.
4. rendt-Nielsen L, Eskehave TN, Egsgaard LL, Petersen KK, Graven-Nielsen T, Hoeck HC, et al. Association between experimental pain biomarkers and serologic markers in patients with different degrees of painful knee osteoarthritis. Arthritis Rheumatol. 2014;66:3317–26.
5. Arendt-Nielsen L, Nie H, Laursen MB, Laursen BS, Madeleine P, Simonsen OH, et al. Sensitization in patients with painful knee osteoarthritis. Pain. 2010;149:573–81.
6. Bjordal JM, Ljunggren AE, Klovning A, Slordal L. Non-steroidal anti-inflammatory drugs, including cyclo-oxygenase-2 inhibitors, in osteoarthritic knee pain: meta-analysis of randomised placebo controlled trials. BMJ. 2004;329:1317.
7. Bjordal JM, Klovning A, Ljunggren AE, Slordal L. Short-term efficacy of pharmacotherapeutic interventions in osteoarthritic knee pain: a meta-analysis of randomised placebo-controlled trials. Eur. J Pain. 2007;11:125–38.
8. Illingworth KD, El BY, Siewert K, Scaife SL, El-Amin S, Saleh KJ. Correlation of WOMAC and KOOS scores to tibiofemoral cartilage loss on plain radiography and 3 Tesla MRI: data from the osteoarthritis initiative. KneeSurgSports TraumatolArthrosc. 2014;22:1649–58.

9. Deere KC, Clinch J, Holliday K, McBeth J, Crawley EM, Sayers A, et al. Obesity is a risk factor for musculoskeletal pain in adolescents: findings from a population-based cohort. Pain. 2012;153:1932–8.
10. Velasquez MT, Katz JD. Osteoarthritis: another component of metabolic syndrome? Metab Syndr Relat Disord. 2010;8:295–305.
11. Bannuru RR, TE MA, Sullivan MC, Wong JB, Kent DM, Schmid CH. Effectiveness and implications of alternative placebo treatments: a systematic review and network meta-analysis of osteoarthritis trials. Ann Intern Med. 2015;163:365–92.
12. Zhang W, Robertson J, Jones a C, Dieppe P a, Doherty M. The placebo effect and its determinants in osteoarthritis: meta-analysis of randomised controlled trials. Ann Rheum Dis. 2008;67:1716–23.
13. Abhishek A, Doherty M. Understanding placebo effects in rheumatology. Jt Bone Spine. 2015;82:222–4.
14. Abhishek A, Doherty M. Mechanisms of the placebo pain reduction in pain in osteoarthritis. Osteoarthr Cartil. 2013;21:1229–35.
15. Arendt-Nielsen L. Central sensitization in humans: assessment and pharmacology. Handb Exp Pharmacol. 2015;227:79–102.
16. Shaygan M, Böger A, Kröner-Herwig B. Clinical features of chronic pain with neuropathic characteristics: a symptom-based assessment using the pain DETECT questionnaire. Eur J Pain. 2013;17:1529–38.
17. Bellamy N, Buchanan WW, Goldsmith CH, Campbell J, Stitt LW. Validation study of WOMAC: a health status instrument for measuring clinically important patient relevant outcomes to antirheumatic drug therapy in patients with osteoarthritis of the hip or knee. J Rheumatol. 1988;15:1833–40.
18. Lo GH, TE MA, Niu J, Zhang Y, Beals C, Dabrowski C, et al. Bone marrow lesions and joint effusion are strongly and independently associated with weight-bearing pain in knee osteoarthritis: data from the osteoarthritis initiative. Osteoarthr Cartil. 2009;17:1562–9.
19. EMA H, Dube B, Kingsbury SR, Tennant A, Conaghan PG. Toward a clinical definition of early osteoarthritis: onset of patient-reported knee pain begins on stairs. Data from the osteoarthritis initiative. Arthritis Care Res. 2015;67:40–7.
20. Stratford PW, Kennedy DM, Woodhouse LJ, Spadoni GF. Measurement properties of the WOMAC LK 3.1 pain scale. Osteoarthr Cart. 2007;15:266–72.
21. Karsdal MA, Byrjalsen I, Alexandersen P, Bihlet A, Andersen JR, Riis BJ, et al. Treatment of symptomatic knee osteoarthritis with oral salmon calcitonin: results from two phase 3 trials. Osteoarthr Cartil. 2015;23
22. Karsdal MA, Bihlet A, Byrjalsen I, Alexandersen P, Ladel C, Michaels M, et al. OA phenotypes, rather than disease stage, drive structural progression - identification of structural progressors from 2 phase III randomized clinical studies with symptomatic knee OA. Osteoarthr Cartil. 2015;23
23. Barnett AG, van der Pols JC, Dobson AJ. Regression to the mean: what it is and how to deal with it. Int J Epidemiol. 2005;34:215–20.
24. Hrobjartsson A. What are the main methodological problems in the estimation of placebo effects? J ClinEpidemiol. 2002;55:430–5.
25. Skou ST, Graven-Nielsen T, Rasmussen S, Simonsen OH, Laursen MB, rendt-Nielsen L. Widespread sensitization in patients with chronic pain after revision total knee arthroplasty. Pain. 2013;154:1588–94.
26. Bedson J, Croft PR. The discordance between clinical and radiographic knee osteoarthritis: a systematic search and summary of the literature. BMCMusculoskeletDisord. 2008;9:116.
27. Conaghan PG, Felson DT. Structural associations of osteoarthritis pain: lessons from magnetic resonance imaging. NovartisFoundSymp. 2004; 260:191–201.
28. Graven-Nielsen T, Wodehouse T, Langford RM, rendt-Nielsen L, Kidd BL. Normalization of widespread hyperesthesia and facilitated spatial summation of deep-tissue pain in knee osteoarthritis patients after knee replacement 2012;64:2907–16.
29. Skou ST, Roos EM, Laursen MB. A randomized, controlled trial of Total knee replacement. NEnglJ Med. 2016;374:692.
30. Wylde V, Hewlett S, Learmonth ID, Dieppe P. Persistent pain after joint replacement: prevalence, sensory qualities, and postoperative determinants. Pain. 2011;152:566–72.
31. Bastick AN, Wesseling J, Damen J, SPJ V, Emans PJ, PJE B, et al. Defining knee pain trajectories in early symptomatic knee osteoarthritis in primary care: 5-year results from a nationwide prospective cohort study (CHECK). Br J Gen Pract. 2016;66:e32–9.
32. de Craen AJ, Kaptchuk TJ, Tijssen JG, Kleijnen J. Placebos and placebo effects in medicine: historical overview. J RSocMed. 1999;92:511–5.
33. Whittle R, Jordan KP, Thomas E, Peat G. Average symptom trajectories following incident radiographic knee osteoarthritis: data from the osteoarthritis initiative. RMD Open. 2016;2:e000281.
34. Nicholls E, Thomas E, van der Windt DA, Croft PR, Peat G. Pain trajectory groups in persons with, or at high risk of, knee osteoarthritis: findings from the knee clinical assessment study and the osteoarthritis initiative. Osteoarthr Cartil. 2014;22:2041–50.
35. Karsdal MA, Bihlet A, Byrjalsen I, Alexandersen P, Ladel C, Michaels M, et al. OA phenotypes, rather than disease stage, drive structural progression - identification of structural progressors from 2 phase III randomized clinical studies with symptomatic knee OA. Osteoarthr Cartil. 2015;23:550–8.
36. Felson D, Niu J, Sack B, Aliabadi P, McCullough C, Nevitt MC. Progression Of osteoarthritis as a state of inertia. Ann Rheum Dis. 2012:1–6.

12

Understanding knee osteoarthritis from the patients' perspective

Victoria Carmona-Terés[1†], Jenny Moix-Queraltó[1], Enriqueta Pujol-Ribera[2,3], Iris Lumillo-Gutiérrez[4], Xavier Mas[5], Enrique Batlle-Gualda[6], Milena Gobbo-Montoya[7], Lina Jodar-Fernández[8] and Anna Berenguera[2,3*†]

Abstract

Background: No studies of Health Coach Interventions for knee OA sufferers that include patients' perspectives have been published. The study assesses current clinical practice and primary care professionals' advice from the patients' perspective, in order to obtain a participative design for a complex intervention based on coaching psychology. Moreover, wants to analyse the experiences, perceptions, cognitive evaluation, values, emotions, beliefs and coping strategies of patients with knee osteoarthritis, and secondly the impact of these factors in the Self-management of this condition.

Methods: It is an interpretative qualitative study. The study included patients with diagnosis of knee osteoarthritis (OA) from 4 primary health care centres in Barcelona. A theoretical sampling based on a prior definition of participants' characteristics was carried out. Ten semi-structured interviews with knee OA patients were carried out. A content thematic analysis was performed following a mixed-strategy text codification in Lazarus framework and in emerging codes from the data.

Results: The results are structured in two blocks: Experiences and perceptions of informants and Experiences of knee osteoarthritis according to the Lazarus model. Regarding experiences and perceptions of informants: Some participants reported that the information was mostly provided by health professionals. Informants know which food they should eat to lose weight and the benefits of weight loss. Moreover, participants explained that they like walking but that sometimes it is difficult to put into practice. Regarding experiences of knee osteoarthritis according Lazarus model: Cognitive evaluation is influenced by cognitive distortions such as obligation, guilt, dramatization and catastrophism. Values: Family is the value most associated with wellbeing. Helping others is another recurring value. Emotions: Most participants explain that they feel anxiety, irritability or sadness. Beliefs: To some, physiotherapy helps them feel less pain. However, others explain that it is of no use to them. Participants are aware of the association overweight– pain. Coping strategies: The strategies for coping with emotions aim to reduce psychological distress (anxiety, sadness, anger) and some are more active than others.

Conclusions: The study highlights that patients with knee osteoarthritis require a person-centered approach that provides them with strategies to overcome the psychological distress caused by this condition.

Keywords: Lifestyle, Knee osteoarthritis, Qualitative research, Health coaching, Primary health care, Interviews

* Correspondence: aberenguera@idiapjgol.org; http://www.idiapjgol.org
†Equal contributors
[2]Primary Care University Research Institute (IDIAP Jordi Gol), Gran Via Corts Catalanes, 587, àtic, Barcelona 08007, Spain
[3]Universitat Autònoma de Barcelona, Bellaterra, Cerdanyola del Vallès, Spain
Full list of author information is available at the end of the article

Background

Clinical guidelines for knee osteoarthritis (OA) recommend non-pharmacological first-line management which should include weight loss, healthy eating habits, physical activity (PA), Self-management of pain, information-education and orthoses [1]. In particular, they recommend the education of patients even if current evidence remains inconclusive [2–4]. Indeed, non-pharmacological recommendations frequently lack precision regarding contents, duration, intensity and frequency and might result in the suboptimal care of OA patients observed in several studies [4].

Based on personal living experiences with the disease, the interactions with health professionals and the treatments received, the informants have identified various elements to take into account in the design, contents and format of a new intervention for knee OA implemented in Primary Health Care [5]. The impact of knee OA can be profound on self-esteem [6], it limits daily activity, causes a feeling of loss [7] and decreases work productivity. These effects could be mitigated if the health services provided more information on the disease and on how to manage it self-efficiently [8]. Moreover, taking into consideration the beliefs and expectations of patients can contribute to improve the interventions [9].

The theoretical foundation of Health Coaching (HC) is linked to the theoretical-conceptual framework of behavioural change [10] and has been defined as a behavioural intervention to facilitate the establishment and achievement of health promotion objectives, modify behaviours, reduce harmful habits, improve self-management of chronic conditions and increase health related quality of life [11].

Health Coaching (HC) can improve quality of life, change attitudes, decrease unhealthy habits, treatment adherence, self-management and pain in chronic patients [12–19] and also promote healthy eating and PA [20]. In order to live with knee OA, patients use coping strategies that are determined by their values, emotions and beliefs. These categories define the key components that knee OA sufferers perceive as important for the design of a coaching intervention [5].

No studies of HC interventions for knee OA sufferers that include patients' perspectives have been published. The Medical Research Council has established a methodology for the development of complex interventions that consists of several phases and uses qualitative and quantitative methods [21, 22]. The first phase of this methodology aims at identifying the contextual factors that shape the theories of how the intervention works and might affect implementation, the modelling process and outcomes.

The objectives of this study were:

1. To identify current practice and advice of primary care professionals from the patients' perspective in order to achieve a participative design of a complex intervention based on coaching psychology
2. To further understand the experiences, perceptions, cognitive evaluation, values, emotions, beliefs and coping strategies of patients with knee OA and the influence of all these factors in the Self-management of this condition.

Methods

Design

We conducted an interpretative qualitative study [23] to further our understanding of the phenomenon as experienced by the individual living with knee OA. The study also looked for patient related factors that could facilitate or restrict the implementation of the intervention (acceptability, adequacy, feasibility, integration within other programs, location, schedule and duration).

Conceptual framework of the study: Lazarus stress model

The Lazarus stress coping model [24, 25] has been used to understand stressful life events. This framework is adequate for our research when we consider knee OA as a potential stressful factor. The level of distress and well-being of people are determined by their coping strategies.

A growing body of studies stresses the importance of psychological factors in the pain process. The Lazarus stress model has been transferred to the chronic pain field to study these factors. This model suggests that when there is a potentially stressful event, anxiety levels depend on the cognitive evaluation of pain stimulus and the strategies used to cope with it. Psychological pain factors which have recently appeared in the literature are analysed from the perspective of the Lazarus model [26].

The Lazarus model includes the following variables:

Cognitive Evaluation: process that determines the consequences that a particular event will generate in an individual.
Values: Values convey what is important for the individual and determine what is at stake in a particular stressing situation.
Emotions: Lazarus enumerates the following emotions: anger, envy, jealousy, anxiety-horror, guilt, shame, relief, hope, sadness-depression, gratefulness, compassion, happiness-joy, pride and love [27].
Beliefs: cognitive configurations created individually or culturally shared. They are pre-existing notions of reality that can be used as a perceptual lens.
Coping Strategies: constantly changing cognitive and behavioural efforts developed to manage specific external and/or internal demands that are evaluated as excessive or overwhelming for the resources of the individual.
Social Support: coping resource whereby we have somebody that provides emotional, informative and/or tangible support.

Participants: The study included symptomatic knee OA patients, with clinical and radiographic OA grades 1–3 in the Kellgren-Lawrence classification, selected from four primary health care centres (PHCC) in Barcelona. Participants were recruited by the general practitioners in each PHCC between February and April 2015.

Sampling and participant selection strategy

A theoretical sampling based on a prior definition of participants' characteristics was carried out to obtain optimal variety and discursive wealth [28]. Patients with knee OA living in the metropolitan area of Barcelona were selected in accordance to *a priori* defined profiles. We took the following variables into account: gender, age, number of years with knee OA, employment status, household and relevant health problems.

Patients with knee OA were recruited by their general practitioner or nurse, who explained the study and suggested the participation.

Techniques to generate information

Face to face individual Interviews were conducted by the first author, a specialist in this technique, in the PHCC of the participants, and lasted from 30 to 60 min. The interview guide followed five sequences (impact of knee OA; interaction with health professionals, physiotherapists and social workers; coping strategy; recommendations toward the design of the intervention; and use of information technology techniques - ICTs) (Additional file 1). The interviewer used open, non-directive formulation consistent with the participant's language. Observational field notes that included contextual characteristics, atmosphere and relevant non-verbal expressions were produced. Ten patients with knee OA were invited to participate, all of them accepted and data saturation was reached (Table 1).

Data analysis

All interviews were recorded and transcribed literally and systematically by trained personnel. After successive readings of the transcriptions, researchers reached preanalytical intuitions. A content thematic analysis was performed [24, 25]. Next, the following analytical steps were carried out: a) identification of the relevant texts; b) fragmentation of the text in units of meaning; c) a mixed-strategy text codification in Lazarus categories and in emerging codes from the data; d) creation of categories grouping the codes by the criterion of analogy; e) analysis of each category; and f) elaboration of a new text with the results. These results were subsequently discussed with the whole research team and, after careful deliberation and exchanges of findings, consensus was reached.

The following procedures were performed to improve rigour [29]: triangulation of analysis by four researchers; and comparison of findings with the original data.

Results

The results are structured in two blocks: Experiences and perceptions of informants and Experiences of knee osteoarthritis according to the Lazarus model.

Experiences and perceptions of informants

1) ***Experiences and perceptions in patients' interactions with health professionals* (General Practitioner and nurse), physiotherapists and social workers** The following subcategories emerged from the informants' discourses:

Information-education on knee osteoarthritis Some participants reported that the information was mostly provided by their family doctors, who

Table 1 Sociodemographic characteristics of participants with knee OA

Code	Gender	Age (years)	Years since onset knee osteoarthritis	Employment status	Household size	Relevant health problems
M1_CR	Female	60	16	Housewife	Partner	Haemophilia and Depression
H2_CR	Male	84	14	Retired (building)	Partner	Silicosis, vascular problem in one leg
H3_CR	Male	58	20	Disabled (graphic design)	Partner	Pain in lower limbs
H4_SA	Male	85	6	Retired (factory)	Alone (widower)	Diabetes, bladder cancer (operated)
M5_U	Female	66	16	Disabled (cleaning)	Alone (divorced)	Polyarthritis, anxiety
M6_U	Female	62	15	Housewife	Partner	Polyarthritis, anxiety symptoms, high blood pressure
M7_U	Female	67	5	Retired	Partner	Knee prosthesis, carpal tunnel
M8_VR	Female	75	3	Housewife	Grandson	Knee prosthesis and breast cancer
M9_VR	Female	83	<1	Housewife	Alone (widow)	High blood pressure
M10_VR	Female	67	17	Retired	Alone (single)	Diabetes and depression

explained the repercussions of knee OA, the progression of the disease and also provided some advice. However, a participant told that sometimes she did not understand the information provided. Others were not satisfied with the information received, in particular by specialists; they considered that it amounted practically to nothing and that the interaction was limited to prescribing painkillers and to referring them for diagnostic tests.

Do you feel that the professionals of the health centre have provided enough information on knee osteoarthritis?. . No, they just prescribe painkillers. And I cannot take strong painkillers because I have a large hernia and they prescribe paracetamol, which is useless. M9_VR

None of the participants received materials on these issues, and some said it would be useful for them to have this information *although they did not specify which type of materials they expected. The patients' expectations aimed to obtain more information on their condition, prognosis and treatment".*

Professional advice on diet and weight

Advice on losing weight was mentioned by most participants. Informants are aware that they are overweight, they know which food they should eat to lose weight and the benefits of weight loss. Some explained that they take care of their weight, but that putting on weight comes very easy to them. They find it difficult to modify behaviours, mainly because of lack of discipline and because of the food they love. They emphasized the difficulty of sustaining a healthy weight, they had lost weight with the help of dieticians, endocrinologists and acupuncture and have again put it on.

"...I'm very strict ...You tell me "take this list: Monday this, Tuesday that,.." and I will do it... don't give me anything ambiguous for me to plan between 5 possible first courses, 5 possible second courses.. no. H4_SA

Some had received leaflets about diets to help them achieve weight loss.

Professional advice on physical activity

Participants explained that health professionals tell them to walk. They explained that they like it and they walk even if it is difficult, because if they move they feel better.

Some receive positive feedback for exercising in water to reduce impact on the joints,

"Aguagym? Yesyesyes, it's wonderful. I go twice a week, and then I feel so relaxed, because I leave the swimming pool, I have a shower...and such, I then feel so relaxed ..." M1_CR

and others use the stationary bicycle. They explained that they would feel more motivated if they could exercise in a group.

Experiences with the different treatments provided

Informants mentioned painkillers and non-steroidal anti-inflammatory agents, usually prescribed by health professionals. They are anxious about the side effects of these medications.

"I avoid taking pills...I have some, in case one day it hurts too much...." M5_U

Depending on the situation, they choose to take paracetamol, NSAIDs, sometimes with a "gastric protection agent", or bear the pain without taking any tablets.
Gels and creams are well accepted by participants, but they complained that the public health system does not cover this type of treatment; they also complain about (the) long waiting times for local injections.
Some participants had also had physiotherapy with mostly positive results on the short and medium term. In general, they complained about the long waiting lists to access these services.
One informant explained a positive experience with magnesium supplements. They did not comment on the opinions of professionals on alternative therapies.
Two participants have a knee prosthesis and they evaluate them positively. Most consider that prosthesis is the best option in the long term although they leave it for when their condition is unsustainable. The youngest participants explained that in this case the health professionals recommend to wait and to bear the condition. Two participants expressed the need for research in this area.

"in November 2011 they were about to give me a prosthesis, I had the day of admission, for the operation and everything, but in the preoperative stage, the last person you talked to is the anaesthetist, and he really scared me he told me you are very young and the average duration of the prosthesis is 10 years, and there is more rejection in the second...and I didn't do it," H3_CR
"Well, if some people need the operation, they don't want to suffer more then, explain, tell him to not be

afraid, that the operation no no... My experience of the operation is very positive..." M8_VR

2) **Experiences of knee osteoarthritis according to the Lazarus model (Fig. 1)**
   We have used the Lazarus Stress Model for a structured analysis of the patients' experiences. This model explains that when faced with a potentially stressing event, people respond with different levels of stress and emotions. This response depends basically on two factors: cognitive evaluation (where according to Beck cognitive distortion takes place) and coping strategies. In summary, emotions depend on how the person evaluates the situation and which behaviours and thoughts does she use to manage this situation. However, this model also includes two additional cognitive variables of a more static nature that determine the other: beliefs and values. Consequently, based on their beliefs and personal values, individuals will evaluate and cope with a particular situation with different degrees of stress. An outline of the model can be found in Fig. 1.

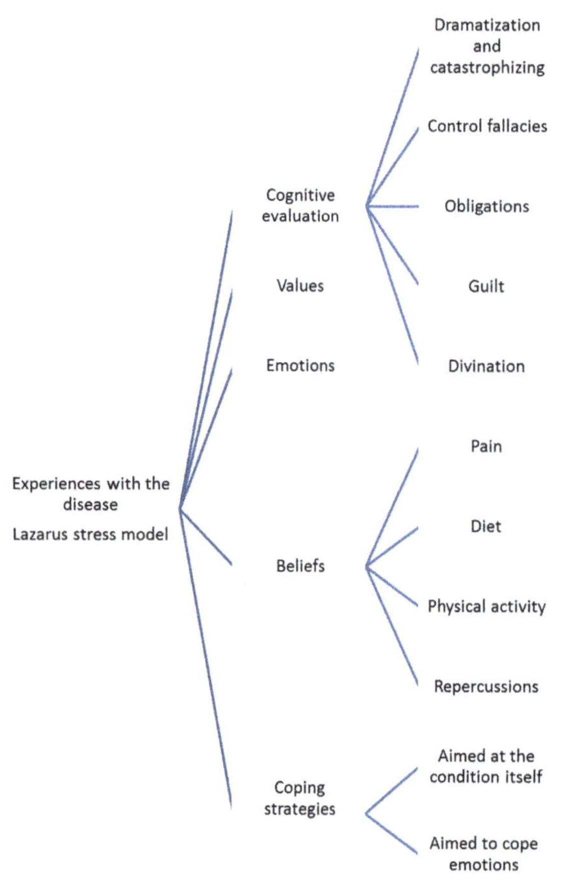

Fig. 1 Lazarus theoretical model applied to knee osteoarthritis

This model can be applied in this study, since knee osteoarthritis is a potentially stressing condition.

A. ***Cognitive evaluation***
   Different cognitive distortions bias the cognitive evaluation of participants. For instance:
   Within the distortion *"obligations"*, the concept of helping those around them is the most used.

"I have to do the shopping, I have to do the housework to my family" M7_U

In relation to *guilt*, they feel guilty about not following the advice on diet and PA and for not meeting the expectations of the people closest to them.

"I feel bad when I eat something forbidden". M6_U

Dramatization and catastrophizing are observed when participants refer to pain and they label it as terrible, as greatly affecting them, etc.

"... Terrible, terrible. But in 1998 it was less painful, I think that because I still had my house and was busy with my children, but since I came here, in 2001, uyy, this has been terrible" M10_VR

The *control fallacies* are conveyed in verbalisations such as lack of time or putting on armour to protect themselves from being hurt.

" until now I went swimming, but lately I had to quit due to family problems, I don't have time " "I know many thin women that have bad arthritis" M6_U

The *divination of thought* usually focuses on the feelings of the loved ones (they think they know what their family members think about them).

"... For me it's not a trauma or anything, people should see that ... people are very nosey, they like to ask; there she is with the bad knee.. you have to explain, otherwise ..." M1_CR

B. ***Values***
   Values are compromises that express what is important for the person. Family is the main answer to the question of what makes them happy and the value most associated with wellbeing.
   Helping others is another recurring value.
   Some of them prioritize the needs of others over their own needs, which they associate with the importance of the family.

"And most of all not being in much pain, because I have things to do, ... help my daughter, ... help my mother...". M1_CR

They lose sight of self-care. Another important value is *filling time.*

"Being busy the whole day!! I spend cleaning ... cleaning here and there... It does not even hurt.. M10_VR

The absence of "occupation" takes them back to dejection and sadness thoughts and emotions and feelings of uselessness.
The value of *autonomy*, being physically independent and not needing canes and crutches; it is essential to help the family, others and to be busy.

"It makes me sad because it limits me, it limits me a lot, I cannot do what I would do". M8_VR

All participants mention self-demand (overcoming personal frontiers) and discipline by action (following medical recommendations) or by omission (neglecting to follow these recommendations). They consider themselves demanding in relation to their values and to the important aspects of their life. Prevention of knee OA was not considered a priority.

C. *Emotions*

Most participants explain that they feel *anxiety, irritability* or *sadness*. Anxiety affects them differently: in some the diet is affected, in others it increases ruminative thoughts. In most cases, and even if not directly articulated, the low mood status is enhanced by the lack of acceptance of the aging process. They feel nostalgia for the activities they could do "before the arthrosis", which in fact were activities they carried out in their youth. Indeed, knee osteoarthritis represents a "mourning process" for the participants.
Fear takes place when someone in their immediate environment had been seriously disabled as a consequence of osteoarthritis. In these cases, we observed a keener interest for prevention.

"I had my mother sitting in a chair for many years as a result of arthrosis. That's what I fear most" M8_VR

Participants find *happiness* in small things related to their values: housework, since it signifies *autonomy*; helping others; and spending time with the family.

D. *Beliefs*

Beliefs are cognitive configurations individually created or culturally shared, pre-existing concepts of reality that act as a perceptual lens.

Beliefs on pain

To some, physiotherapy helps them feel less pain. However, others explain that it is of no use to them.

"No... Because when I'm doing physiotherapy it hurts even more, and when physiotherapy finishes it goes on hurting. It doesn't work for me". M1_CR

Patients believe that physiotherapy is useful when they are doing it and are aware that when they stop physiotherapy the pain comes back. Only one participant explained that he consistently practices the exercises daily because he believes that it is key to improve pain. For some, the pain of knee OA hinders the practice of physical activity because of the belief that it can increase the pain.
Another shared belief on pain is "that it must be borne", possibly related to some Judeo-Christian values of sacrifice, be it as acceptance (coping strategy) or some resignation (negative emotion). To cope with pain, patients choose as a first option looking for distractions, secondly they prefer to bear it and lastly they take medication.

Beliefs on diet

Participants are aware of the association overweight– pain. The impossibility of losing weight is one of the most common beliefs amongst women with knee OA. They attribute this impossibility to menopause, age and other factors unrelated to the quality and amount of food intake. Anxiety surrounding food is another factor related to the difficulty in losing weight. Most participants believe that the dieting recommendations are not effective for their particular case. They pointed out that the leaflets with standard advice are of no use to them.

"He gave me some paper, but I don't follow it because it's bad for me. However, him and another one have insisted that I should not put on weight " M5_U

Beliefs on PA

Participants believe that PA is positive. When they are more active they feel better and their mood improves. The most common PA are walking and Aqua gym.

"In water you can do any exercise" "outside water no". M1_CR

The main limitations for being physically active were knee pain and in some cases negative emotions.

Beliefs on OA

Participants explain that OA is a chronic disease and that professionals have told them that it cannot be cured. Beliefs on the possibilities of a cure for knee OA emerge in the interviews, whereas at a conscious level participants are aware that no cure exists yet. However, they mention hope and the need to find a curative treatment.

"I think that everything but death has a cure". M10_VR

Patients need to translate the medical indications into something practical in their daily lives. Resignation when faced with knee OA has a strong emotional impact and generates sadness, anger and anxiety. Some patients talked about acceptance with a resigned face and non-verbal signs of negative emotions.

E. Coping strategies

The coping strategies aim either at emotions or at the condition itself.

The strategies for *coping with emotions* aim to reduce psychological distress (anxiety, sadness, anger) and some are more active than others. Amongst the most active we highlight looking for distractions, for social support (more emotional than practical). Other patients use strategies to avoid thinking about their problem and being surrounded by family to feel better (one of the most commonly used strategies) such as praying or counting to 10 to calm down.

"I spoil myself with a latte". M8_VR
"I wake up around 10 a.m. First thing I drink lukewarm water with lemon, eh, I have breakfast after half an hour, and I make my beds, clean the floor, sweep the apartment, I do, I prepare lunch.. and in the afternoon I get out. " H3_CR
"Mm.. little things, then you understand, how can I explain it.. look, right now I'm enjoying the tablet and my husband with the ball and me with the tablet is no problem at all " M6_U.
"I get it out of my mind" (referring to the disease of the daughter). M8_VR

The most commonly reported strategy is acceptance or resignation.

"If you accept it your attitude changes" H3_CR

Whereas for some acceptance is a negative concept, others assert that when you accept your condition you change your attitude for the better. The strategies for the condition (chronic and without a lasting solution) aim at reducing the deterioration and the pain (taking medication, walking, cold, rubs, rest and exercise.

"When it's very painful I take ibuprofen or naproxen". M7_U
"Walking at my pace is very relaxing for me". H3_CR
"And I rub it with wasps' poison" M8_VR
" if you join a gym, whether you believe it or not it's super positive for the brain " M10_VR)

They learn to pace activities so that the pain does not increase, and to "say no" to avoid being overloaded with obligations. Not all strategies are equally used. Some patients never learn to say "no" or to pace efforts. The strategies aimed at the condition can also be used for the emotions (the calming effect of exercise).

II-Recommendations for the design of the coaching psychology intervention (Table 2)

Reference framework

Participants pointed out that even within a group intervention there is a need for a holistic, person-centered approach that does not just focus on arthrosis. They underlined the community aspect and the need to be made aware of the resources of the neighbourhood.

"To help us know what's in there, in this neighbourhood there is nothing to do. Things like aqua gym and such" M7_U

On the other hand, they highlighted the relevance of a participative design that allows sharing experiences and improvement proposals. In their opinion, sharing makes people feel more involved in the activities and it implies more consistency in relation to learning and implementing what they have learned. However, some participants

Table 2 Recommendations for the coaching intervention – barriers and facilitators

Barriers in the management of knee osteoarthritis	
Result	Contributions
Difficulty for translating theory into practice	Strategies and techniques to take action
Difficulties in sustaining a healthy diet	Indications and recommendations for a healthy diet
	To facilitate simple menus
	To facilitate healthy menus
	Techniques to control stress (anxiety)
	Motivation strategies to implement a healthy diet and make it sustainable over time
Pain associated with physical activity	Techniques to manage pain
	Indications and recommendations to carry out physical activity
	Motivation strategies to start and sustain physical activity
Fear	Strategies to overcome fears
Facilitators in the management of knee osteoarthritis	
Result	Contributions
Holistic Vision	Holistic vision focused on individual needs
Lack of individualisation	Taking into account the person within the group
Physiotherapy to reduce pain	Include physiotherapy exercises in the intervention
	Strategies to sustain the practice of these exercises
They would like to have more information	To provide information on the disease, its repercussions and advice on how to live with it
Learning to say "no"	Assertiveness strategies
Social support	To offer space for participants to talk about their particular situation
	To offer the possibility of continuity of contact between participants at the end of the intervention (WhatsApp, phone, etc.)
Self-care	To provide strategies for the patient to have time for him/herself
Learning to calm down	Strategies to control stress
	Mindfulness
	Breathing and relaxation techniques
Acceptance	Work with acceptance and differentiating it from resignation
Values	The patients' most important values will be used to motivate and to generate change in the participants (family, autonomy, discipline)

think that they might feel uncomfortable within a group. They also mentioned the importance of working with cultural and socioeconomic sensitivity.

Participants accepted and were open to the proposal of having a health psychologist as coach because they believed it is a professional trained to listen to and solve needs related to their disease.

> *"I'm happy, because it's working well with the doctor, and now with you, and if there are things to do for no, to slow down a bit the arthritis, then fantastic....". M7_U*

None of the participants manifested that they wanted another type of professional to conduct the Health Coaching.

Contents/components

Participants emphasized the need to translate theory into practice for behavioural change. In general, they proposed to encourage the strengths of individuals and to promote strategies to live with a more positive, problem-solving attitude.

> *"We need to cheer up people that feels down, teach them that they have to move even if they are in pain. Because I also have pain, eh?" M8_VR*

Participants also expressed the need to learn to say "no" to be able to focus on self-care. In relation to diet, they explained that they need to learn how to prepare restrictive diets and how to combine foods with nutrients. In relation to PA, they wanted to know the activities most suited to their financial, practical and health needs. With regard to pain, they wanted to know how to channel thoughts toward more positive attitudes.

Use of TICs

Most participants mentioned the regular use of smartphones, tablets and computers. They knew how to use messaging apps and were open to work using these technologies.

> *"Whatsapp yes. My friend in Italy, I will show you, that I have a friend in Italy, that friend I mentioned from Italy. Whatsapp yes and gmail too... Let's see, Nicoletta... Every day or every night, "good night", "", "bon giorno" "#italiano#" "#italiano#". M5_U.*

Location, schedule and duration and frequency

In relation to location, they consider that activities should take place in any community site that is close and accessible (libraries, schools, Primary Health Care Centre, community and sports centres, parks). Moreover, with the use of different locations more people gets to know the resources and participation is enhanced.

With regard to schedule, they point out that arrangements are generally more difficult for working people, more so since the financial crisis. They suggest schedules that include morning and afternoon. As regards duration and frequency, they propose weekly frequency during 5–6 weeks, duration around 2–2.5 h.

Discussion

In relation to interaction with professionals, participants acknowledged that even though they received advice on health behaviours for the management of knee OA and other conditions, adherence to this advice is difficult. They expressed fear and ambivalence in relation to surgical and pharmacological treatments and suggested that professionals should focus on the needs of the patients, on alleviating pain and on delaying the progression of the disease. These results coincide with various studies that indicate that patients and health professionals felt that OA should receive more attention and better consistency of care, with more emphasis on self-management to help patients manage their condition more effectively and appropriately [8, 30]. Indeed, patient information and education are considered core treatments for OA in evidence-based clinical guidelines. Patients should then use this information to implement changes and for decision-taking regarding treatment [31–34].

Similarly to other qualitative studies, patients explained that knee OA affects the whole body and their lives on many levels [35]. The symptoms experienced illustrate a diversity of problems that represented a major concern for many participants in our study: knee pain, stiffness, difficulties in daily activities, reduction of work, instability, weakness, lack of mobility and psychological impact. Patients with knee osteoarthritis often suffer from obesity/overweight (90%), hypertension (40%), depression (30%) and diabetes (15%), resulting in a decreased quality of life [36]. However, most patients can differentiate when the pain is due to knee osteoarthritis or other conditions.

With regard to psychological impact, we should highlight that most questionnaires that evaluate knee OA and its treatment do not include this factor, probably because there was no involvement of knee OA patients in its design [34]. In this study, participants mentioned the need for research in this area. Indeed, research projects should plan their agendas working with those that should benefit from that research [33]. Since they are best placed to reflect on their experience of an illness, it is essential to collect their opinions to build evidence about their priorities [37] and to enhance the relevance of research. A strength of our study is that we take into account patients' perspectives. The study protocol [5] explains that the integral management of the patient is paramount in the treatment of knee osteoarthritis. Accordingly, the design of the coaching intervention takes into account other factors such as associated diseases, environment and personal circumstances, all of which are considered during the sessions.

Patients explained that translating theory into practice and modifying behaviour is difficult. They request a holistic vision from professionals, based on their needs and not only on their health problems [38]. The person-centered approach model involves being an active agent for change and a non-directive role of the professional; it is based on unconditional acceptance, empathy and authenticity [39, 40]. Including the patient-centered context in complex interventions implies reflection on how to support optimal health and provision of care by means of reflecting on the patient's history [41].

The Lazarus [24, 25, 27] model used in the analysis is useful to detect cognitive evaluations and stress coping strategies. Acceptance is one of the key facilitators for coping with different situations [42–44] such as knee osteoarthritis. Working toward acceptance through HC can help patients improve the self-management.

Our findings point at the various difficulties for participants to follow dietary advice: lack of individualisation, anxiety, and prioritizing other aspects of their lives, in particular the people closest to them [30]. Some studies have shown that HC helps people achieve dietary objectives [45–47]. Also in agreement with other studies and despite a positive attitude in relation to PA, we have found barriers to their implementation such as pain, PA habits prior their current condition, lack of social support and lack of acceptance to their current situation [48–50]. According to various authors, HC provides strategies to start and sustain PA levels appropriate to the conditions of individuals [19, 51–56]. Another main result of our study is the importance that participants attach to mood, a key element for setting in motion their internal resources, also observed in previous investigations [34, 57–59]. In summary, health coaching, which originates within the framework of behavioural change, can help people increase their quality of life, their self-efficacy (a determinant factor of behavioural change), their perception of self-control and to reduce stress [30, 60].

Strengths and weaknesses

This research investigates the experiences of patients with mild to moderate knee OA. These experiences constitute an essential information toward the design and implementation of a complex intervention that will be acceptable, adequate, feasible, integrated within other programs, and appropriate in relation to location, schedule and duration. This article corresponds to Phase 1 or Modelling Phase of the MRC framework; the results have been used to design a HC intervention in knee OA intervention [61, 62].

Most participants in our research have suffered from knee OA for long time, are extremely familiar with this condition, understand available interventions and resources and have developed effective coping strategies. Participants spoke extensively about their problems, so that the data obtained were rich and diverse. The theoretical sample was successful in achieving diversity in age, gender, number of years since onset of disease, employment status, treatment modalities and multimorbidity. We should underscore that the mean age of participants in this study is older than the mean age found in the literature. This is a qualitative study that aims to achieve maximum plurality of discourse (minimum age 58 years, maximum age 85). Although the average age in experimental studies on knee osteoarthritis is 62 years of age, the electronic medical records of primary care centres in Barcelona reveal that the mean age of most patients that consult for this condition is closer to 70, the age group most represented in this study.

Nevertheless, the results of our study have been limited because no adults in the pre-diagnostic phase were included and the immigrant population, which might have different experiences, was not represented. The coaching group sessions with a participative strategy could be useful in case of proactive participants and volunteers but not for other profiles. This is a common characteristic of many intervention studies that require voluntary participation. This issue is worth exploring in depth during a qualitative study (phase 3). Further studies should include their discourses. Therefore, caution is needed before transferring these results to other settings and populations. However, the similarity with other studies with people from other origins and cultures suggests its applicability [7–9]. The rigour procedures used (in-depth-description of the context, theoretical sample design, audio-taping transcription, saturation, triangulation of analysis and reflexivity) have ensured the reliability of the findings in our setting.

Conclusions

This study analyses the experiences of patients that suffer from knee OA. Their discourses have been extremely useful for the modelling of the second phase of this study, a clinical trial to compare current treatment with the HC intervention.

Amongst the findings we should highlight the need for a holistic, person-centered approach that takes into account the characteristics and needs of patients and that includes the physical, psychological, social and practical aspects of knee OA.

These patients need empathy in relation to their suffering and psychological distress caused by their condition. They also explain their concern and ambivalence in relation to the use of medicines to control pain and request more research to obtain pharmacological treatment that is more effective and produces less side effects.

Health coaching should emphasize acceptance as a coping strategy. Acceptance is a key factor toward the improvement of quality of life and to decrease the impact of knee OA.

Acknowledgements
We would like to thank all those who participated in this study and took the time to share their experiences; and we would like to the reviewers of this manuscript for their very helpful comments and suggestions.

Funding
The project received a research grant from the Carlos III Institute of Health, Ministry of Economy and Competitiveness (Spain), awarded on the 2014 call under the Health Strategy Action 2013–2016, within the National Research Program oriented to Societal Challenges, within the Technical, Scientific and Innovation Research National Plan 2013–2016, with reference PI14/00585, co-funded with European Union ERDF funds. The role of this funding source is only to provide the funds.

Authors' contributions
VCT, JMQ, EPR, ILG, XM, EBG, MGM, LJF and AB contributed to the conception and design of the study. AB is the scientific director of the project. VC, JM, ILL, EPR and AB did the fieldwork and the triangulation of the analysis. VCT, JMQ, EPR, ILG, XM, EBG, MGM, LJF and AB participated in the interpretation of the final results. VCT, JMQ, EPR, ILG, XM, EBG, MGM, LJF and AB developed the draft manuscript, and read and approved the final manuscript.

Competing interests
The author(s) declared no conflicts of interest with respect to the authorship and/or publication of this article.

Consent for publication
The participants sign the consent form in order to consent to publish the data guaranteeing the confidentiality and anonymity of their data

Author details
[1]Department of Basic, Evolutionary and Educational Psychology, Universitat Autònoma de Barcelona; Psychology Faculty, Building B. UAB Campus, Bellaterra, Barcelona 08193, Spain. [2]Primary Care University Research Institute (IDIAP Jordi Gol), Gran Via Corts Catalanes, 587, àtic, Barcelona 08007, Spain. [3]Universitat Autònoma de Barcelona, Bellaterra, Cerdanyola del Vallès, Spain. [4]Primary Care Centre Can Bou, Ciutat de Màlaga, 18-20, Castelldefels, Barcelona 08860, Spain. [5]Primary Care Centre Amadeu Torner, Amadeu Torner, 63, l'Hospitalet de Llobregat, Barcelona 08902, Spain. [6]San Juan de

Alicante University Hospital; Rheumatology Unit, Ctra N-332, Sant Joan d'Alacant, Alicante-Valencia 03550, Spain. [7]Psychology of pain and rheumatological diseases, Av. Presidente Carmona, 10 bis 1°A, Madrid 28020, Spain. [8]Primary Care Centre Sant Ildefons, Avda República Argentiana s/n, Cornellà de Llobregat, Barcelona 08940, Spain.

References

1. Mas X, Barraquer ME. Gonalgia. Actualización en Medicina de Familia 3[5]. 2013. p. 249–58.
2. Pagès-Castellà, A., Muñoz Ortego, J., Prieto-Alhambra, D. Guía artrosis [http://www.ics.gencat.cat/3clics/main.php]. Barcelona: [updated January 25, 2013; Accessed 26 Jan 2013]. At http://www.ics.gencat.cat/3clics/main.php?page=GuiaPage&idGuia=238. 2013.
3. Bennell KL, Hunter DJ, Hinman RS. Management of osteoarthritis of the knee. BMJ. 2012;345:e4934.
4. Fernandes L, Hagen KB, Bijlsma JW, Andreassen O, Christensen P, Conaghan PG, et al. EULAR recommendations for the non-pharmacological core management of hip and knee osteoarthritis. Ann Rheum Dis. 2013;72:1125–35.
5. Carmona-Teres V, Lumillo-Gutierrez I, Jodar-Fernandez L, Rodriguez-Blanco T, Moix-Queralto J, Pujol-Ribera E, et al. Effectiveness and cost-effectiveness of a health coaching intervention to improve the lifestyle of patients with knee osteoarthritis: cluster randomized clinical trial. BMC Musculoskelet Disord. 2015;16:38.
6. Maly MR, Krupa T. Personal experience of living with knee osteoarthritis among older adults. Disabil Rehabil. 2007;29:1423–33.
7. Nyvang J, Hedstrom M, Gleissman SA. It's not just a knee, but a whole life: a qualitative descriptive study on patients' experiences of living with knee osteoarthritis and their expectations for knee arthroplasty. Int J Qual Stud Health Well -being. 2016;11:30193.
8. Kao MH, Tsai YF. Illness experiences in middle-aged adults with early-stage knee osteoarthritis: findings from a qualitative study. J Adv Nurs. 2014;70:1564–72.
9. Pouli N, Das NR, Lincoln NB, Walsh D. The experience of living with knee osteoarthritis: exploring illness and treatment beliefs through thematic analysis. Disabil Rehabil. 2014;36:600–7.
10. Michie S. Designing and implementing behaviour change interventions to improve population health. J Health Serv Res Policy. 2008;13 Suppl 3:64–9.
11. Linden A, Butterworth SW, Prochaska JO. Motivational interviewing-based health coaching as a chronic care intervention. J Eval Clin Pract. 2010;16:166–74.
12. Huffman MH. HEALTH COACHING: a fresh, new approach to improve quality outcomes and compliance for patients with chronic conditions. Home Healthc Nurse. 2009;27:490–6.
13. Thom DH, Hessler D, Willard-Grace R, DeVore D, Prado C, Bodenheimer T, et al. Health coaching by medical assistants improves patients' chronic care experience. Am J Manag Care. 2015;21:685–91.
14. Liddy C, Johnston S, Irving H, Nash K, Ward N. Improving awareness, accountability, and access through health coaching: qualitative study of patients' perspectives. Can Fam Physician. 2015;61:e158–64.
15. McGloin H, Timmins F, Coates V, Boore J. A case study approach to the examination of a telephone-based health coaching intervention in facilitating behaviour change for adults with Type 2 diabetes. J Clin Nurs. 2015;24:1246–57.
16. Thom DH, Ghorob A, Hessler D, De VD, Chen E, Bodenheimer TA. Impact of peer health coaching on glycemic control in low-income patients with diabetes: a randomized controlled trial. Ann Fam Med. 2013;11:137–44.
17. Varney JE, Weiland TJ, Inder WJ, Jelinek GA. Effect of hospital-based telephone coaching on glycaemic control and adherence to management guidelines in type 2 diabetes, a randomised controlled trial. Intern Med J. 2014;44:890–7.
18. Wayne N, Perez DF, Kaplan DM, Ritvo P. Health coaching reduces HbA1c in type 2 diabetic patients from a lower-socioeconomic status community: a randomized controlled trial. J Med Internet Res. 2015;17:e224.
19. Willard-Grace R, DeVore D, Chen EH, Hessler D, Bodenheimer T, Thom DH. The effectiveness of medical assistant health coaching for low-income patients with uncontrolled diabetes, hypertension, and hyperlipidemia: protocol for a randomized controlled trial and baseline characteristics of the study population. BMC Fam Pract. 2013;14:27.
20. O'Hara BJ, Phongsavan P, Venugopal K, Eakin EG, Eggins D, Caterson H, et al. Effectiveness of Australia's Get Healthy Information and Coaching Service(R): translational research with population wide impact. Prev Med. 2012;55:292–8.
21. Craig P, Dieppe P, Macintyre S, Michie S, Nazareth I, Petticrew M. Developing and evaluating complex interventions: the new Medical Research Council guidance. BMJ. 2008;337:a1655.
22. Craig P, Dieppe P, Macintyre S, Michie S, Nazareth I, Petticrew M. Developing and evaluating complex interventions: the new Medical Research Council guidance. Int J Nurs Stud. 2013;50:587–92.
23. Reeves S, Albert M, Kuper A, Hodges BD. Why use theories in qualitative research? BMJ. 2008;337:a949.
24. Lazarus RS, Folkman S, Folkman S: Estrés y procesos cognitivos. Barcelona: Martínez Roca; 1986.
25. Lazarus RS. Emotions and interpersonal relationships: toward a person-centered conceptualization of emotions and coping. J Pers. 2006;74:9–46.
26. Moix J. Análisis de los factores psicológicos moduladores del dolor crónico benigno. Anuario de Psicología. 2005;36:37–60.
27. Lazarus FS. Estrés y emoción. Manejo e implicaciones en nuestra salud. Bilbao: Desclée de Brower; 2000.
28. Tuckett AG. Qualitative research sampling: the very real complexities. Nurse Res 2004. 2004;12:47–61.
29. Tong A, Sainsbury P, Craig J. Consolidated criteria for reporting qualitative research (COREQ): a 32-item checklist for interviews and focus groups. Int J Qual Health Care. 2007;19:349–57.
30. Mann C, Gooberman-Hill R. Health care provision for osteoarthritis: concordance between what patients would like and what health professionals think they should have. Arthritis Care Res (Hoboken). 2011;63:963–72.
31. Moe RH, Haavardsholm EA, Grotle M, Steen E, Kjeken I, Hagen KB, et al. Development of a brief multidisciplinary education programme for patients with osteoarthritis. BMC Musculoskelet Disord. 2011;12:257.
32. Chard J, Dickson J, Tallon D, Dieppe P. A comparison of the views of rheumatologists, general practitioners and patients on the treatment of osteoarthritis. Rheumatology (Oxford). 2002;41:1208–10.
33. Tallon D, Chard J, Dieppe P. Relation between agendas of the research community and the research consumer. Lancet. 2000;355:2037–40.
34. Tallon D, Chard J, Dieppe P. Exploring the priorities of patients with osteoarthritis of the knee. Arthritis Care Res. 2000;13:312–9.
35. Sociedad Española de Medicina de Familia y Comunitaria. E, Mas Lodo N, Martín Blázquez M, Raja Casillas M, Izquierdo Zamarriego M, Valles Fernández N, Metola Gómez M. What underlies goalgia in general population? Atención Primaria. 2017;215–219.
36. Hunter DJ. Ostheoarthritis: Managing this chronic disease. Sidney: New Agency for Clinical Innovation. 2013.
37. Royle J, Oliver S. Consumer involvement in the health technology assessment program. Int J Technol Assess Health Care. 2004;20:493–7.
38. Codern-Bove N, Pujol-Ribera E, Pla M, Gonzalez-Bonilla J, Granollers S, Ballve JL, et al. Motivational interviewing interactions and the primary health care challenges presented by smokers with low motivation to stop smoking: a conversation analysis. BMC Public Health. 2014;14:1225.
39. Alharbi TS, Carlstrom E, Ekman I, Jarnebom A, Olsson LE. Experiences of person-centred care - patients' perceptions: qualitative study. BMC Nurs. 2014;13:28.
40. Astin F, Horrocks J, Closs SJ. Managing lifestyle change to reduce coronary risk: a synthesis of qualitative research on peoples' experiences. BMC Cardiovasc Disord. 2014;14:96.
41. Constand MK, MacDermid JC, Dal Bello-Haas V, Law M. Scoping review of patient-centered care approaches in healthcare. BMC Health Serv Res. 2014;14:271.
42. Clarke SP, Poulis N, Moreton BJ, Walsh DA, Lincoln NB: Evaluation of a group acceptance commitment therapy intervention for people with knee or hip osteoarthritis: a pilot randomized controlled trial. Disabil Rehabil. 2017;39:663–70.
43. Trompetter HR, Bohlmeijer ET, Lamers SM, Schreurs KM. Positive psychological wellbeing is required for online self-help acceptance and commitment therapy for chronic pain to be effective. Front Psychol. 2016;7:353.
44. Veehof MM, Trompetter HR, Bohlmeijer ET, Schreurs KM. Acceptance- and mindfulness-based interventions for the treatment of chronic pain: a meta-analytic review. Cogn Behav Ther. 2016;45:5–31.
45. Martin LA, Critelli JW, Doster JA, Powers C, Purdum M, Doster MR, et al. Cardiovascular risk: gender differences in lifestyle behaviors and coping strategies. Int J Behav Med. 2013;20:97–105.
46. Somers TJ, Blumenthal JA, Guilak F, Kraus VB, Schmitt DO, Babyak MA, et al. Pain coping skills training and lifestyle behavioral weight management in patients with knee osteoarthritis: a randomized controlled study. Pain. 2012;153:1199–209.
47. Deasy C, Coughlan B, Pironom J, Jourdan D, Mcnamara PM. Psychological distress and lifestyle of students: implications for health promotion. Health Promot Int. 2015;30:77–87.

48. Ekkekakis P, Vazou S, Bixby WR, Georgiadis E. The mysterious case of the public health guideline that is (almost) entirely ignored: call for a research agenda on the causes of the extreme avoidance of physical activity in obesity. Obes Rev. 2016;17:313–29.
49. Murphy SL, Kratz AL, Williams DA, Geisser ME. The association between symptoms, pain coping strategies, and physical activity among people with symptomatic knee and hip osteoarthritis. Front Psychol. 2012;3:326.
50. Hendry M, Williams NH, Markland D, Wilkinson C, Maddison P. Why should we exercise when our knees hurt? a qualitative study of primary care patients with osteoarthritis of the knee. Fam Pract. 2006;23:558–67.
51. Bennell KL, Egerton T, Bills C, Gale J, Kolt GS, Bunker SJ, et al. Addition of telephone coaching to a physiotherapist-delivered physical activity program in people with knee osteoarthritis: a randomised controlled trial protocol. BMC Musculoskelet Disord. 2012;13:246.
52. Brodin N, Lohela-Karlsson M, Swardh E, Opava CH. Cost-effectiveness of a one-year coaching program for healthy physical activity in early rheumatoid arthritis. Disabil Rehabil. 2015;37:757–62.
53. Demmelmaier I, Lindkvist A, Nordgren B, Opava CH. "A gift from heaven" or "This was not for me". A mixed methods approach to describe experiences of participation in an outsourced physical activity program for persons with rheumatoid arthritis. Clin Rheumatol. 2015;34:429–39.
54. Hinman RS, Delany CM, Campbell PK, Gale J, Bennell KL. Physical Therapists, Telephone Coaches, and Patients With Knee Osteoarthritis: Qualitative Study About Working Together to Promote Exercise Adherence. Phys Ther. 2015.
55. Knittle K, De Gucht V, Hurkmans E, Peeters A, Ronday K, Maes S, et al. Targeting motivation and self-regulation to increase physical activity among patients with rheumatoid arthritis: a randomised controlled trial. Clin Rheumatol. 2015;34:231–8.
56. Sahlen KG, Johansson H, Nystrom L, Lindholm L. Health coaching to promote healthier lifestyle among older people at moderate risk for cardiovascular diseases, diabetes and depression: a study protocol for a randomized controlled trial in Sweden. BMC Public Health. 2013;13:199.
57. DeLongis A, Folkman S, Lazarus RS. The impact of daily stress on health and mood: psychological and social resources as mediators. J Pers Soc Psychol. 1988;54:486–95.
58. Cheng C, Lau HP, Chan MP. Coping flexibility and psychological adjustment to stressful life changes: a meta-analytic review. Psychol Bull. 2014;140:1582–607.
59. Folling IS, Solbjor M, Helvik AS. Previous experiences and emotional baggage as barriers to lifestyle change - a qualitative study of Norwegian Healthy Life Centre participants. BMC Fam Pract. 2015;16:73.
60. McKenzie SH, Harris MF. Understanding the relationship between stress, distress and healthy lifestyle behaviour: a qualitative study of patients and general practitioners. BMC Fam Pract. 2013;14:166.
61. Jagosh J, Bush PL, Salsberg J, Macaulay AC, Greenhalgh T, Wong G, et al. A realist evaluation of community-based participatory research: partnership synergy, trust building and related ripple effects. BMC Public Health. 2015;15:725.
62. Prufer F, Joos S, Miksch A. What do resource-oriented approaches mean to general practitioners and how can they be facilitated in primary care? a qualitative study. Evid Based Complement Alternat Med. 2013;2013:187641.

Impact of treatment strategy and physical performance on future knee-related self-efficacy in individuals with ACL injury

Vala Flosadottir[1*], Richard Frobell[2], Ewa M. Roos[3] and Eva Ageberg[1]

Abstract

Background: In people with anterior cruciate ligament (ACL) injury, high self-efficacy facilitates recovery, indicated by improved muscle function, reduced knee symptoms and increased physical activity. Impact of treatment on future self-efficacy is however not well investigated. The aims of the study were to 1) investigate knee-related self-efficacy 6 years after acute ACL injury in patients treated with exercise therapy alone or in combination with either early or the option of delayed ACL reconstruction (ACLR), and 2) to investigate associations between single-leg physical performance at various time points after ACL injury and knee self-efficacy at 6 years after injury.

Methods: Participants (n = 121) originated from the KANON-study (ISRCTN84752559), a treatment RCT including active adults with acute ACL injury treated with structured exercise therapy combined with early or the option of delayed ACLR. In this ancillary study, participants with knee self-efficacy data at 6 years (n = 89) were analyzed as treated; exercise therapy alone (n = 20), exercise therapy plus early ACLR (n = 46), and exercise therapy plus delayed ACLR (n = 23). The participants performed physical performance tests (hop, strength and balance) at the end the of exercise therapy (mean 10 (SD 6) months), and at 5 years, and rated their knee self-efficacy using Knee Self-Efficacy Scale (K-SES) questionnaire (0 to 10, worst to best) at 6 years.

Results: Median K-SES score for the total group (n = 89) was 7.8 (IQR 5.9–9.0). There were no differences between treatment groups in K-SES scores at 6 years nor in physical performance at any time point ($p \geq 0.097$). Worse knee flexion strength LSI ($r_{sp} = 0.341$, $p = 0.042$) at the end of the exercise therapy, and worse LSI for single-leg hop test ($r_{sp} = 0.310$, $p = 0.005$) at the end of the exercise therapy and at 5 years, correlated moderately with worse knee-related self-efficacy at 6 years. Low associations were observed between the remaining physical performance tests and K-SES scores ($r_{sp} \leq 0.265$, $p \geq 0.045$).

Conclusion: Knee-related self-efficacy at 6 years after ACL injury did not differ between those treated with ACLR, performed early or as a delayed procedure, or exercise therapy alone. Good physical performance at the end of the exercise therapy, and at 5 years, appears to have a positive, yet small, impact on future knee-related self-efficacy.

Keywords: Knee, Patient outcome assessment, Performance-based measures, Psychological factors

* Correspondence: vala.flosadottir@med.lu.se
[1]Department of Health Sciences, Lund University, Box 157, 221 00 Lund, Sweden
Full list of author information is available at the end of the article

Background

In recent years, there has been increased focus on psychosocial factors and their association to recovery and return to sport (RTS) after anterior cruciate ligament (ACL) injury [1, 2]. The expectations of good recovery of knee function and RTS are high among individuals with ACL injury [3, 4]. However, despite treatment, with or without surgical reconstruction, impairments in patient-reported outcome measures (PROMs) [5, 6] and in physical performance often persist [7]. Only 81% return to any sport and 55% return to competitive level sports following an ACL injury or anterior cruciate ligament reconstruction (ACLR) [8].

The way in which a person reacts to an sport injury, i.e., the psychosocial response, includes cognitive, affective and behavioral aspects [9]. Negative psychological responses following an ACL injury or ACLR include pain and anxiety response, depression, and loss of athletic identity [10–12]. Positive psychological responses, on the other hand, include high motivation, high confidence and low fear of reinjury [1, 2] in addition to high self-efficacy [13]. These positive psychological responses interact both with each other and with the outcomes of the treatment [9]. In those with ACL injury, studies show that positive psychological responses, including high self-efficacy (cognitive response), facilitate recovery, in terms of improved muscle function, reduced knee symptoms and increased physical activity and that these are associated with higher return to pre-injury level of sports [1, 2]. However, we are not aware of any studies with the reverse design that evaluate whether modifiable treatment factors influence future self-efficacy.

Self-efficacy has been defined as the perception of one's capability to perform a specific task, irrespective of whether one actually does or can perform it [14]. The level of self-efficacy can influence one's initiative for action, level of effort and resilience to setbacks [14]. Previous experience of failure and success, including one's own and through observation of others, can conversely effect one's self-efficacy. [14] Commonly used measures evaluating knee-related self-efficacy after ACL injury, are the ACL-Return to Sports after Injury scale (ACL-RSI) [15], the Modified Self-Efficacy for Rehabilitation Outcome Scale (SER) [16], knee confidence with the single item Q3 from the Knee injury and Osteoarthritis Outcome Score subscale quality of life (KOOS item Q3) [17], and the Knee Self-Efficacy Scale (K-SES).

Low knee-related self-efficacy, in terms of low K-SES scores, has been reported in the early stages of treatment after ACL injury or reconstruction but is suggested to improve during the course of rehabilitation [18, 19]. One reason for this improvement in knee-related self-efficacy could be associated with decreased knee-related symptoms and the improvements in physical performance that are achieved during rehabilitation, however, to our knowledge this has not been studied. Another potential contributing factor for achieving high self-efficacy may be the treatment strategy, i.e., exercise therapy plus ACLR or exercise therapy alone. Thomeé et al. [20] investigated the role of knee-related self-efficacy in ACL-injured patients, undergoing exercise therapy with or without ACLR, and concluded that self-efficacy increased during the first year after injury and ACLR. The influence of self-reported knee function, age, gender and physical activity on the patients' perceived knee self-efficacy was investigated [20]. However, the possible impact of different treatment strategies on future knee-related self-efficacy following ACL injury has not been reported.

Therefore, the aims of this study were to 1) report knee-related self-efficacy 6 years after acute ACL injury in patients treated with exercise therapy alone or in combination with either early or the option of delayed ACLR, and to 2) investigate associations between objectively measured single-leg physical performance at various time points after ACL injury and self-reported knee self-efficacy at 6 years after injury.

Methods

Participants

The participants in the present study originate from the Knee Anterior Cruciate Ligament, Nonsurgical versus Surgical Treatment (KANON) study (ISRCTN84752559) [5], a randomized controlled trial including 121 physically active adults with an acute ACL injury to a previously un-injured knee. The KANON-trial compared two treatments strategies: structured exercise therapy combined with an early ACLR (n = 62) or exercise therapy with the option of a delayed ACLR performed if needed (n = 59) [5]. The exercise therapy program was consistent with consensus in the literature [21]. At 2 and 5 years, there were no differences between the groups as randomized or as treated in knee-related outcomes, health status, return to preinjury activity level [5], or knee osteoarthritis (OA) frequency [6].

In this ancillary study all participants with available results on the K-SES (n = 89, Table 1) were included and analyzed according to treatment actually received: exercise therapy alone (ACL-D, n = 20), exercise therapy plus early reconstruction (ACL-R n = 46), and exercise therapy plus delayed reconstruction (ACL-X n = 23). Of the included participants, 62 performed the physical performance tests at the end of the exercise therapy period (mean 10 (SD 6) months after injury) [22] and 85 participants performed the physical performance test at 5 years after ACL injury; knee related self-efficacy was self-reported by mail at

Table 1 Baseline characteristics of the study participants (*n* = 89)

	ACL-D (*n* = 20)	ACL-R (*n* = 46)	ACL-X (*n* = 23)	*p*-value
Age (y), mean (SD)	25.7 (4.8)	26.7 (5.4)	25.7 (4.8)	0.673
Female gender, n (%)	7 (35)	11 (24)	7 (30)	0.672
BMI (kg/m^2), mean (SD)*	23.4 (2.4)	24.2 (3.3)	23.4 (2.0)	0.789
Tegner activity score, median (IQR)	9 (7–9)	8.5 (7–9)	8 (7–9)	0.934
Participating in sports when injured, n (%)	19 (95)	46 (100)	22 (96)	0.331
Right knee injured, n (%)	12 (60)	25 (54)	12 (52)	0.868
MRI-findings				
Total ACL-rupture, n (%)	19 (95)	46 (100)	23 (100)	0.175
Meniscal injury, n (%)**	12 (60)	32 (70)	9 (39)	0.052
Autograft type				
Patella tendon (%)		17 (37)	11 (48)	0.386
Hamstring tendon, n (%)		29 (63)	12 (52)	0.386
Supervised exercise therapy sessions[a], mean (SD)	34 (23.2)	67 (32.3)	70 (38.1)	0.000

*n = 87, **n = 88, [a]Number of supervised session until 2 yrs. follow-up
SD standard deviation, *IQR* inter-quartile range, *BMI* body mass index, *MRI* magnetic resonance imaging, *ACL* anterior cruciate ligament, *ACL-D* exercise only, *ACL-R* exercise plus early reconstruction, *ACL-X* exercise plus delayed reconstruction

6 years (Fig. 1). There were no differences in the physical performance tests between the groups as treated (ACL-D, ACL-R, ACL-X). The KANON study was approved by the Research Ethics Committee at Lund University, Sweden (LU 535–01) and all participants gave their written informed consent.

Physical performance

Physical performance was assessed at two time points; at the end of the exercise therapy and at 5 years follow-up. Seven single-leg physical performance tests, as described in Ericsson et al. [22] were assessed at the end of the exercise therapy when all goals of the exercise protocol

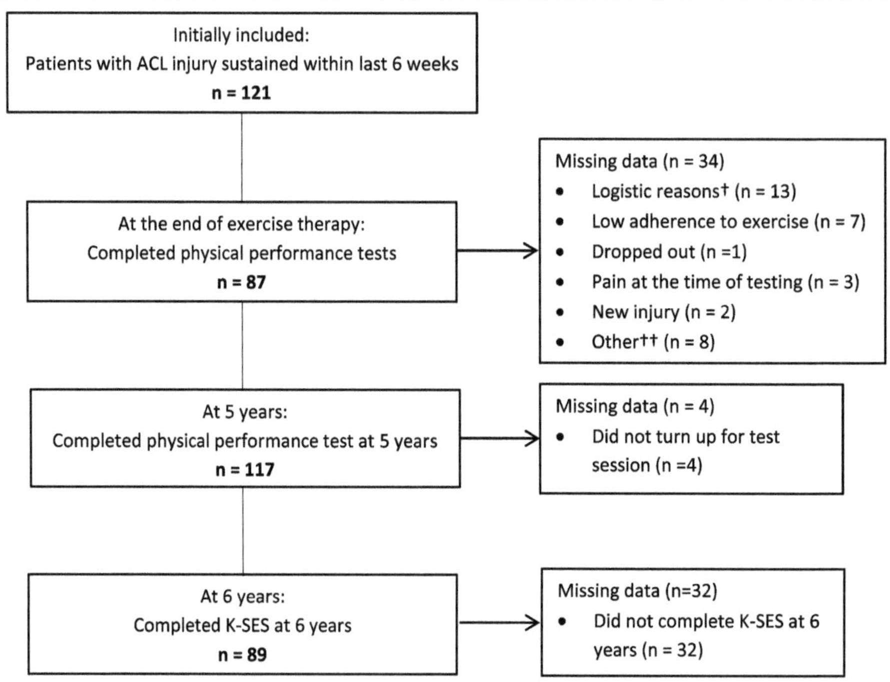

Fig. 1 Flow chart of participants and follow-ups with physical performance tests and the Knee Self-Efficacy Scale (K-SES). †Long-distance relocation or transferal to a physical therapist (PT) not involved in the study. ††Pregnancy (*n* = 1), disc herniation (n = 1), advised against performing test by PT (*n* = 3), missing test protocols (n = 3). Participants with K-SES data and physical performance test data were included in the analyses

were considered to be met [22]. The tests included the single-leg hop for distance, vertical hop, square hop, single-leg rise, single-leg balance test, knee extension strength, and knee flexion strength (Table 2). At mean 5 (SD 0.5) years after injury, performance was only assessed by the single-leg hop test for distance. The change in single-leg hop performance between the end of the exercise therapy and at 5 years was also calculated.

The Limb Symmetry Index (LSI) was used for all analyses of physical performance. The LSI was calculated by dividing the result for the injured leg by that of the uninjured leg and multiplying by 100 [23].

Thirty-four participants (9 women, 25 men) did not complete the physical performance tests at the end of the exercise therapy (Fig. 1), and, were excluded from the correlation analyses. These participants did not differ from those who completed the physical performance tests with respect to age ($p = 0.41$), gender ($p = 0.99$), BMI ($p = 0.24$), activity level ($p = 0.96$), treatment randomized ($p = 0.30$), or number of supervised exercise therapy sessions ($p = 0.32$). Depending on data normality and type, the χ^2 test or the Mann-Whitney test were used for the between-group comparisons, as appropriate.

Knee-related self-efficacy

Perceived knee-related self-efficacy was self-reported at mean 6 (SD 1) years after injury using the K-SES. K-SES consists of four sections; A – daily activities, B – sports and leisure activities, C – knee function tasks and D – future knee function. The full K-SES includes 22 items and the individual rates the certainty about the capability of performing an activity on an 11-point Likert scale, ranging from 0 (not at all certain) to 10 (very certain). Item scores are summarized and divided by the number of items for each section (A-D), yielding a total K-SES score ranging from 0 to 10 [24]. Two subscores, K-SES Present and Future, are also calculated each with a range of 0 to 10 [24]. In sections A through C, the participants report their perception about their present capability of performing knee-related tasks, yielding the subscore K-SES Present. In section D, they report their perception about their future knee function capability, such as return to preinjury level sport and fear of reinjury (plus decreasing knee function if undergoing ACLR), yielding the subscore K-SES Future. [24] The K-SES has been assessed for the following measurement properties; internal consistency, test-retest reliability, face validity, content validity and construct validity [20, 24]. The K-SES is reliable and valid for measuring perceived self-efficacy in patients with an ACL injury [24].

Statistical analysis

Data were analyzed on a post-hoc as-treated basis. The one-way ANOVA test was used for the comparison of age at baseline between the treatment groups, and, the Kruskal-Wallis test was used for between-group comparisons of the BMI, the performance tests and the K-SES scores in the three treatment groups. Spearman's, and partial Spearman's, rank-order correlation analyses were used to assess associations between physical performance and K-SES, controlling for age, gender and treatment. Correlation coefficients thresholds suggested by Cohen [25] were used as follows; ≥ 0.10 to 0.29 denote low association, ≥ 0.30 to 0.49 moderate association and coefficients ≥0.50 large association. *P*-values less than or equal to 0.05 were considered statistically significant.

Table 2 Single-leg physical performance at the end of the exercise therapy at 10 months and at 5 years after ACL injury or reconstruction ($n = 33–85$) [a]

	ACL-D $n = 7–18$	ACL-R $n = 16–46$	ACL-X $n = 10–21$	*p*-value
At the end of the exercise therapy, at mean 10 months (SD 6)				
Single-leg hop LSI, n = 62	101.4 (5.7)	99.8 (10.5)	100.5 (4.0)	0.588
Vertical hop LSI, n = 33	101.1 (9.4)	91.8 (27.3)	101.1 (9.4)	0.144
Square hop LSI, n = 61	106.7 (12.2)	103.4 (11.7)	98.9 (16.8)	0.563
Single-leg rise LSI, *n* = 61	99.5 (5.9)	97.6 (6.5)	98.1 (5.2)	0.264
Single-leg balance LSI, n = 61	116.8 (50.0)	130.6 (67.3)	126.3 (74.8)	0.863
Knee extension, LSI (*n* = 49)	98.2 (8.3)	97.8 (9.3)	100.1 (5.1)	0.484
Knee flexion, LSI (n = 33)	93.7 (11.3)	98.4 (8.9)	107.7 (16.7)	0.097
At mean 5 years (SD 1)				
Single-leg hop LSI, *n* = 85	97.5 (11.5)	95.2 (12.0)	94.8 (12.7)	0.586
Change between 10 months and 5 years				
Single-leg hop LSI, n = 61	−4.2 (13.9)	−1.8 (12.6)	6.6 (13.3)	0.556

Values are the mean (SD)
LSI Limb Symmetry Index, *ACL-D* exercise only, *ACL-R* exercise plus early reconstruction, *ACL-X* exercise plus delayed reconstruction
[a]Missing values due to equipment problems or patients declining to perform a test

Statistical analyses where performed using IBM SPSS for Windows, version 23.0 (IBM corp., Armonk, NY, USA).

Results

The median K-SES scores at 6 years for all participants ($n = 89$) were K-SES 7.8 (IQR 5.9–9.0), K-SES present 8.7 (IQR 6.8–9.6) and K-SES future 4.8 (IQR 2.5–7.5). There were no differences between the three treatment groups in K-SES scores 6 years after injury ($p \geq 0.501$, Fig. 2).

There were no differences between treatment groups in single-leg physical performance at any time point ($p \geq 0.097$, Table 2). Therefore, the correlation analyses were performed with data from all patients combined. Worse LSI for knee flexion strength ($r_{sp} = 0.341$, $p = 0.042$) at the end of the exercise therapy, as well as worse LSI on the single-leg hop test at 5 years ($r_{sp} = 0.310$, $p = 0.005$), correlated moderately with worse knee-related self-efficacy at 6 years after injury (Table 3). Low associations were observed between the remaining physical performance tests at the end of the exercise therapy and K-SES, ranging from $r_{sp} = 0.148$ ($p = 0.264$) for the LSI for the single-leg hop test to $r_{sp} = 0.265$ ($p = 0.045$) for the LSI in the square hop test.

Discussion

Knee-related self-efficacy at 6 years after acute ACL injury was not associated with treatment strategy, in terms of exercise therapy alone or combined with early or

Table 3 Spearman's rank-order correlations (r_s) and rank-order partial correlations (r_{sp}) between physical performance at the end of the exercise therapy and at 5 years after ACL injury/ACLR and K-SES scores at 6 years

	K-SES (n = 33–85)			
	r_s	p-value	r_{sp}^a	*p*-value
At the end of the exercise therapy, at 10 months				
Single-leg hop LSI	0.150	0.244	0.148	0.264
Vertical hop LSI	−0.142	0.431	−0.236	0.210
Square hop LSI	0.267	0.037	0.265	0.045
Single-leg rise LSI	0.163	0.209	0.190	0.153
Single-leg balance LSI	0.237	0.066	0.238	0.072
Knee extension LSI	0.130	0.375	0.167	0.267
Knee flexion LSI	0.286	0.078	**0.341**	0.042
At 5 years				
Single-leg hop LSI	0.298	0.006	**0.310**	0.005
Change between 10 months and 5 years				
Single-leg hop LSI	0.201	0.120	0.196	0.139

Bold numbers represent moderate correlations. Regular numbers represent low correlations. Correlation coefficients: ≥ 0.10 to 0.29 denote low association, ≥ 0.30 to 0.49 moderate association and coefficients ≥0.50 large association
K-SES Knee Self-Efficacy Scale, *LSI* Limb Symmetry Index
[a]Physical performance effect independent of age, gender and treatment

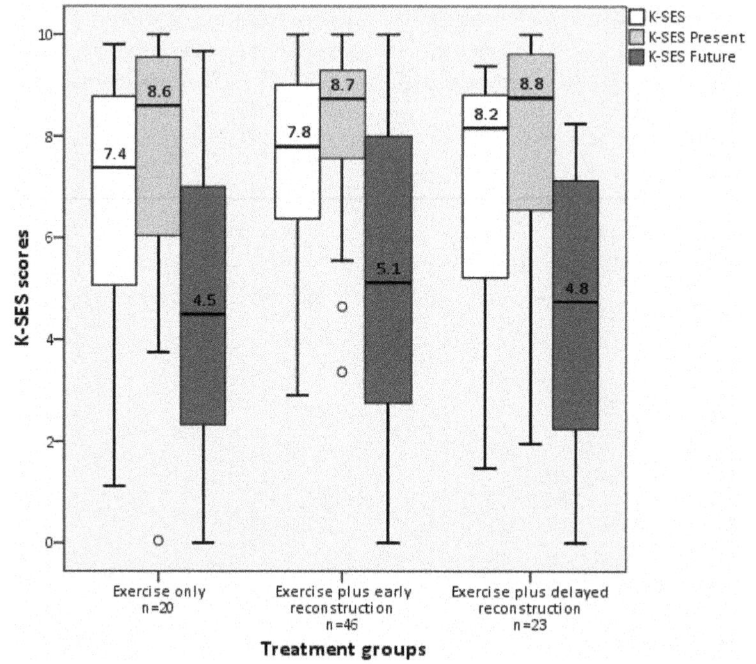

Fig. 2 Distribution of Knee Self-Efficacy (K-SES) scores in the different treatment groups (total $n = 89$) at 6 years after injury. The bar in the box represents the median, the box represents the interquartile range (IQR) and the whiskers extend to the minimum or the maximum values within 1.5 IQR from the lower and the higher edges of the box. Circles represent cases with values between 1.5 and 3 IQR from the lower edge of the box

optional delayed ACLR. Worse LSI in knee flexion strength at the end of the exercise therapy and worse LSI in the single-leg hop test for distance, at 5 years, were moderately associated with worse knee-related self-efficacy at 6 years.

The K-SES scores (median 7.4–8.2) for our cohort were comparable, or better, than K-SES scores previously reported from other Swedish cohorts: mean 6.8 and 7.6 at 12 months after ACL injury and ACLR, respectively [20]; mean 7.3 at 12 months after ACL injury or ACLR [26]; and median 6.7 at 1–12 month after ACL injury and 3–12 months after ACLR [24].

In a previous study, similar levels of K-SES scores (mean 6.9–8.3), have been shown to be associated with greater likelihood of satisfaction with knee function, at mean 3 years after ACLR [27]. In the present study, the K-SES Present scores (perception about one's present capability of performing knee-related tasks) can be considered to be high, whereas the K-SES Future scores (perception about one's return to preinjury level sports and fear of reinjury plus decreasing knee function if undergoing ACLR) were remarkably low, for all three treatment groups. In contrast, previous studies report that the K-SES Future scores correspond to or are higher than the K-SES Present scores [18, 20, 24, 26]. One explanation for this could be that previous studies investigated knee-related self-efficacy within one month after ACL injury or before ACLR and up to 1 year after injury or ACLR [18, 20, 24, 26], whereas in the present study we assessed knee-related self-efficacy at 6 years after ACL injury or ACLR. The K-SES Future score refers to perceptions about return to preinjury level sports, fear of reinjury and decreasing knee function. Previous reports have shown, that less than 50% return to sports, at preinjury or competitive level, at 2–7 years after ACLR [28]. In the KANON-trial, only about 20% of the participants were active at their preinjury activity level or higher at 5 years after structured rehabilitation with or without the addition of ACLR [6]. Thus, it may be assumed that no more than 20% of participants in the present cohort were active at their preinjury activity level at 6 years. This may be reflected by the low K-SES Future scores presented in the present study. Fear of reinjury, despite the perception of good knee function, has been shown to be the most common hindrance for return to sports [29, 30]. This may explain the discrepancy between the high K-SES Present (perception of good knee function capability) and the low K-SES Future (uncertainty about return to preinjury level sports and reinjury) scores. In addition, the expectations and motivation of return to preinjury level sports and the perception of acceptable knee function may change over time. High, and potentially unrealistic, expectations of return to sports and knee function have been reported by patients prior to surgery for an ACL or a meniscus injury [3, 4, 31]. As in the current study, lower, and perhaps more realistic, expectations may be expressed several years later. Therefore, other potentially relevant explanations for the low K-SES Future scores may be natural changes, including increasing age or changes in social commitments. A longitudinal study is required to further investigate these potential explanations for change in future knee self-efficacy in individuals after ACL injury.

The lack of differences in K-SES scores between groups as treated (ACL-D, ACL-R and ACL-X) is in line with previous observations for various outcomes of the KANON-trial, in terms of self-reported outcomes [5] and osteoarthritis (OA) [5, 6] at 2 or 5 years, and muscle function [7] evaluated at 3 years after ACL injury. All participants followed the same exercise therapy protocol regardless of treatment strategy. The as treated group, receiving exercise therapy alone, progressed faster and needed fewer exercise sessions than the two groups who had early or delayed ACLR in addition to exercise therapy. The exercise program was goal-based and progression to a more strenuous level was allowed when the goals for range of motion, muscle function, and functional performance, respectively, were met [5]. As a result, the exercise program was based on functional goals rather than a pre-determined number of sessions. This approach was chosen to ensure that all treatment groups would achieve a similar and good level of physical function. Thus, the extensive exercise therapy program, rather than the early or the optional delayed ACLR, may be the common factor explaining our findings of similar K-SES scores across all treatment groups.

To our knowledge, our study is the first to investigate the influence of physical performance on knee-related self-efficacy after ACL injury. In contrast, previous studies have the reverse design, focusing on the influence of psychological responses on physical function and performance [32]. Higher knee-related self-efficacy, in terms of higher K-SES score, before ACLR has been reported to be associated with good physical performance (LSI ≥ 90 in single-leg hop and muscle power tests) and improved self-reported knee function (KOOS) at 1-year follow-up after ACLR [33]. Our results indicate that greater (better) LSI for knee flexion strength at the end of exercise therapy after ACL injury, correlated with better knee-related self-efficacy (higher K-SES scores) at 6 years. Although these associations were only moderate, our findings are supported by results from previous longitudinal studies, indicating that symmetry between legs in single-leg physical performance after exercise therapy, or within one year after ACL injury or ACLR, is one contributing factor for good future self-reported outcomes, such as, self-reported knee function and high return to pre-injury sports [34–36].

We observed that worse LSI in single-leg physical performance at 5 years correlated moderately with worse knee-related self-efficacy at 6 years. Longitudinal results have previously shown that worse single-leg physical performance after ACL injury or ACLR was associated with worse knee confidence, a construct similar to knee-related self-efficacy. Lower (worse) LSI for single-leg hop performance at 3 years after ACL injury has been shown to be associated with worse knee confidence (KOOS item Q3) at 5 years [37]. These moderate associations between single-leg physical performance and knee confidence found in a previous study [37] and in our present longitudinal study, suggest that good single-leg physical performance is one factor contributing to better psychological outcome after ACL injury or ACLR. Further studies are required to evaluate the relative contribution of physical performance, as well as other factors, that may play a role for the psychological response after injury.

The level of knee-related self-efficacy is important after ACL injury and surgery as it can influence one's initiative for action, level of effort and resilience to setbacks. Surgical treatment in addition to exercise therapy after ACL injury does not appear to influence later knee-related self-efficacy. The findings of the current study show that after ACL injury, patients may benefit from training that targets symmetry between legs, specifically, in knee flexion muscle strength and in single-leg hop performance.

The main strength of the current study is that data originates from the KANON-trial, a high quality RCT. Another strength is that there were no differences between participants and non-participants in baseline characteristics. There are some limitations to the present ancillary study. The completion rates for the physical performance tests at the end of the exercise therapy were between 33% and 70% and only 74% of the participants of the KANON-trial completed the K-SES questionnaire at 6 years after injury. These low completion rates may be explained by equipment problems at the test sites, or participants declining to perform test at the end of the exercise therapy, and that the K-SES was sent out by mail instead of being filled out at a clinical visit at 6 years. However, the majority of the participants included in this study completed the physical performance test at 5 years (96%). Additional limitations are that several testers assessed the physical performance tests at the end of the exercise therapy [22]. However, all assessors were experienced and similar written instructions were used at all centers and for all tests. The use of LSI for the analyses of the physical performance tests may be considered a limitation. Despite the LSI being a common measure, it may misrepresent the performance of the injured leg [38]. Bilateral deficiencies in hop tests have been reported in individuals after ACLR [39]. Since the LSI represents the level of limb symmetry, a high (good) LSI may be the result of either a good, or poor, performance of both legs. Lastly, K-SES was only assessed at 6 years after injury, not allowing adjustment for baseline scores or analyses of change in K-SES scores.

Conclusions

Knee-related self-efficacy at 6 years after an acute ACL injury did not differ between patients treated with ACL reconstruction, performed early or as a delayed procedure, or those treated with exercise therapy alone. At 6 years after injury, the self-efficacy for present knee function capability (K-SES subscore present) was higher than the self-efficacy for return to preinjury level sport and not being reinjured (K-SES subscore Future). Worse single-leg physical performance at the end of the exercise therapy period, and at 5 years, was weakly to moderately associated with worse knee self-efficacy at 6 years. Targeted training to improve the symmetry between legs in knee flexion muscle strength and in the single-leg hop for distance may have a positive, yet small, long-term impact on knee-related self-efficacy after ACL injury.

Abbreviations

ACL: Anterior cruciate ligament; ACL-D: exercise therapy alone; ACLR: Anterior cruciate ligament reconstruction; ACL-R: exercise therapy plus early reconstruction; ACL-RSI: the ACL-Return to Sports after Injury scale; ACL-X: exercise therapy plus delayed reconstruction; BMI: Body mass index; IQR: Inter-quartile range; KANON: the Knee Anterior Cruciate Ligament, Nonsurgical versus Surgical Treatment; KOOS item Q3: the single item Q3 from the Knee injury and Osteoarthritis Outcome Score subscale quality of life; KOOS: the Knee injury and Osteoarthritis Outcome Score; K-SES: the Knee Self-Efficacy Scale; LSI: Limb symmetry index; MRI: Magnetic resonance imaging; OA: Osteoarthritis; PROMs: in patient-reported outcome measures; PT: Physical therapist; r_s: Spearman's rank-order correlations; r_{sp}: Spearman's rank-order partial correlations; RTS: Return to sports; SD: Standard deviation; SER: the Modified Self-Efficacy for Rehabilitation Outcome Scale

Acknowledgements

Not applicable.

Funding

This research was funded by the Swedish Research Council (2009–1447), the Crafoord Foundation, the Swedish Rheumatism Association, the Swedish National Centre for Research in Sports and the Faculty of Medicine of Lund University. The original KANON study, from which the patients were included, was additionally supported by the Faculty of Medicine of Lund University, Region Skåne, Sweden, Pfizer Global Research, the Swedish Research Council, the Swedish National Centre for Research in Sports, the Swedish Rheumatism Association, Thelma Zoegas Fund, and the Stig & Ragna Gorthon Research Fund.

Authors' contributions

VF, EA and RF contributed to the study design. RF and EMR were in charge of data collection. VF was responsible for the analysis and interpretation of the data, and wrote the first draft of the manuscript. EA contributed in analysis and interpretation of data, contributed in writing the manuscript and provided feedback on drafts of this manuscript. RF and EMR contributed in interpretation of data and critically revised the manuscript for important intellectual content. All authors approved the final manuscript.

Consent for publication
Not applicable.

Competing interests
The authors declare that they have no competing interests.

Author details
[1]Department of Health Sciences, Lund University, Box 157, 221 00 Lund, Sweden. [2]Department of Clinical Sciences, Lund University, Lund, Sweden. [3]Department of Sports Science and Clinical Biomechanics, Musculoskeletal Function and Physiotherapy, University of Southern Denmark, Odense, Denmark.

References

1. Ardern CL, Taylor NF, Feller JA, Webster KE. A systematic review of the psychological factors associated with returning to sport following injury. Br J Sports Med. 2013;47(17):1120–6.
2. te Wierike SCM, van der Sluis A, van den Akker-Scheek I, Elferink-Gemser MT, Visscher C. Psychosocial factors influencing the recovery of athletes with anterior cruciate ligament injury: a systematic review. Scand J Med Sci Sports. 2013;23(5):527–40.
3. Feucht MJ, Cotic M, Saier T, Minzlaff P, Plath JE, Imhoff AB, Hinterwimmer S. Patient expectations of primary and revision anterior cruciate ligament reconstruction. Knee surgery, sports traumatology, arthroscopy: official journal of the ESSKA. 2016;24(1):201–7.
4. Sonesson S, Kvist J, Ardern C, Osterberg A, Silbernagel KG. Psychological factors are important to return to pre-injury sport activity after anterior cruciate ligament reconstruction: expect and motivate to satisfy. Knee surgery, sports traumatology, arthroscopy: official journal of the ESSKA. 2017; 25(5):1375–84.
5. Frobell RB, Roos EM, Roos HP, Ranstam J, Lohmander LS. A randomized trial of treatment for acute anterior cruciate ligament tears. N Engl J Med. 2010; 363(4):331–42.
6. Frobell RB, Roos HP, Roos EM, Roemer FW, Ranstam J, Lohmander LS. Treatment for acute anterior cruciate ligament tear: five year outcome of randomised trial. BMJ (Clinical research ed). 2013;346:f232.
7. Ageberg E, Thomee R, Neeter C, Silbernagel KG, Roos EM. Muscle strength and functional performance in patients with anterior cruciate ligament injury treated with training and surgical reconstruction or training only: a two to five-year followup. Arthritis Rheum. 2008;59(12):1773–9.
8. Ardern CL, Taylor NF, Feller JA, Webster KE. Fifty-five per cent return to competitive sport following anterior cruciate ligament reconstruction surgery: an updated systematic review and meta-analysis including aspects of physical functioning and contextual factors. Br J Sports Med. 2014;48(21): 1543–52.
9. Wiese-bjornstal DM, Smith AM, Shaffer SM, Morrey MA. An integrated model of response to sport injury: psychological and sociological dynamics. Journal of Applied Sport Psychology. 1998;10(1):46–69.
10. Tripp DA, Stanish WD, Coady C, Reardon G. The subjective pain experience of athletes following anterior cruciate ligament surgery. Psychol Sport Exerc. 2004;5(3):339–54.
11. Podlog L, Dimmock J, Miller J. A review of return to sport concerns following injury rehabilitation: practitioner strategies for enhancing recovery outcomes. Physical therapy in sport: official journal of the Association of Chartered Physiotherapists in Sports Med. 2011;12(1):36–42.
12. Garcia GH, Wu HH, Park MJ, Tjoumakaris FP, Tucker BS, JDt K, Sennett BJ. Depression symptomatology and anterior cruciate ligament injury: incidence and effect on functional outcome–a prospective cohort study. Am J Sports Med. 2016;44(3):572–9.
13. Hamrin Senorski E, Samuelsson K, Thomee C, Beischer S, Karlsson J, Thomee R. Return to knee-strenuous sport after anterior cruciate ligament reconstruction: a report from a rehabilitation outcome registry of patient characteristics. Knee surgery, sports traumatology, arthroscopy: official journal of the ESSKA. 2017;25(5):1364–74.
14. Bandura A. Self-efficacy: toward a unifying theory of behavioral change. Psychol Rev. 1977;84(2):191–215.
15. Webster KE, Feller JA, Lambros C. Development and preliminary validation of a scale to measure the psychological impact of returning to sport following anterior cruciate ligament reconstruction surgery. Physical therapy in sport: official journal of the Association of Chartered Physiotherapists in Sports Med. 2008;9(1):9–15.
16. Chmielewski TL, Zeppieri G, Jr., Lentz TA, Tillman SM, Moser MW, Indelicato PA, George SZ: Longitudinal changes in psychosocial factors and their association with knee pain and function after anterior cruciate ligament reconstruction. Phys Ther 2011, 91(9):1355–1366.
17. Ageberg E, Roos EM. The association between knee confidence and muscle power, hop performance, and postural orientation in people with anterior cruciate ligament injury. The Journal of orthopaedic and sports physical therapy. 2016:1–16.
18. Thomee P, Wahrborg P, Borjesson M, Thomee R, Eriksson BI, Karlsson J. A randomized, controlled study of a rehabilitation model to improve knee-function self-efficacy with ACL injury. J Sport Rehabil. 2010;19(2):200–13.
19. Chmielewski TL, George SZ, Tillman SM, Moser MW, Lentz TA, Indelicato PA, Trumble TN, Shuster JJ, Cicuttini FM, Leeuwenburgh C. Low- versus high-intensity plyometric exercise during rehabilitation after anterior cruciate ligament reconstruction. Am J Sports Med. 2016;44(3):609–17.
20. Thomee P, Wahrborg P, Borjesson M, Thomee R, Eriksson BI, Karlsson J. Self-efficacy, symptoms and physical activity in patients with an anterior cruciate ligament injury: a prospective study. Scand J Med Sci Sports. 2007;17(3): 238–45.
21. Arna Risberg M, Lewek M, Snyder-Mackler L. A systematic review of evidence for anterior cruciate ligament rehabilitation: how much and what type? Physical Therapy in Sport. 2004;5(3):125–45.
22. Ericsson YB, Roos EM, Frobell RB. Lower extremity performance following ACL rehabilitation in the KANON-trial: impact of reconstruction and predictive value at 2 and 5 years. Br J Sports Med. 2013;47(15):980–5.
23. Engelen-van Melick N, van Cingel RE, Tijssen MP, Nijhuis-van der Sanden MW. Assessment of functional performance after anterior cruciate ligament reconstruction: a systematic review of measurement procedures. Knee surgery, sports traumatology, arthroscopy: official journal of the ESSKA. 2013; 21(4):869–79.
24. Thomee P, Wahrborg P, Borjesson M, Thomee R, Eriksson BI, Karlsson J. A new instrument for measuring self-efficacy in patients with an anterior cruciate ligament injury. Scand J Med Sci Sports. 2006;16(3):181–7.
25. Cohen J. Statistical power analysis for the behavioral sciences, 2nd ed. edn. New Jersey: Lawrence Erlbaum Associates, Inc; 1988.
26. Thomee P, Wahrborg P, Borjesson M, Thomee R, Eriksson BI, Karlsson J. Determinants of self-efficacy in the rehabilitation of patients with anterior cruciate ligament injury. Journal of rehabilitation medicine: official journal of the UEMS European Board of Physical and Rehabilitation Medicine. 2007; 39(6):486–92.
27. Ardern CL, Osterberg A, Sonesson S, Gauffin H, Webster KE, Kvist J: Satisfaction With Knee Function After Primary Anterior Cruciate Ligament Reconstruction Is Associated With Self-Efficacy, Quality of Life, and Returning to the Preinjury Physical Activity. *Arthroscopy : the journal of arthroscopic & related surgery: official publication of the Arthroscopy Association of North America and the International Arthroscopy Association* 2016, **32**(8):1631–1638.e1633.
28. Ardern CL, Taylor NF, Feller JA, Webster KE. Return-to-sport outcomes at 2 to 7 years after anterior cruciate ligament reconstruction surgery. Am J Sports Med. 2012;40(1):41–8.
29. Ardern CL. Anterior cruciate ligament reconstruction-not exactly a one-way ticket back to the preinjury level: a review of contextual factors affecting return to sport after surgery. Sports health. 2015;7(3):224–30.

30. Langford JL, Webster KE, Feller JA. A prospective longitudinal study to assess psychological changes following anterior cruciate ligament reconstruction surgery. Br J Sports Med. 2009;43(5):377–81.
31. Pihl K, Roos EM, Nissen N, JoRgensen U, Schjerning J, Thorlund JB. Over-optimistic patient expectations of recovery and leisure activities after arthroscopic meniscus surgery. Acta Orthop. 2016;87(6):615–21.
32. Everhart JS, Best TM, Flanigan DC. Psychological predictors of anterior cruciate ligament reconstruction outcomes: a systematic review. Knee surgery, sports traumatology, arthroscopy: official journal of the ESSKA. 2015; 23(3):752–62.
33. Thomee P, Wahrborg P, Borjesson M, Thomee R, Eriksson BI, Karlsson J. Self-efficacy of knee function as a pre-operative predictor of outcome 1 year after anterior cruciate ligament reconstruction. Knee surgery, sports traumatology, arthroscopy: official journal of the ESSKA. 2008;16(2):118–27.
34. Grindem H, Logerstedt D, Eitzen I, Moksnes H, Axe MJ, Snyder-Mackler L, Engebretsen L, Risberg MA. Single-legged hop tests as predictors of self-reported knee function in nonoperatively treated individuals with anterior cruciate ligament injury. Am J Sports Med. 2011;39(11):2347–54.
35. Logerstedt D, Grindem H, Lynch A, Eitzen I, Engebretsen L, Risberg MA, Axe MJ, Snyder-Mackler L. Single-legged hop tests as predictors of self-reported knee function after anterior cruciate ligament reconstruction: the Delaware-Oslo ACL cohort study. Am J Sports Med. 2012;40(10):2348–56.
36. Ardern CL, Taylor NF, Feller JA, Whitehead TS, Webster KE. Sports participation 2 years after anterior cruciate ligament reconstruction in athletes who had not returned to sport at 1 year: a prospective follow-up of physical function and psychological factors in 122 athletes. Am J Sports Med. 2015;43(4):848–56.
37. Flosadottir V, Roos EM, Ageberg E. Muscle function is associated with future patient-reported outcomes in young adults with ACL injury. BMJ Open Sport Exerc Med. 2016;2(1):e000154.
38. Wellsandt E, Failla MJ, Snyder-Mackler L. Limb symmetry indexes can overestimate knee function after anterior cruciate ligament injury. The Journal of orthopaedic and sports physical therapy. 2017;47(5):334–8.
39. Gokeler A, Welling W, Benjaminse A, Lemmink K, Seil R, Zaffagnini S. A critical analysis of limb symmetry indices of hop tests in athletes after anterior cruciate ligament reconstruction: a case control study. Orthopaedics & traumatology, surgery & research: OTSR. 2017;103(6):947–51.

14

Association of malalignment, muscular dysfunction, proprioception, laxity and abnormal joint loading with tibiofemoral knee osteoarthritis

Joyce A. C. van Tunen[1*], Andrea Dell'Isola[2], Carsten Juhl[1,3], Joost Dekker[4], Martijn Steultjens[2], Jonas B. Thorlund[1] and Hans Lund[5]

Abstract

Background: To investigate (1) the association of specific biomechanical factors with knee osteoarthritis and knee osteoarthritis development, and (2) the impact of other relevant risk factors on this association.

Methods: MEDLINE, EMBASE, CINAHL and SPORTDiscus were searched up until April 2017. Studies were included if they fulfilled the following criteria: the study 1) assessed the association of a biomechanical factor with knee osteoarthritis, or knee osteoarthritis development; 2) reported on skeletal malalignment, muscular dysfunction, impaired proprioception, laxity and abnormal loading during gait; 3) was a cohort study with participants developing knee osteoarthritis and participants not developing knee osteoarthritis, or a case-control or cross-sectional study with participants with knee osteoarthritis and without knee osteoarthritis. Risk of bias was assessed with the QUIPS tool and meta-analyses were performed using random effects models.

Results: Of 6413 unique studies identified, 59 cross-sectional studies were eligible for meta-analyses (9825 participants, 5328 with knee osteoarthritis). No cohort studies fulfilled the inclusion criteria. Compared with healthy controls, patients with knee osteoarthritis have higher odds of having lower muscle strength, proprioception deficits, more medial varus-valgus laxity and less lateral varus-valgus laxity. Patients with medial knee osteoarthritis have higher odds of having a higher knee adduction moment than healthy controls. Level of evidence was graded as 'very low' to 'moderate' quality. Due to large between study differences moderation of other risk factors on biomechanical risk factors could not be evaluated.

Conclusions: Patients with knee osteoarthritis are more likely to display a number of biomechanical characteristics. The causal relationship between specific biomechanical factors and the development of knee osteoarthritis could not be determined as no longitudinal studies were included. There is an urgent need for high quality, longitudinal studies to evaluate the impact of specific biomechanical factors on the development of knee osteoarthritis.

Keywords: Osteoarthritis, Knee, Biomechanics, Systematic review, Meta-analysis

* Correspondence: jvtunen@health.sdu.dk
[1]Research Unit for Musculoskeletal Function and Physiotherapy, Department of Sports Science and Clinical Biomechanics, Faculty of Health Sciences, University of Southern Denmark, Campusvej 55, 5230 Odense, Denmark
Full list of author information is available at the end of the article

Background

Tibiofemoral knee osteoarthritis (OA) is mainly considered a mechanically driven disease [1] and numerous interventions such as braces, insoles and exercise therapy aim at modifying potential biomechanical drivers to prevent development or stall progression [2]. Biomechanical knee joint-related factors that often are subject to research in relation to knee OA are skeletal malalignment, muscular dysfunction, impaired proprioception, laxity and abnormal loading during gait [3]. The association of those biomechanical factors and other relevant risk factors (e.g. age, gender, obesity, knee injury) with knee OA and its onset have been reported in many individual studies. Such studies describing biomechanical factors' association with the presence or development of knee OA are often used to justify specific research questions but may not necessarily be representative of the available literature. Systematic reviews and meta-analyses give an overview the complete evidence of relevant biomechanical factors and their association with knee osteoarthritis.

Some previous reviews have attempted to summarize the evidence for the association between malalignment, muscular dysfunction, impaired proprioception, and laxity with knee OA. However, several of these reviews are not up-to-date and no attempts were made to estimate the magnitude of association of these biomechanical factors with knee OA [4–8]. Whereas systematic reviews including meta-analyses on knee extensor strength and knee joint loading (i.e. knee adduction moment) have primarily focussed on biomechanical risk factors for onset and progression of knee OA [9–11], only one study has systematically compared gait biomechanics in knee OA patients with controls quantitatively [12]. Thus, it has recently been emphasized that systematic reviews and meta-analysis to investigate the relationship between different biomechanical risk factors and OA should be performed [13].

In this systematic review and meta-analysis we aimed to (1) investigate the association of skeletal malalignment, muscular dysfunction, impaired proprioception, laxity and abnormal loading during gait with knee OA and knee OA development, and (2) to investigate the impact of other relevant risk factors on this association. Such knowledge is important when framing future research questions and designing targeted biomechanical interventions.

Methods

Registration and ethics

The protocol for this systematic review and meta-analysis [14] has been published previously and has been registered with the International Prospective Register of Systematic Reviews (PROSPERO ID: CRD42015025092). This systematic review and meta-analysis follows the Cochrane Collaboration guideline for preparing systematic review and meta-analysis and are reported according to the Preferred Reporting Items for Systematic Reviews and Meta-analyses (PRISMA) guideline [15].

Definition of biomechanical domains

We defined skeletal malalignment as abnormal alignment between the femur and the tibia in the frontal plane (i.e. varus or valgus alignment) [8]. Muscle dysfunction indicates muscle weakness, loss of muscle endurance or changed muscle activation patterns for the muscles that act on the knee joint [3, 5, 6]. Impaired proprioception refers to deterioration of the ability to detect knee joint position and movement [4]. Laxity is a loss of passive joint stabilisation due to the inability of passive structures in and around the knee (knee ligaments, cruciate ligaments, capsule) to provide an adequate counterbalance to the mechanical forces acting upon the knee during activity [7]. Abnormal loading during gait is often represented by evaluating external knee joint moments or the occurrence of varus or valgus thrust [9].

Search strategy

MEDLINE, EMBASE, SPORTDiscus, and the Cumulative Index to Nursing and Allied Health Literature Database (CINAHL) were searched from their inception until April 2017. Searches used subject headings (MeSH) and text words related to osteoarthritis, biomechanical factors and study types. The complete search strategy can be found in the study protocol [14].

Study selection

Studies were included if they fulfilled the following criteria: 1) the study assessed the association of a biomechanical factor with knee OA or incident knee OA development; 2) the biomechanical factor in the study was a knee joint related factor that interacts with the forces, moments and kinematics in and around a synovial joint (e.g. skeletal malalignment, proprioception, etc.); 3) the study was a cohort study with participants developing knee OA and participants not developing knee OA, or the study was a case-control or cross-sectional study with participants with knee OA and without knee OA. Studies were excluded if: 1) the study only included participants with patellofemoral osteoarthritis; 2) the study did not distinguish between hip osteoarthritis and knee OA; 3) study participants underwent treatment such as rehabilitation or surgery; 4) the study did not define knee OA in accordance to the criteria described in the protocol; 5) the study compared knees from the same participant (i.e. compared one knee with, and one knee without osteoarthritis within the same participant); 6) both knees are assessed in patients with bilateral knee OA. A detailed description of the eligibility criteria can be found in the study protocol [14].

Two reviewers (JT, ADI) independently screened eligibility of titles and abstracts of the studies obtained by the search. Subsequently, the reviewers used a standardized form to select studies eligible for inclusion in the review based on full text. Consensus was reached by discussion.

Assessment of risk of bias

Risk of bias was scored independently by two reviewers (JT, ADI) using the Quality In Prognostic Studies (QUIPS) tool [16] as described in the protocol [14]. Six areas of potential study biases were assessed: study participation, study attrition, prognostic factor measurement, study confounding, outcome measurement, and statistical analysis and reporting. Attrition was not applicable for cross-sectional studies.

Data extraction

Two reviewers (JT, ADI) used a customised, pilot-tested form to extract data from the included studies. The following information was extracted by both reviewers: authors, publication year, number of participants developing and not developing knee OA (in cohort studies) or number of participants in the knee OA and control group (in cross-sectional studies), sex, age, body mass index (BMI in kg/m^2), knee injury, knee OA definition, radiographic disease severity, involved compartment and examined biomechanical factor.

For malalignment and thrust measurements, the number of patients and controls with and without malalignment/thrust were extracted. If only the group mean and standard deviation was reported for malalignment, we transformed this into the number of participants with varus (or valgus) alignment and the number of participants with neutral and valgus (or varus) alignment by use of the normal deviation, where more than 1 degree deviation signifies abnormal alignment. For muscular dysfunction, impaired proprioception, laxity and external knee joint moments, group mean and standard deviation were extracted for patients and controls. For all factors, odds ratios were extracted if this was the only available data.

Data was grouped per study design, and into the five biomechanical domains. To allow for comparison, data for each biomechanical factor was further divided. Skeletal malalignment was subdivided into varus and valgus alignment, and muscle dysfunction was subdivided into extensor and flexor weakness. Impaired proprioception was subdivided into reposition error, and thresholds to detect a passive movement in the sagittal or frontal plane (varus and valgus direction). Laxity was subdivided into varus-valgus laxity measured at the medial and lateral side, and anterior-posterior laxity. Abnormal loading was subdivided into varus thrust, valgus thrust, knee adduction moment (KADM), knee flexion moment (KFM), etc.. One outcome measure per study for knee extensor and flexor strength was selected based on hierarchies described by Hall et al. [17] and Øiestadt et al. [10]. Measurements of abnormal loading during gait had to be reported as the peak or maximal value, or had to be examined during the same time period of the gait cycle. Varus and valgus thrust were assessed during early stance. KADM was assessed during early stance or midstance. KFM was assessed during midstance, while knee extension moment (KEM) was assessed during terminal stance.

Statistical analysis

Mean and standard deviation on continuous scales were transformed to odds ratio (OR) using the Chinn formula as described in the Cochrane Handbook [18]. Meta-analyses using random effects models were applied on the (logarithmic transformed) OR of developing knee OA in participants with the biomechanical factor of interest (cohort studies), or the (logarithmic transformed) OR of the biomechanical factor being present in participants with knee OA compared to the control group (cross-sectional studies). Meta-regression analyses were used to assess the impact of other risk factors (i.e. age, gender, BMI, knee injury) and radiographic severity on the association of biomechanical risk factors with knee OA or knee OA development.

Heterogeneity between studies was examined with standard Q-tests, and calculated as the I^2 statistics. Secondary analyses were described in the protocol [14]. The Grading of Recommendation, Assessment, Development and Evaluation (GRADE) framework was used to evaluate quality of evidence [19].

Results

A total of 6413 unique studies were identified. Eighty-six studies met all eligibility criteria and 59 were included in meta-analyses, as 27 studies did not provide sufficient data for the meta-analysis (Fig. 1).

Only cross-sectional studies were included, as no longitudinal studies fulfilled the in- and exclusion criteria. Therefore, we could not report on the association of specific biomechanical factors and knee OA development. Due to sparse data for most meta-analyses it was not feasible to investigate the impact (moderation) of other relevant risk factors on any associations, thus no meta-regression analyses were performed. Few studies reported data on biomechanical outcomes for different level of radiographic severity, precluding any sub group analysis based on disease severity [20–23]. Therefore, we present a comprehensive overview of the direction and magnitude of associations between knee OA and biomechanical factors. Duplicate data extraction on 86 studies was deemed not reasonable time wise, thus we performed duplicate data extraction on half of the studies (JT/ADI), and single data extraction on the other half (JT).

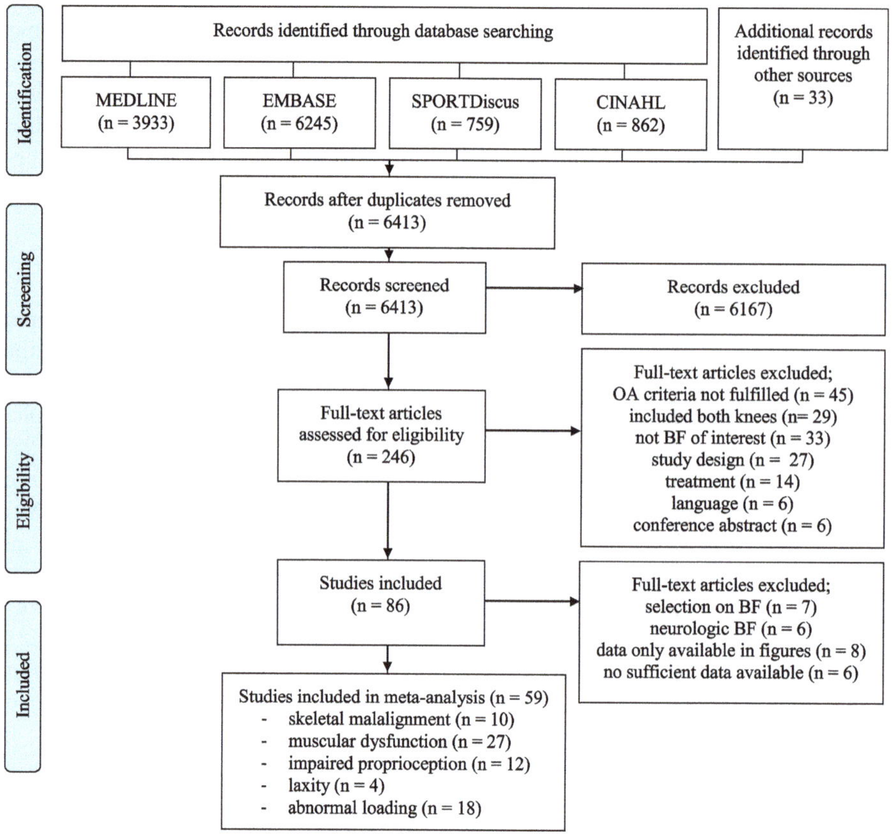

Fig. 1 Flow diagram of study selection. Other sources were reference lists of included papers and suggestions from experts in the field. OA: osteoarthritis, BF: biomechanical factor

Study characteristics

The 59 cross-sectional studies for meta-analyses included a total of 9825 participants (5328 patients with knee OA and 4497 healthy controls). 57% of the knee OA patients and controls were women. Mean age was 63.5 and 61.4 years for knee OA patients and controls, respectively. Mean BMI (kg/m^2) was 29.1 for knee OA patients and 26.5 for controls. As few studies included information on previous knee injury, and knee injury was often used as an exclusion criterion for knee OA patients, healthy controls, or both, we have not included information on this. Sixteen studies reported radiographic severity. Twenty-one studies assessed patients with medial knee OA, 37 with a combination of both compartments or the involved compartment was not specified, and one study assessed patients with medial and lateral knee OA separately.

Skeletal malalignment was assessed in 10 studies ($n = 1051$) [24–33], muscular dysfunction in 27 studies ($n = 6086$) [20, 21, 23–25, 27, 34–54], impaired proprioception in 12 studies ($n = 565$) [34, 37, 46, 54–62], laxity in four studies ($n = 321$) [22, 23, 27, 63], and abnormal loading in 18 studies ($n = 5974$) [25, 27, 50, 64–78] (Table 1). A summary of findings table can be found in Additional file 1, and forest plots of data pooling for each of the domains and the presence of knee OA can be found in Additional file 2.

As the number of included studies for each specific biomechanical factor was lower than expected, we could not perform all secondary analyses suggested in the protocol. We stratified analyses in the domains malalignment and abnormal loading during gait for medial knee OA, lateral knee OA, and medial/lateral knee OA (a combination of both or involved compartment was not reported), as biomechanical mechanisms will differ based on the involved compartment. The involved compartment was assumed to be medial (or lateral) when 80% or more of the participants was reported to have medial (or lateral) knee OA.

Assessment of risk of bias of individual studies and overall quality of evidence

Based on the assessment of risk of bias of individual studies, 32 had a low risk of bias, and 27 studies had a high risk of bias (Table 1). High risk of bias was most often based on a high risk in the areas participation and/

Table 1 Study characteristics

Study	No. OA and control (% female)	Group age, mean ± SD	Group BMI, mean ± SD	Definition OA	Radiographic severity OA	Compartment	Biomechanical factor	Risk of bias
Nordesjö (1983)	OA:14 (85.7) C:96 (47.9)	OA:68 C: NR	NR	Radiographic	NR	Medial / lateral OA	MUSC (extensor weakness; flexor weakness)	High
Hall (1993)	OA:21 (81.0) C:21 (81.0)	OA:62.6 ± 13.9 C:62.2 ± 13.8	OA:29.6 C:25.5	Symptomatic	NR	Medial / lateral OA	MUSC (extensor weakness; flexor weakness)	High
Marks (1993)	OA:10 (100) C:10 (100)	OA: 54.6 ± 9.87 C:48.2 ± 6.97	OA:30.14 C:24.39	Symptomatic	NR	Medial / lateral OA	PROP (reposition error)	High
Marks (1996)	OA:15 (100) C:11 (100)	OA:60.07 ± 10.74 C:48.63 ± 6.77	NR	Symptomatic	NR	Medial / lateral OA	PROP (reposition error)	High
Cooke (1997)	OA:167 (54.4) C:40 (65)	OA:66 ± 12 C:66 ± 8	NR	Radiographic and symptomatic	NR	Medial / lateral OA	MAL (varus)	High
Pai (1997)	OA:30 (73.3) C:29 (58.6)	OA:68.2 ± 8.3 C:71.3 ± 8.3	OA:28.6 ± 4.1 C:24.9 ± 3.9	Radiographic	KL2: 10, KL3: 13, KL4: 7	Medial / lateral OA	PROP (TDPM)	Low
Sharma (1997)	OA:28 (53.6) C:29 (55.2)	OA:65.5 ± 14.5 C:71 ± 11.5	OA:28.9 ± 5.8 C:26.3 ± 5.7	Radiographic	KL2: 7, KL3: 12, KL4: 9	Medial / lateral OA	PROP (TDPM)	Low
Garsden (1999)	OA:20 (50) C:20 (50)	OA:62.8 (R 50–73) C:60.8 (R 51–71)	NR	Radiographic and symptomatic	NR	Medial / lateral OA	PROP (reposition error)	High
Cheing (2001)	OA:66 (86.4) C:10 (50)	OA: women 63.5 ± 7.8; men 63.9 ± 8.9 C: women 57.4 ± 6.6; men 62.4 ± 8.4	OA: women 27.7 ± 4.2; men 26.3 ± 3.5 C: women 24.4 ± 1.8; men 25.5 ± 4.8	Radiographic	NR	Medial / lateral OA	MUSC (extensor weakness; flexor weakness)	Low
Kaufman (2001)	OA:139 (66.2) C:20 (55)	OA:57 ± 12.5 C:30 ± 8	OA:30.48 C:25.06	Radiographic and symptomatic	NR	Medial / lateral OA	LOAD (KEM; KADM; KABM; KIRM; KERM)	Low
Hortobagyi (2004)	OA:20 (75) C:20 (75)	OA:57.5 ± 7.3 C:56.8 ± 5	OA:29.3 ± 3.2 C:28.3 ± 3	Radiographic	NR	Medial / lateral OA	PROP (reposition error)	Low
Lewek (2004)	OA:12 (41.7) C:12 (50.0)	OA:52.6 ± 7.2 C:48.9 ± 4.9	OA:31.3 ± 5.1 C:28.6 ± 5.6	Radiographic and symptomatic	NR	Medial OA	MUSC (extensor weakness)	High
Lewek (2005)	OA:21 (33.3) C:19 (36.8)	OA:49.3 ± 7 C:49.3 ± 5.8	OA:30 ± 4.3 C:28.3 ± 4.9	Radiographic and symptomatic	NR	Medial OA	Laxity (varus-valgus: medial; varus-valgus:lateral)	High
Aoda (2006)	OA:688 (NR) C:568 (NR)	NR	NR	Radiographic	KL2: 510, KL3: 136, KL4: 42	Medial / lateral OA	LOAD (varus thrust)	High
Hall (2006)	OA with pain:36 (61.1) OA without pain:23 (69.6) C: 55 (69.1)	OA with pain: 68.78 ± 7.8 OA without pain: 69.22 ± 5.78 C:67.49 ± 8.45	OA with pain: 29.72 ± 4.4 OA without pain: 28.45 ± 4.69 C:25.89 ± 3.97	Radiographic and symptomatic	NR	Medial / lateral OA	MUSC (extensor weakness); PROP (reposition error)	Low
Zhai (2006)	OA:239 (23.4) C:261 (17.6)	OA:62.7 ± 7.1 C:63.0 ± 7.4	OA:28.7 ± 5.3 C:26.9 ± 4.1	Symptomatic	NR	Medial / lateral OA	MUSC (extensor weakness)	High

Table 1 Study characteristics *(Continued)*

Study	No. OA and control (% female)	Group age, mean ± SD	Group BMI, mean ± SD	Definition OA	Radiographic severity OA	Compartment	Biomechanical factor	Risk of bias
Ling (2007)	OA:17 (NR) C:22 (NR)	NR	NR	Radiographic	KL2: 4, KL3: 9, KL4: 4	Medial / lateral OA	MUSC (extensor weakness)	Low
Petterson (2007)	OA:44 (56.8) C:44 (56.8)	OA:62.3 ± 6.8 C:61.3 ± 7.7	OA:27.9 ± 3.9 C:26.8 ± 4.4	Symptomatic	NR	Medial / lateral OA	MUSC (extensor weakness)	High
Rudolph (2007)	OA:15 (46.7) C:15 (46.7)	OA:49.2 (R 39–57) C:49.2 (R 40–57)	OA:30.7 ± 4.8 C:28.7 ± 5.5	Symptomatic	NR	Medial OA	MAL (varus)	High
Schmitt (2007)	OA:28 (50) C:26 (50)	OA: 60.4 (R 39–78) C: 58.5 (R 38–76)	OA:31.84 C:29.74	Radiographic	NR	Medial OA	MAL (varus); MUSC (extensor weakness); Laxity (varus-valgus: medial; varus-valgus:lateral); LOAD (KFM; KEM: KADM)	Low
Thorp (2007)	OA:52 (73.1) C:37 (73.0)	OA:56.2 ± 10.4 C:53.6 ± 6.1	OA:29.1 ± 3.9 C:26.7 ± 3.9	Radiographic	NR	Medial OA	LOAD (KADM)	Low
Zhai (2007)	OA:56 (NR) C:259 (NR)	NR	NR	Radiographic	NR	Medial / lateral OA	MAL (varus; valgus)	High
Astephen (2008)	OA:61 (54.1) C:60 (61.7)	OA:64.49 ± 7.75 C:50.27 ± 10.09	OA:32.05 ± 5.48 C:25.45 ± 4.04	Radiographic and symptomatic	NR	Medial / lateral OA	LOAD (KFM; KIRM)	High
Janakiramanan (2008)	OA:74 (64) C:128 (78)	OA:59.4 ± 8.5 C:63.8 ± 10	OA:29.4 ± 5.3 C:26.8 ± 4.8	Radiographic	NR	Medial / lateral OA	MAL (valgus)	Low
Liikavainio (2008)	OA:54 (0) C:53 (0)	OA:59 ± 5.3 C:59.2 ± 4.7	OA:29.7 ± 4.7 C:27.1 ± 3.1	Symptomatic	KL1: 12, KL2: 15, KL3: 19, KL4: 8[d]	Medial / lateral OA	MUSC (extensor weakness; flexor weakness)	Low
Lund (2008)	OA:21 (100) C:29 (100)	OA:57.1 ± 12 C:55.3 ± 10.1	OA:28.5 ± 7.4 C:23.3 ± 7.4	Radiographic and symptomatic	NR	Medial / lateral OA	PROP (reposition error; TDPM)	Low
Mohammadi (2008)	OA:30 (100) C:30 (100)	OA:46.4 ± 5.1 C:45.4 ± 4.9	OA:27.1 ± 3.3 C:26.9 ± 4.3	Symptomatic	KL1/2: 5, KL3/4: 26[d, e]	Medial / lateral OA	MUSC (extensor weakness); PROP (reposition error)	Low
Wu (2008)	OA:11 (72.7) C:10 (70.0)	OA:61.1 ± 10.3 C:61.4 ± 6.5	OA:24.4 ± 2.4 C:23.2 ± 2.2	Radiographic	NR	Medial / lateral OA	MUSC (extensor weakness)	High
Heiden (2009a)	OA:54 (55.6) C:27 (66.7)	OA:65.6 ± 7.6 C:64.2 ± 5.1	OA:28.1 ± 4.2 C:24.4 ± 3.6	Radiographic	NR	Medial / lateral OA	LOAD (KEM; KADM)	Low
Heiden (2009b)	OA:54 (55.6) C:27 (66.7)	OA:57 ± 10 C:56 ± 15	OA:29 ± 7 C:25 ± 4	Radiographic	NR	Medial / lateral OA	MUSC (extensor weakness)	Low
Chang (2010)	OA:2026 (57.5) C:1566 (58.7)	OA:63.4 ± 9.1 C:61.0 ± 8.9	OA:29.4 ± 4.8 C:27.6 ± 4.6	Radiographic	NR	Medial / lateral OA	MUSC (extensor weakness); LOAD (valgus and varus thrust)	Low
Cibere (2010)	OA:98 (53) C:33 (52)	OA M:65 C M:47	OA M:26.6 C M:24.1	Symptomatic	NR	Medial / lateral OA	MAL (varus; valgus)	High
Dixon (2010)	OA:37 (62) C:11 (64)	OA: 65.6 ± 9.2 C:57.3 ± 9.5	OA:29.5 ± 4.1 C:25.3 ± 3.1	Radiographic and symptomatic	KL1: 3, KL2: 9, KL3: 10, KL4: 15[d]	Medial OA	LOAD (KEM)	High

Table 1 Study characteristics *(Continued)*

Study	No. OA and control (% female)	Group age, mean ± SD	Group BMI, mean ± SD	Definition OA	Radiographic severity OA	Compartment	Biomechanical factor	Risk of bias
Foroughi (2010)	OA:17 (100) C:17 (100)	OA:66 ± 8 C:51 ± 7	OA:26 ± 3 C:25 ± 4	Symptomatic	NR	Medial OA	MAL (varus); MUSC (extensor weakness); LOAD (KADM)	Low
Linley (2010)	OA:40 (57.5) C:40 (57.5)	OA:63 ± 10 C:64 ± 9	OA:27.4 ± 5.5 C:24 ± 3.2	Radiographic and symptomatic	KL1: 4, KL2: 20, KL3: 9, KL4: 7[d]	Medial OA	LOAD (KADM)	Low
Creaby (2010)	mild OA: 50 (54.0) moderate OA: 45 (44.4) severe OA: 32 (34.4) C:32 (53.1)	mild OA: 61.61 ± 7.12 moderate OA: 65.23 ± 7.72 severe OA: 66.4 ± 9.39 C:59.39 ± 6.92	mild OA: 28.37 ± 4.72 moderate OA: 30.03 ± 4.31 severe OA: 29.72 ± 5.2 C:26.62 ± 2.82	Radiographic and symptomatic	NR	Medial OA	Laxity (varus-valgus: medial; varus-valgus:lateral)	Low
Berger (2011)	OA:8 (50) C:8 (50)	OA:61.3 ± 3.8 C:61.8 ± 5.9	OA:33.4 ± 4.6 C:27.0 ± 27.3[1]	Radiographic and symptomatic	NR	Medial / lateral OA	MUSC (extensor weakness)	High
Butler (2011)	MOA:15 (NR) LOA:15 (NR) C:15 (NR)	MOA:66.2 ± 7.8 LOA:65.7 ± 6.4 C:56.3 ± 10.7	MOA:32.2 ± 7.9 LOA:30.4 ± 7.5 C:27.8 ± 5.7	Radiographic	MOA: KL2: 5, KL3: 4, KL4: 6 LOA: KL2: 3, KL3: 5, KL4: 7	Medial and lateral OA	LOAD (KADM)	Low
Cammarata (2011)	OA:13 (46.2) C:14 (50)	OA:57 ± 10 C:56 ± 15	OA:29 ± 7 C:25 ± 4	Radiographic and symptomatic	NR	Medial / lateral OA	MUSC (extensor weakness; flexor weakness)	Low
Zeni (2011)	OA:30 (NR) C:15 (NR)	OA:63 ± 7 C:58 ± 9	OA:29.75 ± 4.2 C:25.58 ± 3.5	Radiographic	NR	Medial OA	MUSC (extensor weakness, flexor weakness)	High
Cammarata (2012)	OA:13 (46.2) C:14 (50)	OA:57 ± 10 C:56 ± 15	OA:29 ± 7 C:25 ± 4	Radiographic and symptomatic	NR	Medial / lateral OA	PROP (TDPM-varus; TDPM-valgus)	Low
Conroy (2012)	OA with pain: 170 (59) OA without pain: 91 (58) C:334 (58)	OA with pain: 74.1 ± 3.1 OA without pain: 73.7 ± 2.9 C:73.3 ± 2.7	OA with pain: 30.1 ± 4.8 OA without pain: 30.5 ± 5 C:26.4 ± 4.3	Radiographic and symptomatic	NR	Medial / lateral OA	MUSC (extensor weakness)	High
Fallah-Yakhdani (2012)	OA:16 (68.8) C:12 (58.3)	OA:62.3 ± 10.7 C:62.0 ± 12.6	OA:29.7 ± 4.1 C:29.4 ± 4.9	Symptomatic	NR	Medial / lateral OA	MAL (varus; valgus)	High
Levinger (2012)	OA:32 (50) C:28 (53.6)	OA:65.8 ± 7.5 C:65.2 ± 11.4	OA:29.9 ± 5.2 C:25.5 ± 3.9	Radiographic	NR	Medial OA	LOAD (KADM)	Low
Miyazaki (2012)	mild OA: 20 (100) advanced OA:26 (100) C:22 (100)	mild OA: 3.8 ± 9.2 advanced OA: 74.1 ± 7.9 C:71.8 ± 8.3	mild OA: 22.6 ± 2 advanced OA: 23.5 ± 2.9 C:23.6 ± 2.2	Radiographic	KL2: 20, KL3: 16, KL4: 10	Medial OA	MUSC (extensor weakness); Laxity (anterior-posterior)	Low

Table 1 Study characteristics *(Continued)*

Study	No. OA and control (% female)	Group age, mean ± SD	Group BMI, mean ± SD	Definition OA	Radiographic severity OA	Compartment	Biomechanical factor	Risk of bias
Baert (2013a)	OA:24 (100) C:20 (100)	OA:64 ± 7.5 C:62.9 ± 8	OA:27.8 ± 4 C:25.2 ± 3.6	Symptomatic	KL2: 11, KL3: 8, KL4: 5	Medial / lateral OA	MUSC (extensor weakness; flexor weakness); PROP (reposition error)	Low
Baert (2013b)	OA:12 (100) C:14 (100)	OA:68.3 ± 6.8 C:65.8 ± 9.9	OA:28.6 ± 4.1 C: 24.8 ± 3.2	Symptomatic	KL2: 7, KL3: 3, KL4: 2	Medial OA	MAL (varus; valgus); MUSC (extensor weakness)	Low
Kumar (2013)	OA:16 (50) C:12 (50)	OA:65.2 ± 9.5 C:59.5 ± 10.4	OA:28.6 ± 4.3 C:28.4 ± 5.2	Radiographic	NR	Medial OA	MUSC (extensor weakness)	Low
Maly (2013a)[b]	OA:73 (100) C:52 (100)	OA:64.6 ± 6.7 C:60.7 ± 7.1	OA:29.1 ± 4.7 C:26.4 ± 5.0	Radiographic	NR	Medial OA	MUSC (extensor weakness)	Low
Maly (2013b)	OA:31 (29.0) C:30 (53.3)	OA:53.2 ± 6.1 C:33.5 ± 8	OA:30.6 ± 4.3 C:25 ± 4.2	Radiographic and symptomatic	KL2: 14, KL3: 13, KL4: 4	Medial OA	LOAD (KADM)	High
Metcalfe (2013)	OA:20 (45) C:20 (50)	OA:69 ± 7.2 C:68.3 ± 5.9	OA:31.1 ± 3.5 C:26.3 ± 3.6	Radiographic and symptomatic	KL3: 7, KL4: 13	Medial OA	LOAD (KADM)	High
Perry (2013)	OA:19 (52.6) C:17 (47.1)	OA:69.9 ± 6.5 C:66.8 ± 6.4	OA:29.8 ± 3.83 C:28.9 ± 4.7	Symptomatic	NR	Medial / lateral OA	MUSC (extensor weakness)	High
Sagawa (2013)[c]	OA:90 (58.9) C:52 ($n = 26$) (53.8)	OA:68 ± 7 C:66 ± 8	OA:30.4 ± 5.2 C:23.4 ± 2.3	Radiographic and symptomatic	NR	Medial / lateral OA	LOAD (KADM)	Low
Chang (2014)	OA:14 (57) C:14 (57)	OA:60 ± 8.7 C:58.4 ± 9.5	OA:30.5 ± 8 C:23.9 ± 3.1	Radiographic and symptomatic	NR	Medial OA	PROP (TDPM-varus; TDPM-valgus)	Low
Duffell (2014a)	OA:18 (NR) C:18 (NR)	OA:56.4 ± 12.4 C:56.2 ± 13	OA:26.61 C:24.13	Radiographic and symptomatic	NR	Medial OA	LOAD (KADM)	High
Duffell (2014b)	OA:15 (13.3) C:9 (44.4)	OA:54 C:31	OA:25.7 C:22.2	Symptomatic	NR	Medial / lateral OA	MAL (valgus)	High
Favre (2014)	OA:26 (62) C:27 (44)	OA:62 ± 10 C:57 ± 8	OA:29 ± 5 C:27 ± 3	Radiographic and symptomatic	NR	Medial OA	LOAD (KFM; KEM)	Low
Kumar (2014)	OA:30 (50) C:66 (57.6)	OA:57.7 (R:54.3–61.1) C:50.7 (R:48.4–53.1)	OA:26.9 (R:23.5–30.2) C:24.1 (R:23.2–25)	Radiographic and symptomatic	KL2: 10, KL3: 16, KL4: 4	Medial / lateral OA	MUSC (extensor weakness, flexor weakness)	Low
Winters (2014)	OA:26 (46.2) C:23 (47.8)	OA:65.3 ± 7.8 C:63.1 ± 7.7	OA:30.6 ± 4.6 C:25.8 ± 3.8	Radiographic	KL1: 7, KL2: 10, KL3: 10[d, f]	Medial OA	MUSC (extensor weakness); LOAD (KFM; KADM)	High

Legend: *OA* patients with knee osteoarthritis, *C* control group, *NR* not reported, *R* range, *M* median, *SD* standard deviation, *MAL* skeletal malalignment, *MUSC* muscular dysfunction, *PROP* impaired proprioception, *LAX* laxity, *LOAD* abnormal loading, *TDPM* threshold to detect a passive movement, *KFM* knee flexion moment, *KEM* knee extension moment, *KADM* knee adduction moment, *KABM* knee abduction moment, *KIRM* knee internal rotation moment, *KERM* knee external rotation moment, *KL* Kellgren and Lawrence grade. [a] This value seems not realistic, but it was stated in the published report, [b] Muscle strength was assessed for $n = 115$, [c] In controls 52 legs were assessed, [d] Patients with KL 1 were included in the osteoarthritis group as selection was based on other inclusion criteria such as pain, [e] Number of patients calculated from percentage, [f] 27 patients with radiographic severity reported, while 26 osteoarthritis patients are included in the study

or outcome measurement. Details regarding each of the six areas of potential study biases can be found in Additional file 3.

Skeletal malalignment

Low quality evidence was found for the odds of having malalignment in patients with knee OA compared to healthy controls (Fig. 2). Varus malalignment, assessed in four studies examining patients with medial knee OA [24–27], and in four studies examining patients with medial and/or lateral knee OA [28–31], was as prevalent in patients with and without knee OA (medial knee OA: OR = 0.64 [95% CI 0.21, 1.97], medial/lateral knee OA: OR = 0.85 [95% CI 0.54, 1.32]). Five studies assessing valgus malalignment in patients with medial and/or lateral knee OA showed no higher odds of having valgus malalignment in patients with knee OA (OR = 0.80 [95% CI 0.40, 1.61]) [28, 30–33]. One study indicated that patients with knee OA have lower odds of having valgus malalignment compared with healthy controls (OR = 0.16 [95% CI 0.07, 0.37]) [24].

Muscular dysfunction

Low quality evidence was found for the odds of having muscle weakness in patients with knee OA compared to controls (Fig. 3). Studies assessing muscle weakness showed that patients with medial and/or lateral knee OA had four times higher odds of having muscle weakness compared with healthy controls, both for extensor [21, 23–25, 27, 34–54] (OR = 4.02 [95% CI 2.69, 6.00], I^2 = 89.6%, number of studies (k) =27) and flexor muscles [21, 34, 36, 38, 40, 43, 47, 52] (OR = 4.09 [95% CI 1.48, 11.34], I^2 = 86.8%, k = 8). Both analyses showed considerable heterogeneity. Data regarding neurological characteristics (i.e. co-contraction index) had also been extracted, but differences in outcome measures and measurement techniques made it impossible to combine these.

Impaired proprioception

Low to moderate quality evidence was found for the odds of having impaired proprioception in patients with knee OA compared to controls (Fig. 4). Eight studies assessing proprioception as reposition error showed that patients with knee OA have higher odds of having higher reposition error (i.e. poorer proprioception) than healthy controls, with substantial heterogeneity (OR = 3.26 [95% CI 1.73, 6.13], I^2 = 63.1%) [34, 46, 54–59]. The odds of having a higher threshold to detect a passive movement in the sagittal plane was higher in patients with knee OA (OR = 4.44 [95% CI 2.78, 7.10], I^2 = 0.0%, k = 3), indicating poorer proprioception [57, 60, 62]. Two studies examining knee varus-valgus proprioceptive acuity (i.e. in the frontal plane) showed that patients with knee OA are more likely to have higher threshold to detect a passive movement in the varus direction (OR = 5.29 [95% CI 2.00, 13.97], I^2 = 0.0%), again indicating poorer proprioception [37, 61]. This was not observed in the valgus direction (OR = 4.65 [95% CI 0.55, 39.70], I^2 = 78.9%).

Joint laxity

All studies assessing joint laxity described patients with medial knee OA (Fig. 5). Three studies reported that

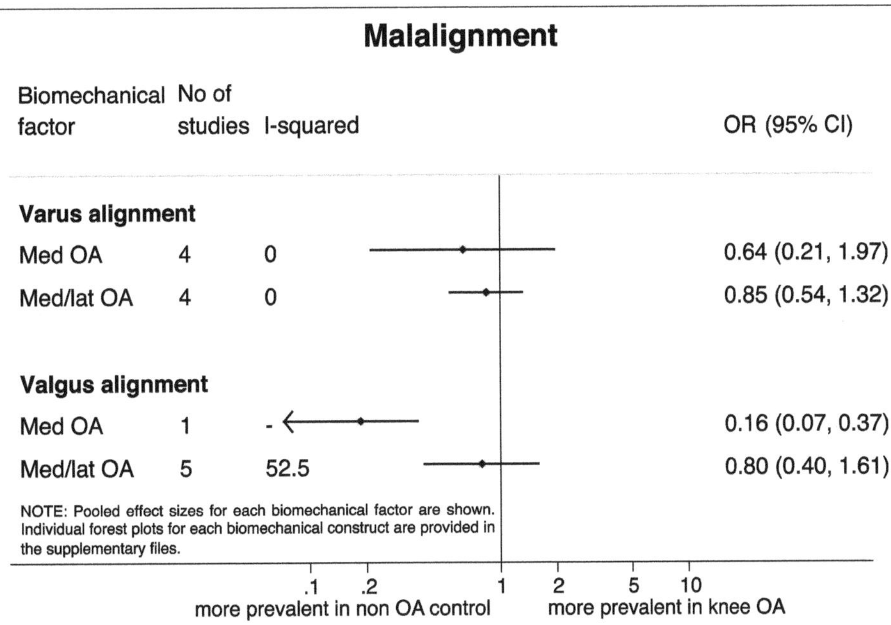

Fig. 2 Results of meta-analyses on skeletal malalignment and the presence of knee osteoarthritis. Results stratified for medial knee OA (Med OA) and a combination of both medial and lateral knee OA (or involved compartment not reported (Med/lat OA))

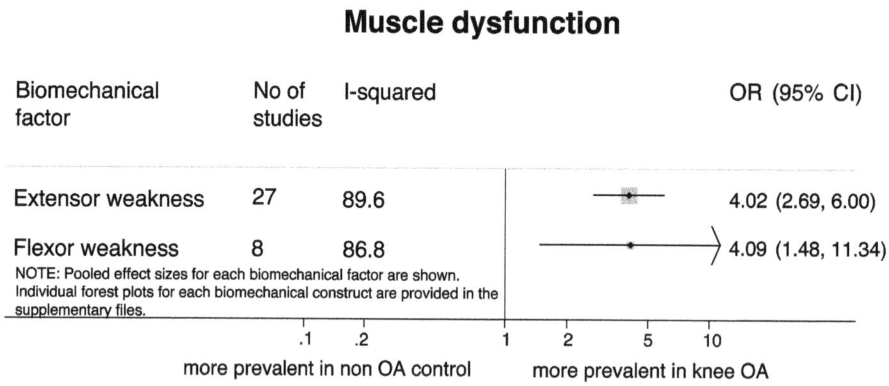

Fig. 3 Results of meta-analyses on muscular dysfunction and the presence of knee osteoarthritis

patients with medial knee OA have four times higher odds of having laxity in varus-valgus direction measured at the medial side of the joint (OR = 4.23 [95% CI 1.34, 13.36], $I^2 = 77.0\%$) [22, 27, 63], however, evidence was of low quality and considerable heterogeneity was present. The same three studies reported that patients with medial knee OA have lower odds of having varus-valgus laxity measured at the lateral side of the joint (OR = 0.42 [95% CI 0.25, 0.69], $I^2 = 0.0\%$). Evidence was of low quality. The only study that assessed laxity in anterior-posterior direction suggested no higher or lower odds for patients with medial knee OA compared to healthy controls [23].

Abnormal loading during gait

Very low to low quality evidence was found for most odds of having abnormal loading in patients with medial and/or lateral knee OA, only moderate quality evidence was found for the odds of having a higher KADM in patients with medial knee OA (Fig. 6). The two studies examining thrust concerned a population with medial and/or lateral knee OA. The odds of having varus thrust was higher in knee OA patients (OR = 1.46 [95% CI 1.00, 2.13], $I^2 = 79.2\%$) [64, 65], while patients with knee OA had no higher odds of having valgus thrust [65]. The odds of having a higher KFM was not higher in patients with medial knee OA [27, 50, 67], while significant higher odds were found for a higher KFM in the healthy controls in one study compared with patients with medial/lateral knee OA [66]. The odds for the presence of a higher knee extension moment (KEM) were not higher in patients with medial and/or lateral knee OA, with considerable heterogeneity [27, 67–70]. Ten studies showed that patients with medial knee OA had higher odds of having a higher knee adduction moment (KADM) (OR = 3.01 [95% CI 1.87, 4.85], $I^2 = 55.5\%$) [25, 27, 50, 71–75, 77, 78]. The only study [71] assessing this in patients with lateral knee OA reported higher odds for having higher KADM values in healthy controls, and

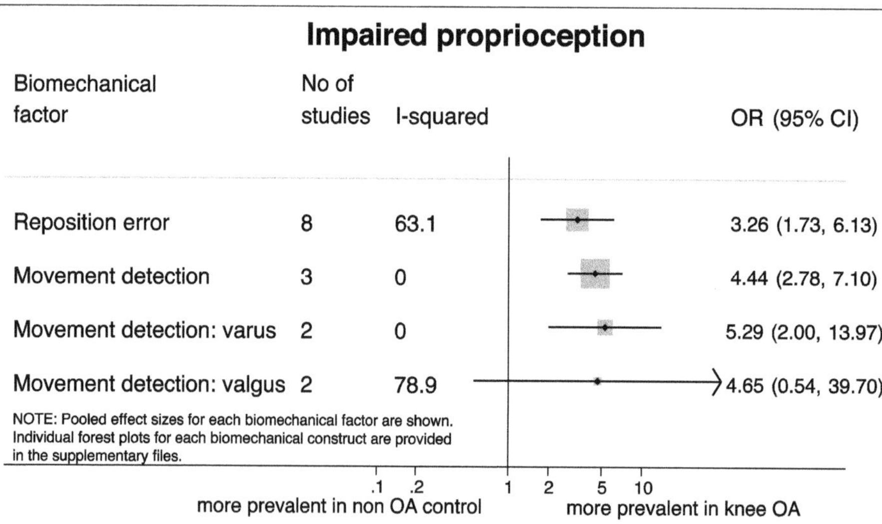

Fig. 4 Results of meta-analyses on impaired proprioception and the presence of knee osteoarthritis. Movement detection refers to the threshold to detect a passive movement in the sagittal or frontal plane

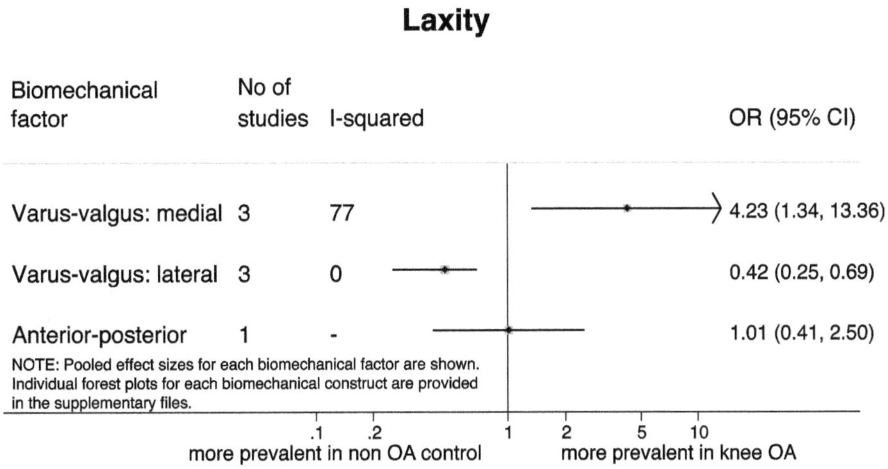

Fig. 5 Results of meta-analyses on laxity and the presence of knee osteoarthritis. Varus-valgus laxity is measured at the medial and lateral side of the knee

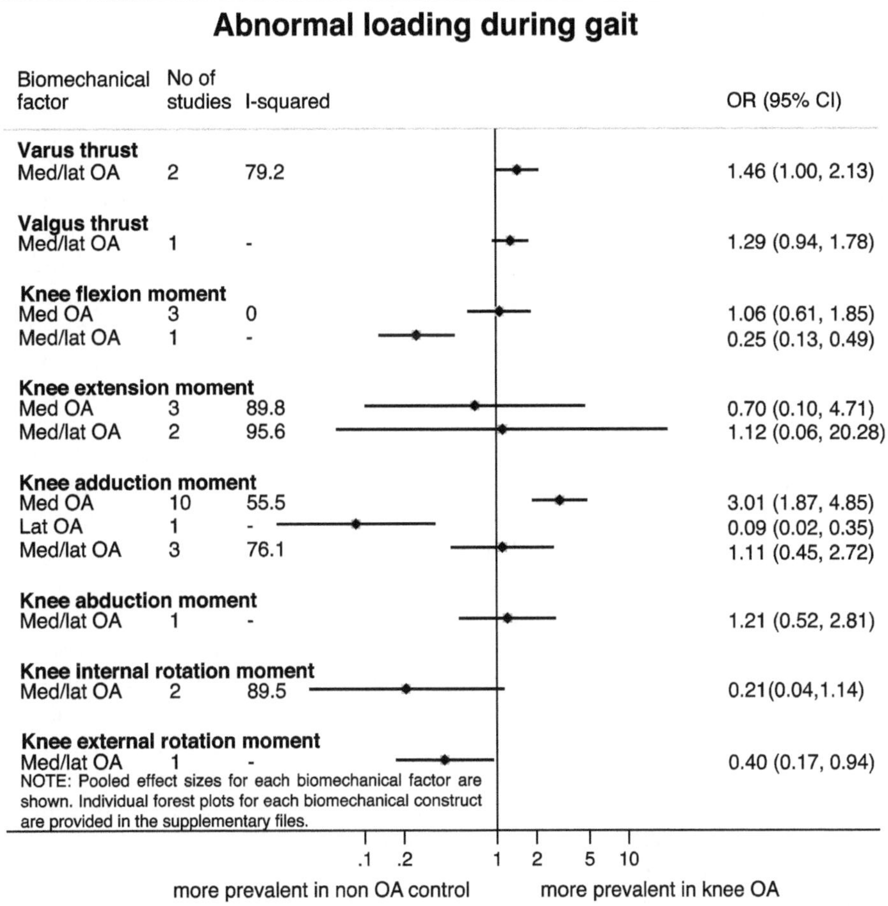

Fig. 6 Results of meta-analyses on abnormal loading during gait and the presence of knee osteoarthritis. Results stratified for medial knee OA (Med OA), lateral knee OA (Lat OA), and a combination of both medial and lateral knee OA (or involved compartment not reported (Med/lat OA))

patients with medial/lateral knee OA had no higher or lower odds than healthy controls (OR = 1.11 [95% CI 0.45, 2.72], $I^2 = 76.1\%$, k = 3) [69, 70, 76]. One study assessing both knee abduction moment (KABM) and knee external rotation moment (KERM) showed only higher odds in patients with medial/lateral knee OA for having a higher KERM [70]. The odds for having a higher knee internal rotation moment (KIRM) was not higher in patients with medial and/or lateral knee OA compared to healthy controls (OR = 0.21 [95% CI 0.04, 1.14], $I^2 = 89.5\%$, k = 2) [66, 70].

Discussion

This systematic review and meta-analyses aimed at investigating the association of specific biomechanical factors with knee OA and knee OA development, and potential effect modification of other relevant risk factors on this association. Based on the predefined selection criteria we did not include any longitudinal studies and sparse data combined with variations in studies for most meta-analyses made precluding any assessment of other relevant risk factors. As a result we could not investigate the association between biomechanical factors and knee OA development, and the impact of other relevant risk factors on any such associations. Thus, this study provides a comprehensive overview of the direction and magnitude of associations between different biomechanical factors and presence of knee OA. Based on mainly low quality evidence following GRADE, the results from this review indicate that patients with knee OA are characterized by lower knee extensor/flexor muscle strength, proprioception deficits, more medial varus-valgus laxity, less lateral varus-valgus laxity, and more varus thrust than healthy controls. Further, patients with medial knee OA are more likely to have a high knee adduction moment compared with healthy controls.

We intended to include longitudinal cohort studies to assess biomechanical risk factors for development of knee OA. However, based on our relative strict inclusion criteria allowing only studies where healthy individuals were available as comparators for assessing biomechanical risk factors, we were not able to include any cohort studies in this review. This was decided because changes in one leg may potentially impact the contralateral leg [4, 57, 79].

Impaired biomechanics is considered to be an important component of knee OA and such characteristics are often the justification of specific research questions. Although there is considerable evidence from individual studies describing those factors, we could not identify any attempts to summarize the association of skeletal malalignment, muscular dysfunction, impaired proprioception and laxity with knee OA by providing pooled estimates of associations. Pooled estimates have only been presented for the association of abnormal loading with knee OA [12]. This study expands this knowledge by providing an overview of the evidence of which biomechanical attributes describe patients with knee OA.

Our findings that decreased extensor/flexor strength and impaired proprioception are associated with knee OA confirm results of earlier narrative reviews [4–6, 80]. In addition, Freisinger et al. also found that patients with medial knee OA have an increased medial, but not lateral laxity [7]. Biomechanical characteristics during level walking have been the subject of a systematic review and meta-analysis by Mills et al. [12]. In agreement with our study, Mills reported conflicting evidence for the association of KFM with knee OA, which might be due to adaptations of walking pattern to reduce pain and instability [81]. In the same study, evidence for an association of KADM with knee OA was found to be inconclusive, whereas we found that patients with medial knee osteoarthritis have a higher KADM. Lack of stratification for the involved joint compartment in the study by Mills and co-workers could influence the results, as biomechanical mechanisms are expected to differ depending on the involved compartment. We were not able to stratify our varus and valgus thrust analysis for the involved compartment. In combination with the low number of included studies for those factors, this might explain why we only found a borderline significant association for varus thrust with knee OA.

Skeletal malalignment is also commonly reported to be present in patients with knee OA. Surprisingly, this was not found in the present study, although evidence was of low quality and methods used to assess malalignment were not uniform. Several individual studies have reported that varus and/or valgus malalignment are risk factors for the development and/or progression of knee OA [82–84], although one study stated that malalignment is not associated with knee OA development, and suggested that it rather is a marker of disease severity or its progression [85]. Those studies were not included in this review. The main reason for excluding studies was that they compared between knees instead of persons (i.e. allowing the contra-lateral leg as control), as evidence suggests that biomechanical factors are also altered in the contralateral knee highlighting the importance of an independent comparator [4, 57]. Another approach for future attempts to summarize such evidence, could be to include all available data and investigate the importance of type of control (i.e. healthy controls or contra-lateral leg) in sensitivity analysis to also be able to include more longitudinal studies. A systematic review and meta-analysis showed limited evidence for an association between knee malalignment and incident knee OA, although it also showed a relationship between varus and valgus alignment and structural progression of knee OA [8].

Limitations of this study warrant consideration. Our findings should be interpreted with caution due to the small number of included studies and the small sample size for most of the biomechanical factors (in particular skeletal malalignment and laxity). As a consequence of the above, and because all studies had a cross-sectional design, we rated most of the quality of evidence to low. Future studies should aim to improve the quality of the evidence.

This systematic review and meta-analysis identified several biomechanical characteristics of patients with knee OA. These findings are important for clinicians, as identification of such biomechanical impairments may help clinicians to better tailor interventions to the individual patient. In fact, the specific biomechanical profile of one patient may mean that some biomechanical interventions could be beneficial and others ineffective or even harmful. Clinical practices may not have the necessary specialized equipment to perform the biomechanical measurements that were performed in the included studies. However, clinical proxy measures exist to examine many of these biomechanical impairments (e.g. manual assessment of laxity or visual assessment of loading during gait by varus or valgus thrust). In addition, longitudinal cohort studies are needed to evaluate the importance of biomechanical factors in the development of knee osteoarthritis. Those studies should aim to evaluate biomechanical factors as risk factors for the development of knee OA. Furthermore, they should focus on the identification of subgroups. This will facilitate identification of persons at high risk of developing knee OA, who might want to be engaged in prevention programs. The longitudinal studies should include healthy persons, who have general risk factors for the development of knee OA, but do not have knee OA at baseline. The presence of knee OA should be assessed at baseline and follow up. General risk factors [86] and at least the biomechanical factors we identified as knee OA characteristics should be assessed. Data of healthy individuals should be compared with data of individuals developing knee OA in one or both knees.

Conclusions

In conclusion, results indicate that patients with knee OA are more likely to display a number of biomechanical characteristics such as lower muscle strength, proprioception deficits, more medial varus-valgus laxity and less lateral varus-valgus laxity and higher knee adduction moment (medial knee OA only) compared with healthy controls. The causal relationship between biomechanical factors and the development of knee OA could not be determined as no longitudinal studies were included. High quality longitudinal studies are needed to evaluate the impact of biomechanical factors on the development of knee OA.

Abbreviations

BMI: Body mass index; C: Control group; CI: Confidence interval; GRADE: Grading of Recommendation, Assessment, Development and Evaluation; k: Number of studies; KABM: Knee abduction moment; KADM: Knee adduction moment; KEM: Knee extension moment; KERM: Knee external rotation moment; KFM: Knee flexion moment; KIRM: Knee internal rotation moment; KL: Kellgren and Lawrence grade; LAX: Laxity; LOAD: Abnormal loading; M: Median; MAL: Skeletal malalignment; MUSC: Muscular dysfunction; n: Number of persons; NR: Not reported; OA: Osteoarthritis; OR: Odds ratio; PRISMA: Preferred Reporting Items for Systematic Reviews and Meta-analyses; PROP: Impaired proprioception; QUIPS tool: Quality In Prognostic Studies tool; R: Range; SD: Standard deviation; TDPM: Threshold to detect a passive movement

Funding

The research leading to these results has received funding form the European Union Seventh Framework Programme (FP7-PEOPLE-2013-ITN; KNEEMO) under grant agreement no. 607510. This funding body had no involvement in the study design, interpretation of data, writing the manuscript or the decision to publish the manuscript.

Authors' contributions

JT, ADI, CJ, JD, MS, and HL made substantial contributions to conception and design of the study. JT performed the data analysis and drafted the manuscript. JT, ADI, CJ, JBT, HL contributed to interpretation of the data. All authors contributed to critical revision of the article for important intellectual content, and read and approved the final version. All authors agreed to be accountable for all aspects for the work in ensuring that questions related to the accuracy or integrity of any part of the work are appropriately investigated and resolved.

Consent for publication

Not applicable.

Competing interests

The authors declare that they have no competing interests.

Author details

[1]Research Unit for Musculoskeletal Function and Physiotherapy, Department of Sports Science and Clinical Biomechanics, Faculty of Health Sciences, University of Southern Denmark, Campusvej 55, 5230 Odense, Denmark. [2]School of Health and Life Sciences, Glasgow Caledonian University, Glasgow, Scotland. [3]Department of Rehabilitation, Copenhagen University Hospital, Herlev and Gentofte, Denmark. [4]Department of Rehabilitation Medicine and Department of Psychiatry, EMGO Insitute for Health and Care Research, VU University Medical Center, Amsterdam, the Netherlands. [5]Centre for Evidence Based Practice, Western Norway University of Applied Sciences, Bergen, Norway.

References

1. Brandt KD, Radin EL, Dieppe PA, van de Putte L. Yet more evidence that osteoarthritis is not a cartilage disease. Ann Rheum Dis. 2006;65:1261–4.
2. Saxby DJ, Lloyd DG. Osteoarthritis year in review 2016: mechanics. Osteoarthr Cartil. 2017;25(2):190–8.
3. Bennell KL, Hunt MA, Wrigley TV, Lim BW, Hinman RS. Role of muscle in the genesis and management of knee osteoarthritis. Rheum Dis Clin N Am. 2008;34(3):731–54.
4. Knoop J, Steultjens MP, van der Leeden M, van der Esch M, Thorstensson CA, Roorda LD, Lems WF, Dekker J. Proprioception in knee osteoarthritis: a narrative review. Osteoarthr Cartil. 2011;19(4):381–8.
5. Bennell KL, Wrigley TV, Hunt MA, Lim BW, Hinman RS. Update on the role of muscle in the genesis and management of knee osteoarthritis. Rheum Dis Clin N Am. 2013;39(1):145–76.
6. Roos EM, Herzog W, Block JA, Bennell KL. Muscle weakness, afferent sensory dysfunction and exercise in knee osteoarthritis. Nat Rev Rheumatol. 2011; 7(1):57–63.
7. Freisinger GM, Schmitt LC, Wanamaker AB, Siston RA, Chaudhari AMW. Tibiofemoral osteoarthritis and varus-valgus laxity. J Knee Surg. 2017;30(5): 440–51.
8. Tanamas S, Hanna FS, Cicuttini FM, Wluka AE, Berry P, Urquhart DM. Does knee malalignment increase the risk of development and progression of knee osteoarthritis? A systematic review. Arthritis Rheum. 2009;61(4):459–67.
9. Henriksen M, Creaby MW, Lund H, Juhl C, Christensen R. Is there a causal link between knee loading and knee osteoarthritis progression? A systematic review and meta-analysis of cohort studies and randomised trials. BMJ Open. 2014;4(7):e005368.
10. Oiestad BE, Juhl CB, Eitzen I, Thorlund JB. Knee extensor muscle weakness is a risk factor for development of knee osteoarthritis. A systematic review and meta-analysis. Osteoarthr Cartil. 2015;23(2):171–7.
11. Culvenor AG, Ruhdorfer A, Juhl C, Eckstein F, Oiestad BE. Knee extensor strength and risk of structural, symptomatic, and functional decline in knee osteoarthritis: a systematic review and meta-analysis. Arthritis Care Res. 2017;69(5):649–58.
12. Mills K, Hunt MA, Ferber R. Biomechanical deviations during level walking associated with knee osteoarthritis: a systematic review and meta-analysis. Arthritis Care Res. 2013;65(10):1643–65.
13. Zhang W. Risk factors of knee osteoarthritis--excellent evidence but little has been done. Osteoarthr Cartil. 2010;18(1):1–2.
14. van Tunen JA, Dell'Isola A, Juhl C, Dekker J, Steultjens M, Lund H. Biomechanical factors associated with the development of tibiofemoral knee osteoarthritis: protocol for a systematic review and meta-analysis. BMJ Open. 2016;6(6):e011066.
15. Moher D, Liberati A, Tetzlaff J, Altman DG. Preferred reporting items for systematic reviews and meta-analyses: the PRISMA statement. PLoS Med. 2009;6(7):e1000097.
16. Hayden JA, van der Windt DA, Cartwright JL, Côté P, Bombardier C. Assessing bias in studies of prognostic factors. Ann Intern Med. 2013;158: 280–6.
17. Hall M, Juhl C, Lund H, Thorlund JB. Knee extensor muscle strength in middle-aged and older individuals undergoing arthroscopic partial meniscectomy: a systematic review and meta-analysis. Arthritis Care Res. 2015;67(9):1289–96.
18. Higgins JPT, Green S: Cochrane Handbook for Systematic Reviews of Interventions. 2011. Version 5.1.0. [http://handbook-5-1.cochrane.org].
19. Guyatt GH, Oxman AD, Schunemann HJ, Tugwell P, Knottnerus A. GRADE guidelines: a new series of articles in the journal of clinical epidemiology. J Clin Epidemiol. 2011;64(4):380–2.
20. Ling SM, Conwit RA, Talbot L, Shermack M, Wood JE, Dredge EM, Weeks MJ, Abernethy DR, Metter EJ. Electromyographic patterns suggest changes in motor unit physiology associated with early osteoarthritis of the knee. Osteoarthr Cartil. 2007;15(10):1134–40.
21. Liikavainio T, Lyytinen T, Tyrvainen E, Sipila S, Arokoski JP. Physical function and properties of quadriceps femoris muscle in men with knee osteoarthritis. Arch Phys Med Rehabil. 2008;89(11):2185–94.
22. Creaby MW, Wrigley TV, Lim BW, Bowles KA, Metcalf BR, Hinman RS, Bennell KL. Varus-valgus laxity and passive stiffness in medial knee osteoarthritis. Arthritis Care Res. 2010;62(9):1237–43.
23. Miyazaki T, Uchida K, Wada M, Sato M, Sugita D, Shimada S, Baba H. Anteroposterior and varus-valgus laxity of the knee increase after stair climbing in patients with mild osteoarthritis. Rheumatol Int. 2012;32(9): 2823–8.
24. Baert IAC, Jonkers I, Staes F, Luyten FP, Truijen S, Verschueren SMP. Gait characteristics and lower limb muscle strength in women with early and established knee osteoarthritis. Clin Biomech. 2013;28(1):40–7.
25. Foroughi N, Smith RM, Lange AK, Baker MK, Fiatarone Singh MA, Vanwanseele B. Dynamic alignment and its association with knee adduction moment in medial knee osteoarthritis. Knee. 2010;17(3):210–6.
26. Rudolph KS, Schmitt LC, Lewek MD. Age-related changes in strength, joint laxity, and walking patterns: are they related to knee osteoarthritis? Phys Ther. 2007;87(11):1422–32.
27. Schmitt LC, Rudolph KS. Influences on knee movement strategies during walking in persons with medial knee osteoarthritis. Arthritis Rheum. 2007; 57(6):1018–26.
28. Cibere J, Zhang H, Thorne A, Wong H, Singer J, Kopec JA, Guermazi A, Peterfy C, Nicolaou S, Munk PL, et al. Association of clinical findings with pre-radiographic and radiographic knee osteoarthritis in a population-based study. Arthritis Care Res. 2010;62(12):1691–8.
29. Cooke DT, Scudamore A, Li J, Wyss U, Bryant T, Costigan P. Axial lower-limb alignment; comparison of knee geometry in normal volunteers and osteoarthritis patients. Osteoarthr Cartil. 1997;5:39–47.
30. Fallah-Yakhdani HR, Abbasi-Bafghi H, Meijer OG, Bruijn SM, van den Dikkenberg N, Benedetti M-G, van Dieën JH. Determinants of co-contraction during walking before and after arthroplasty for knee osteoarthritis. Clin Biomech. 2012;27(5):485–94.
31. Zhai G, Ding C, Cicuttini F, Jones G. A longitudinal study of the association between knee alignment and change in cartilage volume and chondral defects in a largely non-osteoarthritic population. J Rheumatol. 2007;34(1): 181–6.
32. Janakiramanan N, Teichtahl AJ, Wluka AE, Ding C, Jones G, Davis SR, Cicuttini FM. Static knee alignment is associated with the risk of unicompartmental knee cartilage defects. J Orthop Res. 2008;26(2):225–30.
33. Duffell LD, Mushtaq J, Masjedi M, Cobb JP. The knee adduction angle of the osteo-arthritic knee: a comparison of 3D supine, static and dynamic alignment. Knee. 2014;21(6):1096–100.
34. Baert IA, Mahmoudian A, Nieuwenhuys A, Jonkers I, Staes F, Luyten FP, Truijen S, Verschueren SM. Proprioceptive accuracy in women with early and established knee osteoarthritis and its relation to functional ability, postural control, and muscle strength. Clin Rheumatol. 2013;32(9):1365–74.
35. Berger MJ, Chess DG, Doherty TJ. Vastus medialis motor unit properties in knee osteoarthritis. BMC Musculoskelet Disord. 2011;12:199.
36. Cammarata ML, Schnitzer TJ, Dhaher YY. Does knee osteoarthritis differentially modulate proprioceptive acuity in the frontal and sagittal planes of the knee? Arthritis Rheum. 2011;63(9):2681–9.
37. Chang AH, Lee SJ, Zhao H, Ren Y, Zhang LQ. Impaired varus-valgus proprioception and neuromuscular stabilization in medial knee osteoarthritis. J Biomech. 2014;47(2):360–6.
38. Cheing GL, Hui-Chan CW. The motor dysfunction of patients with knee osteoarthritis in a Chinese population. Arthritis Rheum. 2001;45(1):62–8.
39. Conroy MB, Kwoh CK, Krishnan E, Nevitt MC, Boudreau R, Carbone LD, Chen H, Harris TB, Newman AB, Goodpaster BH. Muscle strength, mass, and quality in older men and women with knee osteoarthritis. Arthritis Care Res. 2012;64(1):15–21.
40. Hall KD, Hayes KW, Falconer J. Differential strength decline in patients with osteoarthritis of the knee: revision of a hypothesis. Arthritis Care Res. 1993;6(2):89–96.
41. Heiden TL, Lloyd DG, Ackland TR. Knee extension and flexion weakness in people with knee osteoarthritis: is antagonist cocontraction a factor? J Orthop Sports Phys Ther. 2009;39(11):807–15.
42. Kumar D, Manal KT, Rudolph KS. Knee joint loading during gait in healthy controls and individuals with knee osteoarthritis. Osteoarthr Cartil. 2013; 21(2):298–305.
43. Kumar D, Karampinos DC, MacLeod TD, Lin W, Nardo L, Li X, Link TM, Majumdar S, Souza RB. Quadriceps intramuscular fat fraction rather than muscle size is associated with knee osteoarthritis. Osteoarthr Cartil. 2014;22(2):226–34.
44. Lewek MD, Rudolph KS, Snyder-Mackler L. Control of frontal plane knee laxity during gait in patients with medial compartment knee osteoarthritis. Osteoarthr Cartil. 2004;12(9):745–51.

45. Maly MR, Calder KM, Macintyre NJ, Beattie KA. Relationship of intermuscular fat volume in the thigh with knee extensor strength and physical performance in women at risk of or with knee osteoarthritis. Arthritis Care Res. 2013;65(1):44–52.
46. Mohammadi F, Taghizadeh S, Ghaffarinejad F, Khorrami M, Sobhani S. Proprioception, dynamic balance and maximal quadriceps strength in females with knee osteoarthritis and normal control subjects. Int J Rheum Dis. 2008;11(1):39–44.
47. Nordesjö L-O, Nordgren B, Wigren A, Kolstad K. Isometric strength and endurance in patients with severe rheumatoid arthritis or Osteoarthrosis in the knee joints. Scand J Rheumatol. 1983;12(2):152–6.
48. Petterson SC, Raisis L, Bodenstab A, Snyder-Mackler L. Disease-specific gender differences among total knee arthroplasty candidates. J Bone Joint Surg A. 2007;89(11):2327–33.
49. Perry BD, Levinger P, Serpiello FR, Caldow MK, Cameron-Smith D, Bartlett JR, Feller JA, Bergman NR, Levinger I, McKenna MJ. The effects of osteoarthritis and age on skeletal muscle strength, Na+-K+-ATPase content, gene and isoform expression. J Appl Physiol. 2013;115(10):1443–9.
50. Winters JD, Rudolph KS. Quadriceps rate of force development affects gait and function in people with knee osteoarthritis. Eur J Appl Physiol. 2014;114(2):273–84.
51. Wu S, Chu N, Liu Y, Chen C, Tang SFT, Cheng C. Relationship between the EMG ratio of muscle activation and bony structure in osteoarthritic knee patients with and without patellar malalignment. J Rehabil Med. 2008;40(5):381–6.
52. Zeni JA, Higginson JS. Knee osteoarthritis affects the distribution of joint moments during gait. Knee. 2011;18(3):156–9.
53. Zhai G, Blizzard L, Srikanth V, Ding C, Cooley H, Cicuttini F, Jones G. Correlates of knee pain in older adults: Tasmanian older adult cohort study. Arthritis Care Res. 2006;55(2):264–71.
54. Hall MC, Mockett SP, Doherty M. Relative impact of radiographic osteoarthritis and pain on quadriceps strength, proprioception, static postural sway and lower limb function. Ann Rheum Dis. 2006;65(7):865–70.
55. Garsden LR, Bullock-Saxton JE. Joint reposition sense in subjects with unilateral osteoarthritis of the knee. Clin Rehabil. 1999;13:148–55.
56. Hortobagyi T, Garry J, Holbert D, Devita P. Aberrations in the control of quadriceps muscle force in patients with knee osteoarthritis. Arthritis Rheum. 2004;51(4):562–9.
57. Lund H, Juul-Kristensen B, Hansen K, Christensen R, Christensen H, Danneskiold-Samsoe B, Bliddal H. Movement detection impaired in patients with knee osteoarthritis compared to healthy controls: a cross-sectional case-control study. J Musculoskelet Neuronal Interact. 2008;8(4):391–400.
58. Marks R, Quinney HA, Wessel J. Proprioceptive sensibility in women with normal and osteoarthritic knee joints. Clin Rheumatol. 1993;12(2):170–5.
59. Marks R. Further evidence of impaired position sense in knee osteoarthritis. Physiother Res Int. 1996;1(2):127–36.
60. Pai YC, Rymer WZ, Chang RW, Sharma L. Effect of age and osteoarthritis on knee proprioception. Arthritis Rheum. 1997;40(12):2260–5.
61. Cammarata ML, Dhaher YY. Associations between frontal plane joint stiffness and proprioceptive acuity in knee osteoarthritis. Arthritis Care Res. 2012;64(5):735–43.
62. Sharma L, Pai YC, Holtkamp K, Rymer WZ. Is knee joint proprioception worse in the arthritic knee versus the unaffected knee in unilateral knee osteoarthritis? Arthritis Rheum. 1997;40(8):1518–25.
63. Lewek MD, Ramsey DK, Snyder-Mackler L, Rudolph KS. Knee stabilization in patients with medial compartment knee osteoarthritis. Arthritis Care Res. 2005;52(9):2845–53.
64. Aoda H, Nakamura K, Omori G, Koga Y, Akazawa K, Yamamoto M. Independent predictors of knee osteoarthritis in an elderly Japanese population: a multivariate analysis. Acta Med Biol. 2006;54(2):33–41.
65. Chang A, Hochberg M, Song J, Dunlop D, Chmiel JS, Nevitt M, Hayes K, Eaton C, Bathon J, Jackson R, et al. Frequency of varus and valgus thrust and factors associated with thrust presence in persons with or at higher risk of developing knee osteoarthritis. Arthritis Rheum. 2010;62(5):1403–11.
66. Astephen JL, Deluzio KJ, Caldwell GE, Dunbar MJ. Biomechanical changes at the hip, knee, and ankle joints during gait are associated with knee osteoarthritis severity. J Orthop Res. 2008;26(3):332–41.
67. Favre J, Erhart-Hledik JC, Andriacchi TP. Age-related differences in sagittal-plane knee function at heel-strike of walking are increased in osteoarthritic patients. Osteoarthr Cartil. 2014;22(3):464–71.
68. Dixon SJ, Hinman RS, Creaby MW, Kemp G, Crossley KM. Knee joint stiffness during walking in knee osteoarthritis. Arthritis Care Res. 2010;62(1):38–44.
69. Heiden TL, Lloyd DG, Ackland TR. Knee joint kinematics, kinetics and muscle co-contraction in knee osteoarthritis patient gait. Clin Biomech. 2009;24(10):833–41.
70. Kaufman KR, Hughes C, Morrey BF, Morrey M, An KN. Gait characteristics of patients with knee osteoarthritis. J Biomech. 2001;34(7):907–15.
71. Butler RJ, Barrios JA, Royer T, Davis IS. Frontal-plane gait mechanics in people with medial knee osteoarthritis are different from those in people with lateral knee osteoarthritis. Phys Ther. 2011;91(8):1235–43.
72. Levinger P, Menz HB, Morrow AD, Feller JA, Bartlett JR, Bergman NR. Foot kinematics in people with medial compartment knee osteoarthritis. Rheumatology. 2012;51(12):2191–8.
73. Linley HS, Sled EA, Culham EG, Deluzio KJ. A biomechanical analysis of trunk and pelvis motion during gait in subjects with knee osteoarthritis compared to control subjects. Clin Biomech. 2010;25(10):1003–10.
74. Metcalfe AJ, Stewart C, Postans N, Dodds AL, Holt CA, Roberts AP. The effect of osteoarthritis of the knee on the biomechanics of other joints in the lower limbs. Bone Jt J. 2013;95(3):348–53.
75. Thorp LE, Sumner DR, Wimmer MA, Block JA. Relationship between pain and medial knee joint loading in mild radiographic knee osteoarthritis. Arthritis Rheum. 2007;57(7):1254–60.
76. Sagawa Y Jr, Armand S, Lubbeke A, Hoffmeyer P, Fritschy D, Suva D, Turcot K. Associations between gait and clinical parameters in patients with severe knee osteoarthritis: a multiple correspondence analysis. Clin Biomech. 2013; 28(3):299–305.
77. Duffell LD, Southgate DF, Gulati V, McGregor AH. Balance and gait adaptations in patients with early knee osteoarthritis. Gait Posture. 2014;39(4):1057–61.
78. Maly MR, Robbins SM, Stratford PW, Birmingham TB, Callaghan JP. Cumulative knee adductor load distinguishes between healthy and osteoarthritic knees--a proof of principle study. Gait Posture. 2013;37(3):397–401.
79. Messier SP, Beavers DP, Herman C, Hunter DJ, DeVita P. Are unilateral and bilateral knee osteoarthritis patients unique subsets of knee osteoarthritis? A biomechanical perspective. Osteoarthr Cartil. 2016;24(5):807–13.
80. Wodowski AJ, Swigler CW, Liu H, Nord KM, Toy PC, Mihalko WM. Proprioception and knee Arthroplasty: a literature review. Orthop Clin North Am. 2016;47(2):301–9.
81. Varady NH, Grodzinsky AJ. Osteoarthritis year in review 2015: mechanics. Osteoarthr Cartil. 2016;24(1):27–35.
82. Brouwer GM, Tol AW, Bergink AP, Belo JN, Bernsen RM, Reijman M, Pols HA, Bierma-Zeinstra SM. Association between valgus and varus alignment and the development and progression of radiographic osteoarthritis of the knee. Arthritis Rheum. 2007;56(4):1204–11.
83. Sharma L, Song J, Dunlop D, Felson D, Lewis CE, Segal N, Torner J, Cooke TD, Hietpas J, Lynch J, et al. Varus and valgus alignment and incident and progressive knee osteoarthritis. Ann Rheum Dis. 2010;69(11):1940–5.
84. Felson DT, Niu J, Gross KD, Englund M, Sharma L, Cooke TD, Guermazi A, Roemer FW, Segal N, Goggins JM, et al. Valgus malalignment is a risk factor for lateral knee osteoarthritis incidence and progression: findings from the multicenter osteoarthritis study and the osteoarthritis initiative. Arthritis Rheum. 2013;65(2):355–62.
85. Hunter DJ, Niu J, Felson DT, Harvey WF, Gross KD, McCree P, Aliabadi P, Sack B, Zhang Y. Knee alignment does not predict incident osteoarthritis: the Framingham osteoarthritis study. Arthritis Rheum. 2007;56(4):1212–8.
86. Silverwood V, Blagojevic-Bucknall M, Jinks C, Jordan JL, Protheroe J, Jordan KP. Current evidence on risk factors for knee osteoarthritis in older adults: a systematic review and meta-analysis. Osteoarthr Cartil. 2015;23(4):507–15.

15

Construct validity and reliability of the Finnish version of the Knee Injury and Osteoarthritis Outcome Score

Juhani Multanen[1*], Mikko Honkanen[2], Arja Häkkinen[1,3] and Ilkka Kiviranta[4]

Abstract

Background: The Knee Injury and Osteoarthritis Outcome Score (KOOS) is a commonly used knee assessment and outcome tool in both clinical work and research. However, it has not been formally translated and validated in Finnish. The purpose of this study was to translate and culturally adapt the KOOS questionnaire into Finnish and to determine its validity and reliability among Finnish middle-aged patients with knee injuries.

Methods: KOOS was translated and culturally adapted from English into Finnish. Subsequently, 59 patients with knee injuries completed the Finnish version of KOOS, Western Ontario and McMaster Osteoarthritis Index (WOMAC), Short-Form 36 Health Survey (SF-36) and Numeric Pain Rating Scale (Pain-NRS). The same KOOS questionnaire was re-administered 2 weeks later. Psychometric assessment of the Finnish KOOS was performed by testing its construct validity and reliability by using internal consistency, test-retest reliability and measurement error. The floor and ceiling effects were also examined.

Results: The cross-cultural adaptation revealed only minor cultural differences and was well received by the patients. For construct validity, high to moderate Spearman's Correlation Coefficients were found between the KOOS subscales and the WOMAC, SF-36, and Pain-NRS subscales. The Cronbach's alpha was from 0.79 to 0.96 for all subscales indicating acceptable internal consistency. The test-retest reliability was good to excellent, with Intraclass Correlation Coefficients ranging from 0.73 to 0.86 for all KOOS subscales. The minimal detectable change ranged from 17 to 34 on an individual level and from 2 to 4 on a group level. No floor or ceiling effects were observed.

Conclusion: This study yielded an appropriately translated and culturally adapted Finnish version of KOOS which demonstrated good validity and reliability. Our data indicate that the Finnish version of KOOS is suitable for assessment of the knee status of Finnish patients with different knee complaints. Further studies are needed to evaluate the predictive ability of KOOS in the Finnish population.

Keywords: KOOS, Knee injury, Knee osteoarthritis, Finnish, Reliability, Validity

Background

Knee pain is common complaint affecting people of all ages. In adult populations, the reported prevalence of knee pain has been 25–28% depending on the age of the examined persons and the level of pain chronicity [1–3]. In the younger age groups, knee pain is commonly secondary to increased activity, injury or contact sports [4–6]. In older people, however, knee pain that gets progressively worse over time is often sign of osteoarthritis (OA) [7, 8]. Knee OA in particular is associated with severe disability, owing to the weight-bearing function of the knee and the large range of movements it performs.

To be able to detect and treat individuals with a variety of knee problems effectively requires reliable and valid outcome measures, preferably at low cost. During recent decades, a few well-validated outcome measures have been developed for the assessment of symptoms and function in subjects with knee or hip OA [9–11]. In the elderly population, the Western Ontario and McMaster Osteoarthritis Index (WOMAC) is the

* Correspondence: juhani.multanen@ksshp.fi
[1]Department of Physical Medicine and Rehabilitation, Central Finland Central Hospital, Keskussairaalantie 19, FI-40620 Jyväskylä, Finland
Full list of author information is available at the end of the article

self-administered instrument most commonly used to measure pain, stiffness and function in daily living. However, in younger and/or more physically active subjects, joint injuries cause knee problems more often than primary knee OA per se. Younger patients also often have higher expectations regarding physical functioning. Thus, the WOMAC may not be appropriate for these subjects. Partly for this reason, the Knee injury and Osteoarthritis Outcome Score (KOOS) was developed in the late 1990s as an extension of the WOMAC index to address problems associated with knee injuries and/or knee OA [12].

KOOS is a disease-specific, patient-reported outcome (PRO) measure assessing perceived pain, other symptoms, activities of daily living, sport and recreation functions, and knee-related quality of life. It is freely accessible, and intended for use over the short- and long-term for both research and clinical purposes. KOOS has been found to be a valid, reliable and responsive outcome measure in different patient populations with varying knee injuries (of menisci, ACL or cartilage) [13, 14], knee OA [15–19] and total knee replacement [20]. Currently, KOOS is available in 50 different languages and language variants [21]. However, the validity and reliability of the Finnish version of KOOS in subjects with different knee problems or OA have not been previously reported. Hence, the purpose of this study was to produce a Finnish version of KOOS and to evaluate its construct validity and reliability in a sample of middle-aged patients with knee injuries.

Methods

Cross-cultural adaptation

Prior to the implementation of the KOOS questionnaire, a cross-cultural adaptation of the measure was performed in accordance with the recommendations by Beaton et al. (2000) [22]. The American-English KOOS [12] was translated into Finnish by two translators independently, one translator was an experienced orthopedic surgeon (T1) and the other a professional translator with no medical background or special knowledge of the concepts in question (T2). Both versions were then collated in a consensus meeting. This consensus version was translated back into English independently by two Finnish-speaking translators of English origin (BT1 and BT2) unfamiliar with the original questionnaire or concepts therein. The translations into Finnish and back translations into English were thereafter discussed and collated in a second consensus meeting. This version was then pre-tested with 16 postmenopausal women with mild knee OA to confirm if all the items in the questionnaire were understandable and whether the subjects experienced problems in answering any of them.

Patients and data acquisition

The study population comprised patients with diverse knee problems, including OA, post-traumatic injuries, meniscus and ligament problems. The patients had been referred to the Department of Orthopedics and Traumatology in Helsinki University Hospital from primary health care centers in the Hospital District of Helsinki and Uusimaa, where, based on clinical and radiographic or Magnetic Resonance Imaging findings, they were diagnosed as having OA or Anterior Cruciate Ligament (ACL), meniscus or combined ACL and meniscus injuries. For this study, all the assessed patients had to be in a clinically stable condition and not expected to undergo urgent surgery. The patients were recruited between March 2014 and May 2015 using a systematic sampling technique. The inclusion criteria were age 18 years or over, unresponsive to conservative treatment, and the ability to communicate in written Finnish. Eligible patients were informed about the study, and indicated their willingness to participate by giving their informed consent. For test-retest purposes, the participants were asked to complete KOOS twice: first, during the hospital visit, and then again 2 weeks later at home. During the hospital visit the patients were asked to fill in the KOOS along with the WOMAC, the SF-36 and the Numeric Rating Scale of Pain forms. One hundred thirty-one patients completed all four questionnaires during the hospital visit. Of these patients, 59 returned the KOOS questionnaire 2 weeks later from home by regular mail in a pre-paid envelope, yielding a sample of 59 patients for the study. The local Medical Ethics Committee of Helsinki University Hospital approved the study plan (Approval number 37/13/03/02/2014). Written informed consents were obtained and participants' rights protected.

Questionnaires

KOOS

KOOS is a patient-administered knee-specific questionnaire comprising five subscales: Pain (nine items); Symptoms (seven items); Activities of Daily Living (ADL) (17 items); Sport and Recreation (five items); and Knee-Related Quality of Life (QOL) (four items). Each item is scored from 0 (best) to 4 (worst) using a Likert type scale with 5 boxes. The raw score for each subscale is the sum of the item scores. Scores are then transformed to a 0 to 100 scale. The scores of the five subscales can be expressed as an outcome profile, higher scores indicating fewer problems. A total score has not been validated and is not recommended according to the KOOS Users Guide [21]. When filling the questionnaire the subjects are instructed to consider the previous week when answering the questions. The KOOS has a self-explanatory format and the questionnaire takes about 10 min to complete [12].

WOMAC

The Western Ontario and McMaster Osteoarthritis Index (WOMAC) is a disease-specific, self-administered health status instrument assessing pain, stiffness, and function in subjects with OA of the hip or knee [10]. The index consists of 24 questions in three dimensions: knee pain (5 questions), joint stiffness (2 questions) and functional ability (17 questions). These dimensions are often analyzed and reported separately, but the WOMAC index can also be aggregated into a single score. The original WOMAC is available in two formats: Visual Analog Scales (VAS) and Likert-boxes. In this study, we used the VAS format (0–100 mm), where the sum of the raw scores was transformed to a 0–100 scale. Higher scores indicate a higher level of joint pain, joint stiffness and functional limitation. For this study, however, to allow comparison between the KOOS and WOMAC outcomes, we reversed the scoring direction of the WOMAC outcomes, meaning that higher scores indicate decreased pain, joint stiffness and functional limitation. WOMAC has been extensively tested for reliability, validity and responsiveness in different countries [23]. The Finnish version of WOMAC has been validated for the short- and long-term follow-up of patients scheduled for total knee or hip arthroplasty [24].

SF-36

Health-related quality of life was measured using the Short-Form 36 Health Survey (SF-36) [25]. SF-36 is a generic survey comprising 8 distinct dimensions of health status: Physical Functioning, General Health, Vitality, Mental Health, Role- Physical, Role-Emotional, Social Functioning and Bodily Pain. The scale runs from 0 to 100 in each dimension, with a higher score indicating better health.

Pain-NRS

The subjective intensity of pain in general and in different body regions was measured on the numeric pain rating scale (Pain-NRS). The body regions in this study were neck, back, upper limb, lower limb and knee. The Pain-NRS is an 11-point scale ranging from 0 to 10, where 0 represents "no pain" and 10 represents "the most intense pain imaginable". For this study, however, as with WOMAC we reversed the scoring direction of the Pain-NRS outcomes, meaning that higher scores indicate "no pain" and lower scores indicate "the most intense pain imaginable". When filling the form, patients are asked to select the value that best describes the intensity of pain that they have experienced during the past week.

Background data

During their visit to the outpatient clinic, in addition to demographic data, patients were asked for anamnestic information regarding their knee problem, and to describe the intensity of their habitual physical activity (low = 1, moderate = 2, or high = 3–4).

Assessment of psychometric properties

Construct validity was determined by comparing the first administration of the five KOOS subscales against the five WOMAC subscales, the eight SF-36 subscales, and the six Pain-NRS subscales. On the assumption that the highest correlations can be expected to be observed when comparing scales that are intended to measure the same or similar constructs, we posited a priori sets of hypotheses about convergent relationships between physical health properties which are given in Table 4 in the results section. We defined the construct validity of the KOOS questionnaire as good if at least 75% of the hypotheses could be supported [26]. The *internal consistency* of the first-administered KOOS was determined by defining the degree of inter-relatedness among the items. *Test-retest reliability* was determined by comparing the scores of the first- and second-administered KOOS questionnaires. *Measurement error* is the systematic and random error of a patient's score that is not attributed to true changes in the construct to be measured [27]. The standard error of measurement (SEM) is a measure of the absolute measurement error of how much measured test scores tend to be distributed around a "true" score. SEM is expressed in the unit of measurement of the instrument. The minimal detectable change (MDC), in turn, is the threshold for determining clinical changes outside measurement error. The *floor and ceiling effect* of the KOOS was also examined. We checked each questionnaire for missing values prior to further analysis. The KOOS Users Guide 2012 rule was applied for missing items [21].

Statistical analyses

Quantitative variables are described using mean and standard deviation (SD) or median and interquartile range (IQR) values, and categorical variables are described using frequency and percentage values. Construct validity was calculated by using Spearman's correlation coefficient to assess the relationships between the KOOS subscales and the WOMAC, SF-36 and numeric pain rating scales. Correlation coefficients less than 0.2 were considered very weak, between 0.2 and 0.39 weak, between 0.4 and 0.59 moderate, between 0.6 and 0.79 strong, and above 0.79 very strong [28]. Internal consistency was determined by calculating Cronbach's α coefficient. A Cronbach's α equal to, or greater than, 0.70 is generally regarded as acceptable for internal consistency [29, 30]. Test-retest reliability, indicating the consistency of the KOOS scores between the first and second administration of the questionnaire, was calculated using the two-way random effect model of the intraclass correlation coefficient (ICC) presented with 95% confidence intervals (CI). ICC values above 0.81 were interpreted as excellent, whereas values between 0.80 and 0.61 indicated good, values between 0.60 and 0.41 moderate, values between 0.40 and 0.21 fair, and values below 0.20 low reliability [31]. SEM was calculated using the formula: SEM = $1.96\sqrt{(1\text{-R})}$, where 1.96 derives from the 0.95% CI and R represents the calculated ICC coefficient. MDC was calculated using the formula: MDC = SEM*$1.96\sqrt{2}$, where 2 represents two measurements evaluating the change [32]. For group comparison the MDC can be calculated, depending on the size of the group (n = 59), as follows: $MDC_{group} = MDC_{individual}/\sqrt{n}$ [33]. The floor and ceiling values representing the percentages of the patients who obtained the lowest or highest scores were calculated for each KOOS subscale separately. Floor and ceiling effects are considered present if more than 15% of the respondents achieve the lowest or highest possible scores [26].

Results

Patients

A total of 59 patients were included in the validity, internal consistency, test-retest, measurement error and floor/ceiling effects assessments. Mean participant age was 49 (SD 14), most were women (78%), and the median duration of knee symptoms was 7 months for women (IQR 4, 12) and 6 months for men (IQR 3, 18). Mean self-reported knee pain for all patients was 5.6 (SD 2.6) on a NRS scale of 0 to 10. The characteristics of the study population are presented in Table 1.

Only a few individual items (2%), all from the Pain and Sport and Recreation Function subscales, were missing, and hence a total score for all the subscales was available for all patients (Table 2). The lowest possible scores were reported by 5 (9%) patients for the subscale Sport and Recreation Function and by 4 (7%) patients for the subscale QOL. The best possible scores were reported by one patient (2%) for the subscales Pain and QOL, and by 2 patients (3%) for the subscales ADL and Sport and Recreation Function (Table 2).

Cross-cultural adaptation

The cross-cultural adaptation revealed minor cultural differences. In the subscale Activities of Daily Living, items A9 and A11 ("Putting on socks/stockings", and "Taking off stocks /stockings") the word "stockings" was omitted. In addition, item A13 on the same subscale ("Getting in/out of the bath") the word "shower" was added as an alternative to bath. The Finnish version of the KOOS questionnaire was well received by the sample of 16 postmenopausal women with mild knee OA. All the questions and response options were considered understandable and applicable. The back-translation of the Finnish version of the KOOS questionnaire is available in the additional file [see Additional file 1].

Table 1 Demographic and clinical characteristics of patients

Variables	Values
Women, n (%)	46 (78)
Age, mean (SD)	49 (14)
Body mass index, mean (SD)	26.5 (4.9)
≥30, n (%)	13 (22)
Employment status, n (%)	
Employed	41 (69)
Unemployed	8 (14)
Retired	10 (17)
White collar workers, n (%)	28 (47)
Duration of symptoms, month, median (IQR)	6 (3, 12)
Onset of knee pain, n (%)	
Accidentally	27 (46)
No clear event	32 (54)
Leisure time physical activity, n (%)	
Low	8 (14)
Moderate	27 (46)
High	24 (40)
Numeric Pain Rating Scale (0 to 10 scale)[a], mean (SD)	
General	4.5 (2.3)
Neck	2.6 (2.5)
Back	2.4 (2.5)
Upper limb	1.9 (2.6)
Lower limb	3.9 (3.1)
Knee	5.6 (2.6)

SD Standard Deviation, *IQR* Interquartile Range
[a]negative number indicates less pain

Construct validity

Overall, the highest correlations were found between the KOOS subscales and WOMAC subscales. As shown in Table 3, all the KOOS and WOMAC subscales correlated significantly, with values of r within the range 0.33 to 0.86. The highest correlations were between the subscales intended to measure similar constructs (KOOS ADL vs. WOMAC Physical function, r = 0.86; KOOS Pain vs. WOMAC Pain, r = 0.81). In addition, the KOOS Symptoms and WOMAC Stiffness subscales correlated moderately (r = 0.48). Thus, the set of a priori hypotheses posited for KOOS and WOMAC was supported (Table 4).

Table 2 Mean scores, response rates and floor and ceiling percentages for the Finnish KOOS subscales

	Mean (SD)	Response rate (%)	Floor[a] (%)	Ceiling[b] (%)
Pain	55.4 (22.3)	98	0	2
Symptoms	53.3 (13.4)	100	0	0
Activities of Daily Living	67.4 (23.0)	100	0	3
Sport and Recreation Function	32.9 (25.9)	98	9	3
Knee-related Quality of Life	32.3 (22.5)	100	7	2

100 = no knee problems, 0 = extreme knee problems
KOOS Knee Injury and Osteoarthritis Outcome Score, *SD* Standard Deviation
[a]Worst possible value on the subscale
[b]Best possible value on the subscale

Higher correlations were found for the KOOS scales and the SF-36 scales, indicating their high ability to measure physical health, i.e., Physical Functioning, Role-Physical, and Bodily Pain (Table 3). As with WOMAC, the highest correlation between KOOS and SF-36 was found between the subscales intended to measure similar constructs (KOOS Pain vs. SF-36 Bodily Pain, r = 0.69; KOOS ADL vs. SF-36 Physical Functioning, r = 0.83). The KOOS Sport and Recreation Function and SF-36 Physical Functioning subscales also correlated strongly (r = 0.67), thus supporting the set of a priori hypotheses posited for KOOS and SF-36 (Table 4). The correlations between the KOOS subscales and the SF-36 dimensions of General Health, Vitality, Mental Health, Role-Emotional and Social Functioning, were lower, indicating the KOOS's ability to measure rather physical than mental health.

Table 3 Spearman's correlation coefficients for comparisons of the five KOOS subscales with the three WOMAC subscales, eight SF-36 subscales, and the six Pain-NRS subscales

	KOOS Pain	KOOS Symptoms	KOOS ADL	KOOS Sport/Rec	KOOS QOL
WOMAC					
Pain	0.81	0.37	0.65	0.52	0.54
Stiffness	0.60	0.48	0.79	0.62	0.46
Physical function	0.75	0.33	0.86	0.72	0.63
SF-36					
Physical Functioning	0.70	0.43	0.83	0.67	0.66
General Health	0.11	0.25	0.39	0.13	0.10
Vitality	0.28	0.24	0.43	0.18	0.19
Mental Health	0.12	0.15	0.33	0.06	0.08
Role-Physical	0.39	0.34	0.58	0.36	0.30
Role-Emotional	0,41	0.22	0.60	0.29	0.23
Social Functioning	0.42	0.29	0.64	0.41	0.30
Bodily Pain	0.69	0.46	0.77	0.58	0.51
Pain-NRS					
General	0.42	0.23	0.48	0.44	0.53
Back	0.19	0.17	0.37	0.16	0.33
Lower limb	0.37	0.37	0.61	0.41	0.37
Neck	0.09	0.05	0.35	0.07	0.21
Upper limb	0.18	0.39	0.57	0.28	0.33
Knee	0.66	0.46	0.68	0.50	0.53

All correlations over 0.27 were significant at 0.05 level; N = 59
KOOS Knee Injury and Osteoarthritis Outcome Score, *ADL* Activities of Daily Living, *Sport/Rec* Sport and Recreation Function, *QOL* Quality of Life, *WOMAC* Western Ontario and McMaster Osteoarthritis Index, *SF-36* Short-Form 36 Health Survey, *Pain-NRS* Numeric Pain Rating Scale

The highest correlations between the KOOS and Pain-NRS subscales pertaining to different regions of the body were found for the knee area (r = 0.46–0.68) and lower limbs (r = 0.37–0.61) (Table 3). In addition, overall general pain showed moderate correlations with most of the KOOS subscales. The hypotheses of a strong correlation between KOOS ADL and Pain-NRS Knee (r = 0.68), and moderate correlation between KOOS QOL and Pain-NRS Knee (r = 0.53) were both supported. However, KOOS Pain and Pain-NRS Knee showed strong correlation (r = 0.66) instead of expected very strong correlation (Table 4).

Reliability

The mean change in the second measurement varied from − 0.7 in the Symptoms subscale to 8.7 in the Sport and Recreation Function subscale (Table 5).

Internal consistency

Cronbach's α ranged from 0.79 to 0.96, indicating good internal consistency in all the KOOS subscales (Table 5).

Test-retest reliability

The test-retest reliability of the KOOS was excellent for the Pain, ADL and Knee-related Quality of Life subscales, with ICCs ranging from 0.83 to 0.86. In the Symptoms and Sport and Recreation Function subscales, reliability was good, with ICCs (95% CIs) of 0.73 (0.59 to 0.83) and 0.72 (0.57 to 0.82), respectively (Table 5).

Measurement error

The SEM values ranged from 6.0 to 12.2, with the lowest for the Symptoms subscale and highest for the Sport and Recreation Function subscale (Table 5). Correspondingly,

Table 4 A priori hypotheses of the expected correlations and realized correlations between the KOOS subscales and the subscales of the WOMAC, SF-36 and Pain-NRS. The correlations are given as Spearman's correlation coefficient (r) values

Comparative subscales		Expected correlation	Realized correlation
KOOS Pain	WOMAC Pain	*r* = > 0.79 *(very strong)*	*r* = 0.81, supported
KOOS Symptoms	WOMAC Stiffness	*r* = 0.40 to 0.79 *(moderate - strong)*	*r* = 0.48, supported
KOOS ADL	WOMAC Physical function	*r* = > 0.79 *(very strong)*	*r* = 0.86, supported
KOOS Pain	SF-36 Bodily Pain	*r* = 0.60 to 0.79 *(strong)*	*r* = 0.69, supported
KOOS ADL	SF-36 Physical Functioning	*r* = > 0.79 *(very strong)*	*r* = 0.83, supported
KOOS Sport/Rec	SF-36 Physical Functioning	*r* = 0.60 to 0.79 *(strong)*	*r* = 0.67, supported
KOOS Pain	Knee Pain-NRS	*r* = > 0.79 *(very strong)*	*r* = 0.66, not supported
KOOS ADL	Knee Pain-NRS	*r* = 0.60 to 0.79 *(strong)*	*r* = 0.68, supported
KOOS QOL	Knee Pain-NRS	*r* = 0.40 to 0.59 *(moderate)*	*r* = 0.53, supported

KOOS Knee Injury and Osteoarthritis Outcome Score, *WOMAC* Western Ontario and McMaster Osteoarthritis Index, *SF-36* Short-Form 36 Health Survey, *Pain-NRS* Numeric Pain Rating Scale, *ADL* Activities of Daily Living, *Sport/Rec* Sport and Recreation Function, *QOL* Quality of Life

at the individual level the MDC was lowest (16.6) for the Symptoms subscale and highest (33.8) for the Sport and Recreation Function subscale. At the group level, MDC ranged between 2.2 and 4.4 (Table 5).

Discussion

This study reports on the cross-cultural adaptation and translation of KOOS into Finnish and its reliability, construct validity and floor/ceiling effects in patients with knee injuries and/or OA. The results indicated that the Finnish version of KOOS has good construct validity, and that the questionnaire is a reliable measure of pain, symptoms, activities of daily living, sport and recreation, and quality of life in Finnish-speaking patients with knee injuries of different kinds.

The psychometric properties of the Finnish version of KOOS were in line with those of the original KOOS [13, 34, 35] and with the Persian version of KOOS [14], which studied a group of patients with knee injuries, similar to those in the present study, although not including knee OA. The mean scores for the Sport and Recreation Function and QOL subscales were considerably lower than the scores for the other subscales, as previously reported [12, 15, 16, 34, 36]. The likely reason for these low values, especially for the Sport and Recreation Function, is that knee injury patients tend to avoid risky activities in their daily lives. The present study demonstrated neither floor nor ceiling effects, as the proportion of worst or best possible percentage scores for the KOOS subscale with the highest scores was only 9%. This demonstrates the appropriateness and comprehensiveness of the questionnaire for a patient population with relatively moderate knee pain and other knee injury symptoms.

The construct validity of the KOOS was determined by comparing the KOOS subscales with the subscales of the WOMAC, SF-36 and Pain-NRS. The KOOS subscales are as representative as those of the WOMAC for measuring pain, stiffness and function. It was therefore expected that strong or very strong correlations between the KOOS and WOMAC subscales would be found. However, in interpreting these coefficients it must be acknowledged that all these measurements overlap to a certain extent. The WOMAC Pain items are included in the KOOS subscale of Pain, the WOMAC Stiffness items are included in the KOOS subscale of Symptoms, and the WOMAC Physical Function items are identical to the KOOS ADL items. Thus, in the latter, the subscale

Table 5 Difference between first and second measurement, internal consistency, test-retest reliability, and measurement error of the KOOS subscales

	Change from first to second measurement	Internal consistency	Test-retest reliability	Measurement error		
	Mean (95% CI)	Cronbach's α (95% CI)	ICC (95% CI)	SEM (95% CI)	MDC (95% CI) in individuals	MDC (95% CI) in groups
Pain	2.8 (−0.3 to 5.9)	0.89 (0.84 to 0.94)	0.86 (0.77 to 0.91)	7.7 (5.8 to 9.6)	21.3 (16.5 to 25.1)	2.8 (2.2 to 3.4)
Symptoms	−0.7 (−3.2 to 1.9)	0.79 (0.69 to 0.89)	0.73 (0.59 to 0.83)	6.0 (4.7 to 7.3)	16.6 (13.0 to 20.2)	2.2 (1.7 to 2.6)
Activities of Daily Living	5.1 (1.7 to 8.4)	0.96 (0.95 to 0.98)	0.83 (0.72 to 0.89)	8.7 (6.4 to 11.1)	24.2 (17.7 to 30.7)	3.1 (2.3 to 4.0)
Sport and Recreation Function	8.7 (3.8 to 13.5)	0.88 (0.82 to 0.94)	0.72 (0.57 to 0.82)	12.2 (9.9 to 14.6)	33.8 (27.3 to 40.4)	4.4 (3.6 to 5.3)
Knee-related Quality of Life	4.2 (1.0 to 7.4)	0.90 (0.84 to 0.96)	0.83 (0.73 to 0.89)	8.3 (6.8 to 9.8)	23.1 (19.0 to 27.2)	3.0 (2.5 to 3.5)

KOOS Knee Injury and Osteoarthritis Outcome Score, *ICC* Intraclass Correlation Coefficient, *SEM* Standard Error of Measurement, *MDC* Minimal Detectable Change, *CI* Confidence Interval

response options (VAS vs Likert) are compared rather than the constructs. Due to overlapping subscales between the KOOS and WOMAC, it was essential in this study to compare and correlate the subscales of the KOOS also with other questionnaire's subscales assessing similar constructs than those of the WOMAC.

We found, somewhat surprisingly, that the KOOS subscale of Symptoms and the WOMAC subscale of Stiffness showed "only" a moderate correlation. This may partially be due to fact, as referred to above, that the KOOS Symptoms subscale contains five items in addition to the two original WOMAC items, as it also takes symptoms related to knee movement into account. Also noteworthy, alongside the KOOS subscales of Pain, Symptoms and Activities of Daily Living, were the subscales of Sport and Recreation Function and QOL, which showed a moderate or strong correlation with all the WOMAC subscales.

When the KOOS and SF-36 were compared for construct validity, we found strong correlations between the KOOS subscales and those of the SF-36 that measured similar constructs. The highest correlations were observed between the SF-36 subscale of Physical Functioning and the KOOS subscales of ADL and Pain. The SF-36 subscale of Bodily Pain and the KOOS subscales of Pain and ADL also showed strong correlations. In contrast, the KOOS subscale of Symptoms showed the lowest correlations with all the SF-36 subscales. This is in line with the findings of Salavati et al. (2008) in patients with knee injuries, and of Roos et al. (1998) in subjects with knee OA. In fact, Roos et al. concluded that the KOOS Symptoms subscale is not as important as the other four subscales as a determinate of Physical Health. The authors suggested that symptoms and functional limitations should be reported separately and not aggregated into a single score [13]. All in all, the construct validity for the patients in our study was at more or less the same level as observed in patients with knee injuries [14] and less severe forms of OA [18], but higher than that obtained in elderly patients with advanced OA eligible for total joint replacement [15, 34].

The numeric pain rating scale used in this study measures the intensity of pain experienced in general as well as in specific body regions. It contains subscales that make it possible to explore correlations with the KOOS subscales. As expected, we found strong and moderate correlations between all the KOOS and Pain-NRS subscales, particularly those focusing on the lower extremities and the knee region. These findings, in conjunction with the fact that self-reported knee pain was more severe than pain in any other body region, confirm the utility of the KOOS as a lower-extremity PRO measure in subjects with diverse knee problems. Also of note was the finding of strong correlations between the Pain-NRS Knee and lower limb subscales and the KOOS Activities of Daily Living subscale. This is understandable, given that the knee is a large weight-bearing joint with a large range of movements, and that managing the activities of daily living presumes an extensive repertoire of pain-free weight-bearing movements. However, somewhat surprisingly, the KOOS Pain subscale correlated only strongly instead of, as expected, very strongly with the Pain-NRS Knee subscale. This is most likely due to only partial similarity between the constructs in the two subscales. While the nine-item KOOS Pain subscale is designed to elicit the prevalence and degree of pain during different activities and rest, the Pain-NRS Knee subscale consists of a single item in asking about the intensity of pain experienced during the past week. Nevertheless, the use of the Pain-NRS yielded new information, since to our knowledge no previous KOOS validation studies have investigated the correlations between the KOOS and Pain-NRS subscales. From our pre-defined hypotheses altogether 89% could be confirmed.

Internal consistency was good for all five subscales, exceeding the cutoff value of 0.70. This result is comparable to observations in other languages and patient populations, such as in the Swedish version with preoperative patients [13], the Dutch version with patients with focal cartilage defects [37], the Persian version with patients with knee injuries [14], and the Singapore English and Singapore Chinese [15], Dutch [17], Portuguese [18] and French [16] versions with knee OA patients. Two recent Polish validation studies with test-retest intervals of one to 2 weeks found Cronbach's αs higher than 0.90 in patients undergoing ACL reconstruction [38] and total knee replacement [36]. The authors concluded that this might be due to the relative homogeneity of their patient group. Accordingly, it has been claimed that, for clinical application, high Cronbach's α values, of at least 0.90, are needed [39]. However, given that, our Cronbach's α values were, with the exception of the Symptoms subscale, all around borderline significance, we consider them reasonable for clinical purposes. The result of the item analysis also suggests that all five subscales are acceptable for inclusion in the Finnish version of KOOS.

The ICC values for test-retest reliability for all the KOOS subscales were good, ranging from 0.72 to 0.86, thereby indicating sufficient standardization of the KOOS questionnaire. Overall, our results are comparable to those of previous methodological studies of KOOS [12, 13] and other studies [14, 17–19, 36, 37, 40, 41] where ICC values over 0.70 have indicated good or excellent test-retest reliability. Noteworthy, the ICC value for Sport and Recreation Function in our study was somewhat lower than expected. It is commonly seen that Sport and Recreation Function has higher ICC value than Symptoms [17, 36, 40, 41].We cannot find an exact reason why Sport and Recreation Function had relatively low value, but it is possible that some patients may have changed their activity level during 2 week interval.

The MDC value of 4.4 points at the group level indicates that the Finnish version of the KOOS has an ability to detect a minimum change of 4.5 points between the measurements. The MDC should be smaller than the minimal important change (MIC), which is regarded as the smallest change score needed for the effect to be considered clinically relevant [42]. For the different KOOS subscales a MIC of 8–10 points has been considered to be appropriate [34]. Thus the Finnish version of the KOOS is applicable to detect such a change without difficulties. However, it is important to note that the mentioned MDC values apply to patient groups and not to individual patients. The MDC values at the individual level were considerably higher ranging from 16.6 to 33.8 for the different KOOS subscales. The MDC values in our study are of same magnitude or somewhat higher than those found in two recent studies in people with OA awaiting arthroplasty [36, 43].

We recognize some limitations of this study. First, our sample size was rather small. The response rate for the re-test remained low (~ 45%), meaning that a relatively small number of participants were investigated. The reasons why some subjects did not respond to the second KOOS questionnaire remain unknown. Nevertheless, according to the Consensus-based Standards for the selection of health status Measurement Instruments (COSMIN) group [44], the sample size of 50 to 99 is considered sufficient. Second, participants in the present study may not represent patients with entire spectrum of knee OA and some common knee complaints affecting pain, such as patellofemoral pain syndrome, rheumatoid arthritis, plica syndrome, Bakers cyst and bursitis. However, it must be borne in mind that the KOOS questionnaire is intended to be used particularly for knee injuries that can result for a variety of reasons, including OA. In addition, the initial participant group recruited to this study was representative of their population, as all knee patients attending the outpatient clinic were invited to take part to the study. Third, due to its cross-sectional design, the responsiveness of the questionnaire was not assessed in this study, which may limit the instrument's ability to detect clinically important changes over time. For these reasons, we recommend further validation of this preliminary Finnish version of KOOS and consideration of its responsiveness with a larger number of patients with knee complaints, including patients across the full radiographic spectrum of knee OA.

Conclusions

This research effort produced an appropriately translated and culturally adapted version of KOOS. The Finnish version of KOOS is a reliable and valid measure that can be applied as a self-report and disease-specific questionnaire for use in middle-aged patients with knee injuries. The responsiveness of the Finnish version of KOOS in larger groups of patients with knee complaints remains to be tested.

Abbreviations

ACL: Anterior cruciate ligament; ADL: Activities of daily living; CI: Confidence interval; COSMIN: Consensus-based standards for the election of health status measurement instruments; ICC: Intraclass correlation coefficient; IQR: Interquartile range; KOOS: Knee Injury and Osteoarthritis Outcome Score; LTPA: Leisure time physical activity; MDC: Minimal detectable change; MIC: Minimal important change; OA: Osteoarthritis; Pain-NRS: Pain numeric rating scale; PRO: Patient-reported outcome; QOL: Quality of life; SD: Standard deviation; SEM: Standard error of measurement; SF-36: Short-Form 36 Health Survey; VAS: Visual Analog Scale; WOMAC: Western Ontario and McMaster Osteoarthritis Index

Acknowledgements

The authors thank Michael Freeman for revising the English language of the manuscript. The authors also thank all the participants for their valuable contribution to the study.

Funding

This work was supported by grants from Helsinki University Hospital (HUS) and the Scientific Advisory Board for Defense (MATINE). The first author Juhani Multanen was funded by the Academy of Finland (Project No. 311587) when preparing the manuscript for publication. The funding agencies had no role in the study design, data collection and analysis, decision to publish, or preparation of the manuscript.

Authors' contributions

AH and IK were involved in the conception of the study plan and design. MH gathered the patient data. IK and JM analyzed and interpreted the patient data. JM was a major contributor in writing the manuscript. All authors were involved in revising the article critically for important intellectual content, and all authors approved the final manuscript.

Competing interests

The authors declare that they have no competing interests.

Author details

[1]Department of Physical Medicine and Rehabilitation, Central Finland Central Hospital, Keskussairaalantie 19, FI-40620 Jyväskylä, Finland. [2]Department of

Surgery, Mikkeli Central Hospital, Mikkeli, Finland. [3]Faculty of Sport and Health Sciences, University of Jyväskylä, Jyväskylä, Finland. [4]Department of Orthopaedics and Traumatology, University of Helsinki, and Helsinki University Hospital, Helsinki, Finland.

References

1. Urwin M, Symmons D, Allison T, Brammah T, Busby H, Roxby M, Simmons A, Williams G. Estimating the burden of musculoskeletal disorders in the community: the comparative prevalence of symptoms at different anatomical sites, and the relation to social deprivation. Ann Rheum Dis. 1998;57:649–55.
2. O'Reilly SC, Muir KR, Doherty M. Knee pain and disability in the Nottingham community: association with poor health status and psychological distress. Br J Rheumatol. 1998;37:870–3.
3. Jinks C, Jordan K, Ong BN, Croft P. A brief screening tool for knee pain in primary care (KNEST). 2. Results from a survey in the general population aged 50 and over. Rheumatology (Oxford). 2004;43:55–61.
4. Kujala UM, Kvist M, Osterman K. Knee injuries in athletes. Review of exertion injuries and retrospective study of outpatient sports clinic material. Sports Med. 1986;3:447–60.
5. Maffulli N, Longo UG, Gougoulias N, Loppini M, Denaro V. Long-term health outcomes of youth sports injuries. Br J Sports Med. 2010;44:21–5.
6. Molloy MG, Molloy CB. Contact sport and osteoarthritis. Br J Sports Med. 2011;45(4):275–7.
7. Busija L, Bridgett L, Williams SR, Osborne RH, Buchbinder R, March L, Fransen M. Osteoarthritis. Best Pract Res Clin Rheumatol. 2010;24:757–68.
8. Loeser RF. Age-related changes in the musculoskeletal system and the development of osteoarthritis. Clin Geriatr Med. 2010;26:371–86.
9. Tegner Y, Lysholm J. Rating systems in the evaluation of knee ligament injuries. Clin Orthop Relat Res. 1985;198:43–9.
10. Bellamy N, Buchanan WW, Goldsmith CH, Campbell J, Stitt LW. Validation study of WOMAC: a health status instrument for measuring clinically important patient relevant outcomes to antirheumatic drug therapy in patients with osteoarthritis of the hip or knee. J Rheumatol. 1988;15:1833–40.
11. Lequesne M. Informational indices. Validation of criteria and tests. Scand J Rheumatol Suppl. 1989;80:17–28.
12. Roos EM, Roos HP, Lohmander LS, Ekdahl C, Beynnon BD. Knee Injury and Osteoarthritis Outcome Score (KOOS)–development of a self-administered outcome measure. J Orthop Sports Phys Ther. 1998;28:88–96.
13. Roos EM, Roos HP, Ekdahl C, Lohmander LS. Knee Injury and Osteoarthritis Outcome Score (KOOS)–validation of a Swedish version. Scand J Med Sci Sports. 1998;8:439–48.
14. Salavati M, Mazaheri M, Negahban H, Sohani SM, Ebrahimian MR, Ebrahimi I, Kazemnejad A, Salavati M. Validation of a Persian-version of Knee Injury and Osteoarthritis Outcome Score (KOOS) in Iranians with knee injuries. Osteoarthr Cartil. 2008;16:1178–82.
15. Xie F, Li SC, Roos EM, Fong KY, Lo NN, Yeo SJ, Yang KY, Yeo W, Chong HC, Thumboo J. Cross-cultural adaptation and validation of Singapore English and Chinese versions of the Knee Injury and Osteoarthritis Outcome Score (KOOS) in Asians with knee osteoarthritis in Singapore. Osteoarthr Cartil. 2006;14:1098–103.
16. Ornetti P, Parratte S, Gossec L, Tavernier C, Argenson JN, Roos EM, Guillemin F, Maillefert JF. Cross-cultural adaptation and validation of the French version of the Knee Injury and Osteoarthritis Outcome Score (KOOS) in knee osteoarthritis patients. Osteoarthr Cartil. 2008;16:423–8.
17. de Groot IB, Favejee MM, Reijman M, Verhaar JA, Terwee CB. The Dutch version of the Knee Injury and Osteoarthritis Outcome Score: a validation study. Health Qual Life Outcomes. 2008;6:16. https://doi.org/10.1186/1477-7525-6-16.
18. Goncalves RS, Cabri J, Pinheiro JP, Ferreira PL. Cross-cultural adaptation and validation of the Portuguese version of the Knee Injury and Osteoarthritis Outcome Score (KOOS). Osteoarthr Cartil. 2009;17:1156–62.
19. Nakamura N, Takeuchi R, Sawaguchi T, Ishikawa H, Saito T, Goldhahn S. Cross-cultural adaptation and validation of the Japanese Knee Injury and Osteoarthritis Outcome Score (KOOS). J Orthop Sci. 2011;16:516–23.
20. Collins NJ, Prinsen CA, Christensen R, Bartels EM, Terwee CB, Roos EM. Knee Injury and Osteoarthritis Outcome Score (KOOS): systematic review and meta-analysis of measurement properties. Osteoarthr Cartil. 2016;24:1317–29.
21. Knee Injury and Osteoarthritis Outcome Score. http://www.koos.nu/index.html. Accessed 15 Mar 2018.
22. Beaton DE, Bombardier C, Guillemin F, Ferraz MB. Guidelines for the process of cross-cultural adaptation of self-report measures. Spine. 2000;25:3186–91.
23. WOMAC 3.1 Index. Knee and Hip Osteoarthritis Index. http://www.womac.org/womac/index.htm. Accessed 15 Mar 2018.
24. Soininen JV, Paavolainen PO, Gronblad MA, Kaapa EH. Validation study of a Finnish version of the Western Ontario and McMasters University osteoarthritis index. Hip Int. 2008;18:108–11.
25. Ware JE, Kosinski M, Keller SK. SF-36 physical and Mental health summary scales: a user's manual. Boston: The Health Institute; 1994.
26. Terwee CB, Bot SD, de Boer MR, van der Windt DA, Knol DL, Dekker J, Bouter LM, de Vet HC. Quality criteria were proposed for measurement properties of health status questionnaires. J Clin Epidemiol. 2007;60:34–42.
27. Mokkink LB, Terwee CB, Patrick DL, Alonso J, Stratford PW, Knol DL, Bouter LM, de Vet HC. The COSMIN study reached international consensus on taxonomy, terminology, and definitions of measurement properties for health-related patient-reported outcomes. J Clin Epidemiol. 2010;63:737–45.
28. Evans JD. Straightforward statistics for the behavioral sciences. Pacific Grove: Brooks/Cole Publishing; 1996.
29. Hays RD, Anderson RT, Revicki D. Assessing reliability and validity of measurement in clinical trials. In: Staquet MJ, Hays RD, Fayers PM, editors. Quality of life assessment in clinical trials methods and practice. Oxford: Oxford University Press; 1998. p. 169–82.
30. Fayers PM, Machin D. Quality of life: assessment, analysis and interpretation. Chichester: Wiley; 2000.
31. Landis JR, Koch GG. The measurement of observer agreement for categorical data. Biometrics. 1977;33:159–74.
32. Atkinson G, Nevill AM. Statistical methods for assessing measurement error (reliability) in variables relevant to sports medicine. Sports Med. 1998;26:217–38.
33. de Vet HC, Bouter LM, Bezemer PD, Beurskens AJ. Reproducibility and responsiveness of evaluative outcome measures. Theoretical considerations illustrated by an empirical example. Int J Technol Assess Health Care. 2001;17:479–87.
34. Roos EM, Toksvig-Larsen S. Knee Injury and Osteoarthritis Outcome Score (KOOS) - validation and comparison to the WOMAC in total knee replacement. Health Qual Life Outcomes. 2003;1:17.
35. Roos EM, Lohmander LS. The Knee Injury and Osteoarthritis Outcome Score (KOOS): from joint injury to osteoarthritis. Health Qual Life Outcomes. 2003;1:64.
36. Paradowski PT, Keska R, Witonski D. Validation of the Polish version of the Knee Injury and Osteoarthritis Outcome Score (KOOS) in patients with osteoarthritis undergoing total knee replacement. BMJ Open. 2015;5:e006947. https://doi.org/10.1136/bmjopen-2014-006947.
37. Bekkers JE, de Windt TS, Raijmakers NJ, Dhert WJ, Saris DB. Validation of the Knee Injury and Osteoarthritis Outcome Score (KOOS) for the treatment of focal cartilage lesions. Osteoarthr Cartil. 2009;17:1434–9.
38. Paradowski PT, Witonski D, Keska R, Roos EM. Cross-cultural translation and measurement properties of the Polish version of the Knee Injury and Osteoarthritis Outcome Score (KOOS) following anterior cruciate ligament reconstruction. Health Qual Life Outcomes. 2013;11:107. https://doi.org/10.1186/1477-7525-11-107.
39. Bland JM, Altman DG. Cronbach's alpha. BMJ. 1997;314(7080):572.
40. Monticone M, Ferrante S, Salvaderi S, Rocca B, Totti V, Foti C, Roi GS. Development of the Italian version of the knee injury and osteoarthritis outcome score for patients with knee injuries: cross-cultural adaptation, dimensionality, reliability, and validity. Osteoarthr Cartil. 2012;20:330–5.
41. Almangoush A, Herrington L, Attia I, Jones R, Aldawoudy A, Abdul Aziz A, Waley A. Cross-cultural adaptation, reliability, internal consistency and validation of the Arabic version of the knee injury and osteoarthritis outcome score (KOOS) for Egyptian people with knee injuries. Osteoarthr Cartil. 2013;21:1855–64.
42. de Vet HC, Ostelo RW, Terwee CB, van der Roer N, Knol DL, Beckerman H, Boers M, Bouter LM. Minimally important change determined by a visual method integrating an anchor-based and a distribution-based approach. Qual Life Res. 2007;16:131–42.

16

Micro-fragmented adipose tissue injection associated with arthroscopic procedures in patients with symptomatic knee osteoarthritis

G. Cattaneo[1*], A. De Caro[1], F. Napoli[1], D. Chiapale[2], P. Trada[2] and A. Camera[1]

Abstract

Background: The social impact of degenerative diseases is steadily increasing, because of the continued rise in the mean age of the active population. Articular cartilage lesions are generally associated with disability and symptoms such as joint pain and reduced function, and remain a challenge for the orthopaedic surgeon. Several non-invasive solution have been proposed, but the results achieved to date are far from being completely satisfactory. Recently, new therapeutic approaches, such as the use of mesenchymal stem cells, have been developed. Among the many sources, the adipose tissue is nowadays considered one of the smartest, due to its abundance and easy access. The aim of this retrospective study is to explore whether patients affected by symptomatic knee osteoarthritis treated with micro-fragmented adipose tissue associated with a chondral shaving procedure experience an improvement in symptoms and function.

Methods: Thirty-eight patients affected by symptomatic knee osteoarthritis were treated in 2015 with an arthroscopic procedure associated with an injection of autologous and micro-fragmented adipose tissue. Micro-fragmented adipose tissue was obtained using a minimal manipulation technique in a closed system. Clinical outcomes were determined at 1, 3, 6, and 12 months follow-up using Knee Injury and Osteoarthritis Outcome Score questionnaire and direct physical examination. Safety of the procedure, recording type and incidence of any adverse event, was also assessed.

Results: A steady and statistically significant improvement of all the clinical scores from pre-operative evaluation to 1, 3, 6, and 12 months follow-up was observed, with KOOS sport and quality of life being the most improved scores. On average, 92% of the patients clinically improved and 100% of them were satisfied with the treatment. No adverse events nor relevant complications were recorded.

Conclusion: The result of the study pointed to micro-fragmented adipose tissue as a safe and beneficial adjuvant in the surgical treatment of degenerative knee chondropathy. The procedure is simple, sustainable, quick, minimally invasive, one-step, and safe. After one year, the results are very satisfactory and promising. A longer follow-up is needed to draw definitive conclusions and enlarge the indications.

Keywords: Knee chondropathy, Osteoarthritis, MSCs, ASCs, Micro-fragmented adipose tissue

* Correspondence: gabrielecattaneo@hotmail.com
[1]Spotorno Foundation c/o San Michele Clinics, Viale Pontelungo, 79, 17031 Albenga, SV, Italy
Full list of author information is available at the end of the article

Background

The social impact of degenerative diseases such as articular cartilage pathology is steadily increasing, because of the continued rise in the mean age of the active population. Articular cartilage lesions are generally, but not always, associated with disability and with symptoms such as joint pain and reduced function, and might progress to end-stage osteoarthritis (OA). Varieties of non-invasive solutions for pain relief, improvement in function and disability, and eventually, modification of the progression of severe cartilage lesions and OA, have been proposed with variable success rates [1–3]. Non-surgical treatments, such as physiokinesitherapy, pharmacological treatments (analgesics/anti-inflammatory agents, glucocorticoids, opioids, nonsteroidal anti-inflammatory drugs - NSAIDs), hyaluronic acid (HA) or its derivatives [4, 5] or platelet-rich plasma (PRP) injections [6, 7], indicated for small or diffused degenerative lesions, temporarily target the symptoms but cannot prevent the degeneration process [8]. Joint-preserving surgical treatments, such as arthroscopic shaving or debridement, laser chondroplasty, and microfractures, provide temporary relief of symptoms, but the clinical findings are highly variable and many authors contraindicated their use for diffused joint degeneration. For these reasons, new therapeutic approaches, such as the use of mesenchymal stem cells (MSCs) have been developed. Through trophic, mitogenic, anti-scarring, anti-apoptotic, immunomodulatory, and anti-microbial actions, produced by a large amount of bioactive elements, growth factors and cytokines, MSCs "sense" and "signal" changes in the microenvironment where they reside [9, 10]. Bone marrow and adipose tissue are the most readily available sources of MSCs, and, in this context, the adipose tissue is nowadays considered the smartest due to its abundance, the easy access and the simple isolation procedure [11, 12]. In addition, of the many cell types contained in the adipose tissue, MSCs (ASCs) comprise up to 2%, whereas only 0.02% of cells in bone marrow are MSCs. The use of ASCs, either culture-expanded or obtained by mechanical or enzymatic treatment as stromal vascular fraction (SVF) [13] have recently created a huge interest in the context of cartilage regeneration and shown promising results [14–18]. However, the studies published to date used a tissue-engineering approach, involving the use of scaffolds, cells, and growth factors, either alone or in any combination [16, 19–21]. In addition to the large number of processing steps, the high economic burden, and the restrictions associated with cell expansion and extensive manipulation [22, 23], the results achieved to date are far from being completely satisfactory. Therefore, availability of a minimally manipulated adipose tissue providing in one-step the key elements to support a natural regenerative response would have remarkable clinical relevance [24]. Based on these considerations, a commercially available technique that intra-operatively provides micro-fragmented and minimally manipulated adipose tissue without expansion or enzymatic treatment [25] was employed in this study. This approach, that has been already shown to be safe and promising in different pathologies [26–33], provides the key elements to support a natural reparative response, that is scaffold (the adipose tissue structure), cells (ASCs), and growth factors (secreted cytokines and chemokines) [34]. The aim of this retrospective study is to explore whether patients affected by symptomatic knee OA treated with micro-fragmented adipose tissue injection associated with a chondral shaving procedure experience an improvement in symptoms and function.

Methods

Study population

The retrospective analysis of the patient data was approved by the Regional Ethics Committee of Liguria - Italy (protocol n° 164REG2016, September 22, 2016). No approval for the initial treatment of the patients was required being the procedure standard clinical practice in our Hospital. In 2015, 38 consecutive patients affected by symptomatic knee OA underwent an arthroscopic procedure associated with an injection of autologous and micro-fragmented adipose tissue. The indication for the treatment was knee chondropathy grade > II (ICRS classification), constant pain and failure of conservative treatments (physiokinesitherapy, corticosteroids, HA and/or PRP) for at least 12 months. Contraindications for the treatment were immune-mediated (non-infectious) synovitis, OA Kellgren-Lawrence grade > 3, axial defects > 10°, metabolic disorders and BMI > 40. Pre-operative assessments included standard X-rays, MRI, direct physical examination, Knee Injury and Osteoarthritis Outcome Score (KOOS) questionnaire. Of these 38 patients, 3 subjects were treated with micro-perforations because of a severe chondral damage and where excluded from the global analysis. The remaining 35 underwent a standard chondral shaving procedure [35]. Those patients having also a meniscal injury no longer repairable (14 patients) underwent an associated meniscectomy to correct the defect.

Harvesting of the adipose tissue

The lower or the lateral abdomen was chosen as donor site for adipose tissue harvesting. Before harvesting the fat, the site was injected with Klein solution (1 vial adrenaline + 50 cm^3 mepivacaine 2% in 250 cm^3 saline) using a disposable 17G blunt cannula connected to a luer-lock 60-cm^3 syringe. The fat was then harvested using a 13G blunt cannula, for a fast and a-traumatic suction, connected to a VacLok® 20-ml syringe.

Processing of the adipose tissue with Lipogems® device and injection in the joint

The harvested fat was immediately processed in the Lipogems® processing kit, a disposable device that progressively reduces the size of the adipose tissue clusters while eliminating oily substances and blood residues with pro-inflammatory properties. The entire process, carried out in one surgical step, was performed in complete immersion in physiological solution minimizing any trauma to the cells. The resulting micro-fragmented fat was collected in a 60-cm^3 syringe and positioned for decanting the excess saline solution. The resulting product was then transferred into several 10-cm^3 syringes to be injected in the patient. Micro-fragmented fat (10 cm^3) was injected intra-articular after the arthroscopic procedure (shaving or shaving + meniscectomy).

Post-op rehabilitation protocol and clinical evaluations

All patients were discharged the day after the procedure with an elastic compression band on the harvesting site, low MW heparin for 3 weeks, 2 weeks of unloading and then full load recovery in the following 7 days. Continuous passive motion from the immediate post-op and active physiokinesitherapy from day 15 post-op.

Standard clinical evaluations at 1, 3, 6, and 12 months post-op included Knee Injury and Osteoarthritis Outcome Score (KOOS) questionnaire and direct physical examination with the evaluation of knee range of motion, patellar subluxation, ability to walk, go up and down the stairs, squatting, muscular strength, stiffness and knee swelling. The Western Ontario and McMaster Universities Osteoarthritis Index (WOMAC) was calculated from the KOOS.

Safety assessment

Safety was assessed by evaluating local adverse events, such as infections, fever, and excessive swelling of the knee at 1, 3, 6, and 12 months post-op.

Statistical analysis

To guarantee standard operating procedures, all the patients were operated by the same surgeon (GC) and the clinical evaluations at any follow-up time were performed by the same surgeon assisted by another surgeon. Considering the relatively small sample size, results are expressed as the mean and standard deviation. For statistical comparisons, the chi-squared test for all categorical data, Student's t-test for unpaired groups for parametric data, and Mann-Whitney test for non-parametric data (calculated with the Kolmogorov-Smirnoff normality test) were used (GraphPad Prism v5.0, La Jolla, USA). A $p < 0.05$ was considered statistically significant. A $p < 0.1$ is reported as a tendency.

Results

Due to the differences in the surgical procedure, the patients that underwent the corrective meniscectomy were analysed separately and indicated in the text with the code "SM"; patients that underwent the chondral shaving only are indicated with the code "SH". Background data of the two sub-populations included in the study are reported in Table 1.

The analysis of the SH category data revealed a steady and statistically significant improvement of all the clinical scores from pre-operative evaluation to 1, 3, 6, and 12 months follow-up (Fig. 1a). At 12 months, the average improvement in KOOS compared to pre-operative condition was 29 in symptoms ($p < 0.0001$), 36 in pain ($p < 0.0001$), 37 in function in daily living ($p < 0.0001$), 51

Table 1 Characteristics of the 2 study populations

	SH group	MS group
Age		
Mean	53 y.o.	55 y.o.
SD	12	11
Gender		
M	13 (62%)	8 (57%)
F	8 (38%)	6 (43%)
BMI		
Mean	27	27
SD	4	4
Smoke		
Smokers/Former	8 (38%)	5 (36%)
Non Smokers	13 (62%)	9 (64%)
Grade Chondropathy (ICRS classification)		
II	5 (24%)	2 (14%)
III	8 (38%)	7 (50%)
IV	8 (38%)	5 (36%)
Grade OA (Kellgren Lawrence)		
1	8 (38%)	1 (7%)
2	4 (19%)	2 (14%)
3	9 (43%)	11 (79%)
Site of Lesion		
FC	10 (48%)	11 (79%)
PF	3 (14%)	3 (21%)
TP	8 (38%)	–
Type of Lesion		
Diffused	16 (76%)	11 (79%)
Focal - mean size	5 (24%) - 10 mm	3 (21%) - 14 mm
Surgery	SH	SM

SD standard deviation, *FC* femoral condyle, *PF* patellofemoral, *TP* tibial plateau, *SH* chondral shaving, *SM* chondral shaving + meniscectomy

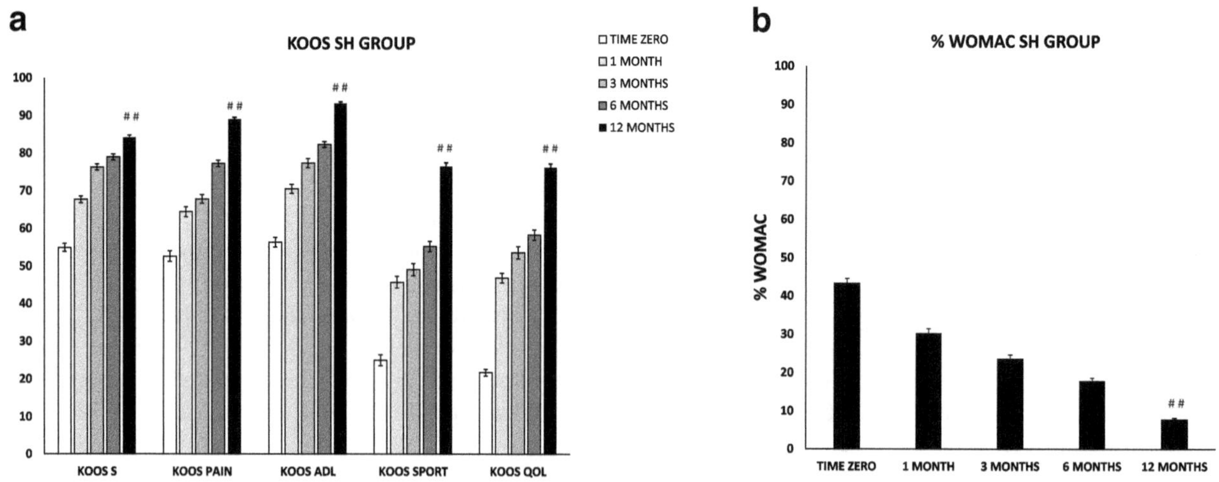

Fig. 1 Trend of functional improvements of the SH group from baseline to 12 months' follow-up. Results are expressed as mean and standard error. A $p < 0.05$ (T12 vs. T0) was considered statistically significant (# #). **a** KOOS score. KOOS S = symptoms; KOOS P = pain; KOOS ADL = activity daily living; KOOS Spt = sport; KOOS QoL = quality of life. **b** WOMAC Index

in sport (p < 0.0001) and 54 in the quality of life ($p <$ 0.0001). Statistically significant differences ($p < 0.0001$) between pre-treatment and follow-up values were found also for the total WOMAC scores. In details, pain, stiffness and functional limitation decreased from an average of 43 at baseline to 30 at 1 month, 24 at 3 months, 18 at 6 months, and 8 at 12 months (Fig. 1b). The physical examination at 6 months revealed that the majority of the patients entered in the category "normal" and, at 12 months, no patients were in the category "symptomatic" except for one patient in squatting (see Table 2 for comparison with the pre-operative condition).

Results of the SM population appeared slightly different, with a steady and statistically significant improvement of all the clinical scores until the 6 months follow-up followed by a slight, but not statistically significant, decrease at 12 months (Fig. 2a). At 12 months, the average improvement in KOOS compared to pre-operative condition was 17 in symptoms ($p = 0.014$), 12 in pain ($p =$ 0.183), 16 in function in daily living ($p = 0.027$), 24 in sport ($p = 0.014$) and 26 in the quality of life ($p = 0.002$). The same trend was found between pre-treatment and follow-up values for the total WOMAC scores ($p <$ 0.0001). In details, pain, stiffness and functional limitation decreased from an average of 40 at baseline to 24 at 1 month, 20 at 3 months, 17 at 6 months, and 24 at 12 months (Fig. 2b). The physical examination at 6 months revealed that the majority of the patients entered in the category "normal" and, at 12 months, no patients were in the category "symptomatic" except for one patient in walking and two patients in squatting (see Table 2 for comparison with pre-operative condition). The comparison of the two populations revealed that SM patients improved less, but still a lot, compared to SH patients (Δ_{t12-t0} KOOS symptoms 17 vs. 29 [p≅0.05], pain 12 vs. 36 [$p < 0.05$], function in daily living 16 vs. 37 [p < 0.05], sport 24 vs. 51 [$p < 0.05$], and quality of life 26 vs. 54 [$p < 0.01$]). Interestingly, despite this finding, the Student's t-test revealed that, besides the meniscectomy, other parameters such as age, sex, type and grade of chondropathy affect specific outcomes at different time points. Due to the small number of patients, this analysis has been performed on the whole population (35 patients). At 1 month, women and patients under 55 years old showed better improvements in the KOOS sport compared to men and elderly patients respectively (31% women vs. 14% men [p < 0.05] and 30% patients < 55 y.o. vs. 9% patients > 55 y.o. [$p < 0.01$]). At 3 months, patients with a chondropathy of grade IV showed higher improvements in the KOOS quality of life compared to patients with a grade II-III (51% grade IV vs. 31% grade II-III, p≅0.05). In addition, patients with a femoral condyle chondropathy showed better improvements in the KOOS pain compared to patients affected by a patellofemoral chondropathy (31% femoral condyle vs. 11% patellofemoral, p≅0.05). At 6 months, patients under 55 years old showed better improvements in the KOOS sport compared to elderly patients (41% vs. 23% respectively, p < 0.05). At 12 months, only the surgical procedure (meniscectomy), as already shown, affects the outcomes. Considering the improvement between the pre-operative scores and the last follow up at 12 months, females showed better improvements in KOOS functional score with respect to males (tendency, $p = 0.077$).

Interestingly, the degree of OA does not significantly affect the outcomes.

On average, 92% of the SH patients and 74% of the SM patients clinically improved (Table 3) and 100% of them were satisfied with the treatment.

Table 2 Knee objective evaluation – summary of the results

	ROM	PAT SUBLUX	Walking	Stairs	Squatting	Strength	Stiffness	Swelling
SH								
Pre-op								
N	43%	86%	76%	71%	5%	90%	95%	57%
S	57%	14%	24%	29%	95%	10%	5%	43%
6 months								
N	100%	100%	100%	100%	71%	100%	100%	100%
S	0%	0%	0%	0%	29%	0%	0%	0%
12 months								
N	100%	100%	100%	100%	95%	100%	100%	100%
S	0%	0%	0%	0%	5%	0%	0%	0%
MS								
Pre-op								
N	36%	100%	86%	43%	0%	100%	100%	36%
S	64%	0%	14%	57%	100%	0%	0%	64%
6 months								
N	100%	100%	100%	92%	77%	100%	100%	100%
S	0%	0%	0%	8%	23%	0%	0%	0%
12 months								
N	100%	100%	93%	100%	86%	100%	100%	100%
S	0%	0%	7%	0%	14%	0%	0%	0%

N normal, *S* symptomatic, *ROM* range of motion, *PAT SUBLUX* patellar subluxation

No adverse events or complications were observed throughout the follow-up period, apart from one case of a temporary and small subcutaneous hematoma that did not require any additional treatment. For the sake of comprehensiveness, we report also the exceptional outcomes of the three patients (ICRS grade III-IV) that underwent the micro-perforations associated with micro-fragmented adipose tissue injection (data not shown). At 12 months, the average improvement for KOOS was 46 in symptoms ($p < 0.0001$), 48 in pain ($p < 0.0001$), 41 in function in daily living ($p < 0.0001$), 28 in sport ($p < 0.0001$) and 25 in the quality of life ($p < 0.0001$). Statistically significant differences ($p < 0.0001$) between pre-treatment and follow-up values were found also for the total WOMAC scores

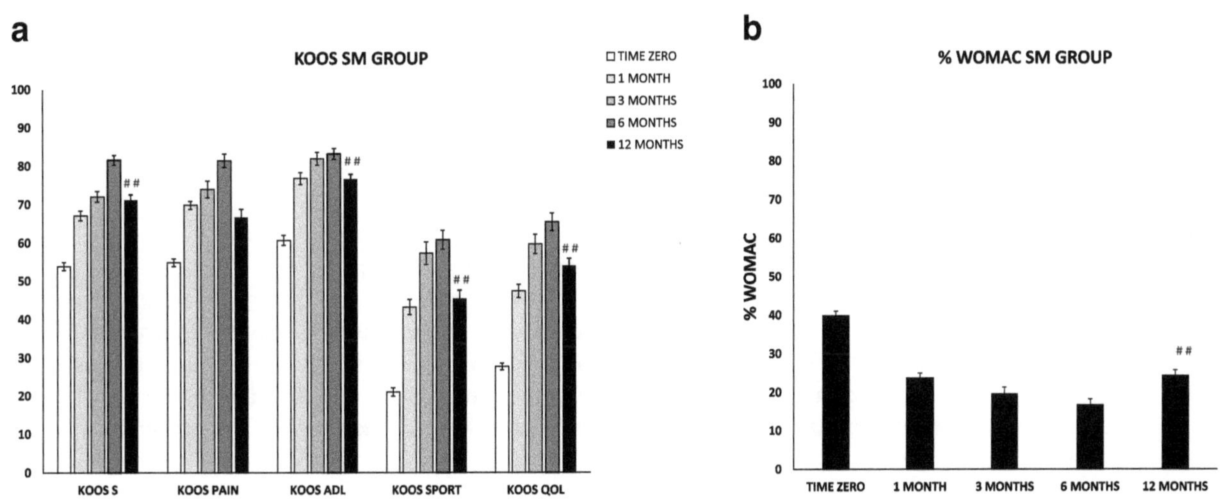

Fig. 2 Trend of functional improvements of the SM group from baseline to 12 months' follow-up. Results are expressed as mean and standard error. A $p < 0.05$ (T12 vs. T0) was considered statistically significant (# #). **a** KOOS score. KOOS S = symptoms; KOOS P = pain; KOOS ADL = activity daily living; KOOS Spt = sport; KOOS QoL = quality of life. **b** WOMAC Index

Table 3 Summary of the results

	Δ KOOS_s	Δ KOOS_p	Δ KOOS_adl	Δ KOOS_spt	Δ KOOS_QoL	Δ WOMAC
SH						
Mean	29	36	37	51	54	−36
SE	1.11	1.45	1.31	1.73	1.32	1.31
% improved patients	90%	86%	95%	90%	95%	95%
SM						
Mean	17	12	16	24	26	−15
SE	2.2	2.4	1.7	2.7	1.7	1.8
% improved patients	64%	57%	86%	71%	86%	79%

Data are expressed as mean Δ (t_{12}-t_0) and standard error (SE)
SH chondral shaving, *SM* chondral shaving + meniscectomy, *s* symptoms, *p* pain, *adl* function in daily living, *spt* sport, *QoL* quality of life

where the pain, stiffness and functional limitation decreased from 56 at baseline to 12 at 12 months follow-up.

Discussion

This study retrospectively analysed the safety and potential benefits of using autologous and micro-fragmented adipose tissue as adjuvant in the surgical treatment of degenerative knee chondropathy. The results demonstrated that, when associated with a shaving procedure, it improves symptoms and function at least until 1-year follow-up, with a trend of steady increase during time. Indeed, a constant and statistically significant improvement of all the clinical scores was observed from pre-op evaluation to the 1, 3, 6, and 12 months follow-up with KOOS sport and quality of life being the most improved scores.

Articular cartilage lesions and degenerations, generally associated with disability and symptoms such as joint pain and reduced function, are hard to treat and remain challenging. Current pharmacologic interventions only temporarily reduce pain and symptoms, but no proven disease-modifying therapy is available [1]. Non-surgical treatments, such as HA or PRP injections target the symptoms but cannot inhibit the degeneration process. Joint-preserving surgical treatments, such as arthroscopic shaving, debridement, laser chondroplasty, and microfractures, provide temporary relief of symptoms, but for the diffused degenerative pathology or chondropathies at the initial stage are contraindicated by many authors. In these cases, regenerative medicine, and, in particular, the use of progenitor cells is preferable. Indeed, besides their multipotency, these cells secrete a variety of bioactive molecules that act in a paracrine manner to prime and sustain angiogenic, anti-fibrotic, anti-apoptotic, anti-microbial and immunomodulatory responses in the target tissue [9, 11, 36].

A very important finding of this study, in addition to the constant improvement of all the clinical scores from baseline evaluation to the 1, 3, 6, and 12 months follow-up, is that no patient worsened compared to the pre-operative condition or underwent additional treatments. Noteworthy, patients who declared to be very active in sport still improved, demonstrating that also high functional demands benefit from the treatment (data not shown). The meniscectomy did not substantially affected the outcomes that were, anyway, very positive, with an average improvements of all the KOOS scores of 20 points and a physical examination positive for all the patients except for 2 in squatting. This is a very important finding, considering reported data showing that meniscectomy in the long term has been shown both experimentally and clinically to exacerbate the osteoarthritic condition [1]. The observed decrease in the scores from 6 to 12 months, although not statistically significant, can be explained by a loss of the functional unit "meniscus" in terms of knee stability leading to a progressive chondral damage. Nevertheless, the MRI at 12 months revealed no signs of bone edema in the treated compartments as index of severe chondral damage. The main limitation of the study is the lack of a control group that does not allow for any definitive conclusion about micro-fragmented adipose tissue effect. Nevertheless, we believe that this approach is very promising since, in our experience, standard chondral shaving did not allow for satisfactory results so far.

Conclusion

The results of this study show the safety and potential benefits of using autologous, micro-fragmented and minimally manipulated adipose tissue injection associated with the arthroscopic chondral shaving for the treatment of diffused knee chondropathy. The procedure is simple, sustainable, quick, minimally invasive, one-step, and safe. After one year, the results are very satisfactory and promising. A longer follow-up and a randomized controlled study on a big number of patients is needed to draw definitive conclusions and enlarge the indications.

Abbreviations
ASCs: Adipose-derived stem cells; FC: Femoral condyle; HA: Hyaluronic acid; KOOS: Knee Injury and Osteoarthritis Outcome Score; MSCs: Mesenchymal stem cells; NSAIDs: Nonsteroidal anti-inflammatory drugs; OA: Osteoarthritis; PF: Patellofemoral; PRP: Platelet-rich plasma; SVF: Stromal vascular fraction; TP: Tibial plateau; VAS: Visual analogue pain scale; WOMAC: Western Ontario and McMaster Universities Osteoarthritis Index

Authors' contributions
GC and ADC contributed equally to the work; they performed surgical procedures, adipose tissue processing, and data collection and wrote the manuscript draft; FN contributed in data collection; DC and PT performed the surgical procedures; AC revised the manuscript and approved the modified text. All the authors read and approved the final manuscript.

Competing interests
The authors declare that they have no competing interests.

Author details
[1]Spotorno Foundation c/o San Michele Clinics, Viale Pontelungo, 79, 17031 Albenga, SV, Italy. [2]Orthopaedic Department, San Paolo Hospital, Savona, SV, Italy.

References
1. Hunziker EB. Articular cartilage repair: basic science and clinical progress. A review of the current status and prospects. Osteoarthr Cartil. 2002;10:432–63.
2. Zhang W, Moskowitz R, Nuki G, et al. OARSI recommendations for the management of hip and knee osteoarthritis, part II: OARSI evidence-based, expert consensus guidelines. Osteoarthr Cartil. 2008;16:137–62.
3. Zhang W, Ouyang H, Dass CR, et al. Current research on pharmacologic and regenerative therapies for osteoarthritis. Bone Res. 2016;4:15040.
4. Bellamy N, Campbell J, Robinson V, et al. Viscosupplementation for the treatment of osteoarthritis of the knee. Cochrane Database Syst Rev. 2005;2:1–59.
5. Filardo G, Kon E, Longo UG, et al. Non-surgical treatments for the management of early osteoarthritis. Knee Surg Sports Traumatol Arthrosc. 2016;24:1775–85.
6. Kon E, Mandelbaum B, Buda R, et al. Platelet-rich plasma intra-articular injection versus hyaluronic acid viscosupplementation as treatments for cartilage pathology: from early degeneration to osteoarthritis. Arthroscopy. 2011;27:1490–501.
7. Shen L, Yuan T, Chen S, et al. The temporal effect of platelet-rich plasma on pain and physical function in the treatment of knee osteoarthritis: systematic review and meta-analysis of randomized controlled trials. J Orthop Surg Res. 2017;12:16.
8. McAlindon TE, Bannuru RR, Sullivan M, et al. OARSI guidelines for the non-surgical management of knee osteoarthritis. Osteoarthr Cartil. 2014;22:363–88.
9. Caplan AI, Correa D. The MSC: an injury drugstore. Cell Stem Cell. 2011;9:11–5.
10. Caplan AI, Dennis JE. Mesenchymal stem cells as trophic mediators. J Cell Biochem. 2006;98:1076–84.
11. Zuk PA, Zhu M, Ashjian P, et al. Human adipose tissue is a source of multipotent stem cells. Mol Biol Cell. 2002;13:4279–95.
12. Gimble JM, Guilak F, Bunnell BA. Clinical and preclinical translation of cell-based therapies using adipose tissue-derived cells. Stem Cell Res Ther. 2010;1:1.
13. Aronowitz JA, Lockhart RA, Hakakian CS. Mechanical versus enzymatic isolation of stromal vascular fraction cells from adipose tissue. Springerplus. 2015;4:713.
14. Caplan AI. Review: mesenchymal stem cells: cell-based reconstructive therapy in orthopedics. Tissue Eng. 2005;11:1198–211.
15. Kristjánsson B, Honsawek S. Current perspectives in mesenchymal stem cell therapies for osteoarthritis. Stem Cells Int. 2014;2014:1–13.
16. Pak J, Lee JH, Kartolo WA, et al. Cartilage regeneration in human with adipose tissue-derived stem cells: current status in clinical implications. Biomed Res Int. 2016;2016:1 12.
17. Pak J, Lee JH, Lee SH. Regenerative repair of damaged meniscus with autologous adipose tissue-derived stem cells. Biomed Res Int. 2014;2014:1–10.
18. Ruetze M, Richter W. Adipose-derived stromal cells for osteoarticular repair: trophic function versus stem cell activity. Expert Rev Mol Med. 2014;16:e9.
19. Mollon B, Kandel R, Chahal J, et al. The clinical status of cartilage tissue regeneration in humans. Osteoarthr Cartil. 2013;21:1824–33.
20. Dhollander AA, Sánchez VRG, Almqvist KF, et al. The use of scaffolds in the treatment of osteochondral lesions in the knee: current concepts and future trends. J Knee Surg. 2012;25:179–86.
21. Emans P, Jansen E, Iersel D, et al. Tissue-engineered constructs: the effect of scaffold architecture in osteochondral repair. J Tissue Eng Regen Med. 2013;7:751–6.
22. Arcidiacono JA, Blair JW, Benton KA. US Food and Drug Administration international collaborations for cellular therapy product regulation. Stem Cell Res Ther. 2012;3:1.
23. Torre ML, Lucarelli E, Guidi S, et al. Ex vivo expanded mesenchymal stromal cell minimal quality requirements for clinical application. Stem Cells Dev. 2014;24:677–85.
24. Smith P, Adams Jr WP, Lipschitz AH, et al. Autologous human fat grafting: effect of harvesting and preparation techniques on adipocyte graft survival. Plast Reconstr Surg. 2006;117:1836–44.
25. Bianchi F, Maioli M, Leonardi E, et al. A new nonenzymatic method and device to obtain a fat tissue derivative highly enriched in pericyte-like elements by mild mechanical forces from human lipoaspirates. Cell Transplant. 2013;22:2063–77.
26. Benzi R, Marfia G, Bosetti M, et al. Microfractured lipoaspirate may help oral bone and soft tissue regeneration: a case report. CellR4. 2015;e1583:3.
27. Cestaro G, De Rosa M, Massa S, et al. Intersphincteric anal lipofilling with micro-fragmented fat tissue for the treatment of faecal incontinence: preliminary results of three patients. Videosurgery and Other Miniinvasive Techniques. 2015;10(2):337–41.
28. Franceschini M, Castellaneta C, Mineo G. Injection of autologous micro-fragmented adipose tissue for the treatment of post-traumatic degenerative lesion of knee cartilage: a case report. CellR4. 2016;e1768:4.
29. Giori A, Tremolada C, Vailati R, et al. Recovery of function in anal incontinence after micro-fragmented fat graft (Lipogems®) injection: two years follow up of the first 5 cases. CellR4. 2015;e1544:3.
30. Grossi P, Giarratana S, Cernei S, et al. Low back pain treated with disc decompression and autologous micro-fragmented adipose tissue: a case report. CellR4. 2016;e1772:4.
31. Raffaini M, Tremolada C. Micro fractured and purified adipose tissue graft (Lipogems®) can improve the orthognathic surgery outcomes both aesthetically and in postoperative healing. CellR4. 2014;e1118:2.
32. Saibene A, Pipolo C, Lorusso R, et al. Transnasal endoscopic microfractured fat injection in glottic insufficiency. B-ENT. 2014;11:229–34.
33. Striano R, Chen H, Bilbool N, et al. Non-responsive knee pain with osteoarthritis and concurrent meniscal disease treated with autologous microfragmented adipose tissue under continuous ultrasound guidance. CellR4. 2015;e1690:3.
34. Tremolada C, Colombo V, Ventura C. Adipose tissue and mesenchymal stem cells: state of the art and Lipogems® technology development. Current Stem Cell Reports. 2016;2:304–12.
35. Ward BD, Lubowitz JH. Basic knee arthroscopy part 4: chondroplasty, meniscectomy, and cruciate ligament evaluation. Arthroscopy techniques. 2013;2:e507–8.
36. Zuk PA, Zhu M, Mizuno H, et al. Multilineage cells from human adipose tissue: implications for cell-based therapies. Tissue Eng. 2001;7:211–28.

17

Footwear for self-managing knee osteoarthritis symptoms: protocol for the Footstep randomised controlled trial

Kade L. Paterson[1*], Kim L. Bennell[1], Tim V. Wrigley[1], Ben R. Metcalf[1], Penny K. Campbell[1], Jessica Kazsa[2] and Rana S. Hinman[1]

Abstract

Background: Knee osteoarthritis (OA) is a leading cause of musculoskeletal pain and disability globally, and abnormal knee loading is central to disease pathogenesis. Clinical guidelines recommend clinicians provide advice regarding appropriate footwear for people with knee OA, yet there is little research comparing the effects of different footwear on knee OA symptoms. Research suggests that wearing flat flexible shoes is associated with lower knee joint loads compared to stable supportive shoe styles. This two-arm pragmatic, comparative effectiveness randomised controlled trial will compare the effects of daily use of flat flexible shoes and stable supportive shoes on knee OA clinical outcomes, over 6 months.

Methods: 164 people with symptomatic medial tibiofemoral OA of moderate to severe radiographic severity (Kellgren and Lawrence Grade 3 & 4) will be recruited from the community. Following baseline assessment, participants will be randomly allocated to receive either i) flat flexible shoes or; ii) stable supportive shoes. Participants will choose two different pairs of shoes from a selection that fulfil the criteria in their allocated shoe class. Limited disclosure will blind participants to group allocation. Participants will be instructed to wear their allocated shoes daily for 6 months (minimum of 6 h/day), after which participants will be reassessed. The primary outcomes are knee pain severity on walking (measured by numerical rating scale) and self-reported physical function (measured by the Western Ontario and McMaster Universities Osteoarthritis Index), assessed at baseline and 6 months. Secondary outcomes include additional measures of knee pain, function, sport and recreation participation and quality-of-life (measured using subscales of the Knee Osteoarthritis Outcome Score), as well as pain at other sites (measured by numerical rating scale), self-reported global ratings of change in pain and physical function (measured by 7-point rating scale), and physical activity levels (measured by Physical Activity Scale for the Elderly).

Discussion: This study will determine whether daily wear of flat flexible shoes improves clinical outcomes in the management of knee OA, compared to stable supportive shoes. Findings will assist clinicians in providing evidence-based advice regarding appropriate footwear for people with knee OA to self-manage symptoms.

Keywords: Osteoarthritis, Knee, Footwear, Shoes, Clinical trial, RCT, Biomechanics, Clinical trial

* Correspondence: kade.paterson@unimelb.edu.au
[1]Centre for Health, Exercise and Sports Medicine, Department of Physiotherapy, School of Health Sciences, Faculty of Medicine Dentistry & Health Sciences, The University of Melbourne, Melbourne, VIC, Australia
Full list of author information is available at the end of the article

Background

Osteoarthritis is the 11th highest contributor to global disability [1]. In 2012, 1.9 million Australians had OA [2], and modelling data estimate a 58% increase in OA by 2032 [2]. The knee joint is commonly affected, and knee OA is extremely debilitating. Pain is dominant, becoming persistent and more limiting as OA progresses. Health expenditure on OA in Australia in 2012 was $3.75 billion AUD [2], with most costs related to conservative and surgical treatments, lost productivity and substantial loss of quality of life. Globally, the annual total direct and indirect cost is estimated to vary between €300 to €19,5000 EUD per patient per year [3].

As OA is a chronic disease with no cure, people with OA have little choice but to self-manage their condition. Accordingly, advice about self-management is the cornerstone of conservative treatment, along with exercise and weight control [4, 5]. As abnormal biomechanics have been implicated in knee OA onset and progression [6, 7], clinical guidelines advocate that clinicians provide advice on "appropriate" footwear to help people with knee OA self-manage their symptoms [4, 8]. However, there is scant evidence from clinical trials to guide footwear choice for this patient group, or indeed, any population with chronic musculoskeletal pain. Guidelines suggest that shoes with thick shock-absorbing soles and arch supports are best for people with OA [8], based largely on expert opinion. Due to the lack of robust clinical trials in this area, footwear trials have been identified as an OA research priority by both the European League Against Rheumatism [8] and the National Institute for Health and Care Excellence (UK) [4].

Abnormal knee joint loading is central to OA pathogenesis [6, 7]. Knee load is typically inferred from three-dimensional gait analysis, usually by parameters of the external peak knee adduction moment. There is some evidence that greater knee load may increase symptoms and risk of structural progression in people with knee OA. For example, an increased knee adduction moment is associated with increased prevalence of medial bone marrow lesions [9] (an important source of pain in knee OA [10]) and medial cartilage defects [11]. The knee adduction moment is also one of the few modifiable factors that predict OA structural progression [7, 12–14]. Reducing knee loads via non-surgical biomechanical treatment strategies is thus an appropriate treatment aim for people with knee OA. Footwear is a promising avenue for self-management, given that foot position and motion influence knee loads.

Biomechanical research shows that wearing shoes significantly increases the knee adduction moment in people with knee OA, compared to barefoot walking [15, 16]. Biomechanical studies also show that some types of footwear increase knee loads more than others [17]. We, and others, have shown that stable supportive shoe styles increase knee loads significantly more compared to flat flexible shoe styles [18–20]. However it is stable supportive shoe styles that are typically recommended by clinicians for people with knee OA, and that are typically worn by people with the condition [21].

There are no high quality clinical trials comparing the effects of flat flexible shoes to stable supportive shoes on knee OA clinical outcomes. Uncontrolled data from the USA show flat flexible shoes reduce knee pain by 36% when worn for 6 h/day over 6 months in 16 people with medial knee OA [22]. In the only randomised controlled trial (RCT) to date [23], a small Brazilian study in 56 women with knee OA compared a standardized flat flexible "Moleca" shoe, worn ≥6 h/day for 6 months, to a control group who wore their own neutral tennis shoes "without characteristics of minimalist footwear". Flat flexible shoes led to greater pain relief compared to the control group, and significant improvements in function were also observed. Although promising, participants in this study were not blinded, which introduces a high risk of bias given that treatment benefits are often over-estimated when using subjective outcomes with unblinded participants [24]. Thus, further research comparing the effects of flat flexible shoes to stable supportive shoes, using robust RCT designs, is warranted.

The primary aim of this study is to determine if flat flexible shoes lead to significantly greater reductions in knee pain with walking, and improvements in physical function, compared to stable supportive shoes when worn daily over six months. We hypothesise that flat flexible shoes will reduce pain and improve self-reported physical function more than stable supportive shoes.

Methods/design

Trial design

This protocol is described according to SPIRIT guidelines for clinical trials ([25]). The trial is a two-arm pragmatic, comparative effectiveness RCT comparing flat flexible shoes to stable supportive shoes. It will be conducted at The University of Melbourne over 3 years. The primary end-point for analysis of outcomes is after 6 months of shoe wear.

Participants

We will recruit 164 participants with medial tibiofemoral OA from the community via advertisements in print/radio/social media, clinicians and our volunteer database. Knee OA will be classified according to the American College of Rheumatology clinical and radiographic criteria for knee OA [26]. Participants will be included if they:

i) are aged ≥50 years;

ii) report knee pain on most days of the past month;
iii) report average pain during walking (over the previous week) of at least 4 on an 11-point numerical rating scale (NRS, with terminal descriptors of 'no pain' and 'worst pain possible');
iv) demonstrate moderate-severe (Grade 3–4) tibiofemoral OA on x-ray as determined by the Kellgren & Lawrence grading system [27], as recent research suggests these patients may represent a subgroup to which biomechanical interventions designed to reduce the KAM may be more effectively targeted; and
v) demonstrate tibiofemoral osteophytes on x-ray.

Participants will be excluded if they:

i) have lateral joint space narrowing greater than or equal to medial joint space narrowing on x-ray;
ii) have had knee pain for < 3 months;
iii) have had recent knee surgery (past 6 months) or planning surgery in next 6 months;
iv) currently use shoe orthoses, customized shoes or ankle braces;
v) primarily wear high heels, thongs or work boots that would restrict ability to wear allocated shoes 6 h/day;
vi) have had a hip or knee joint replacement on either side;
vii) have had a high tibial osteotomy on either leg;
viii)have had any knee injections in the past 3 months or planning injections in next 6 months;
ix) self-report any other muscular, joint or neurological condition affecting lower limb function,
x) self-report any systemic or inflammatory joint disease (e.g. rheumatoid arthritis);
xi) currently use, or plan to use, a gait aid in the next 6 months;
xii) do not understand written/spoken English; or
xiii)are unable to commit to study requirements (e.g. wearing shoes, attending appointments, completing outcomes, do not have foot size in the range of 8 to 13US for men, and 6 to 11US for women).

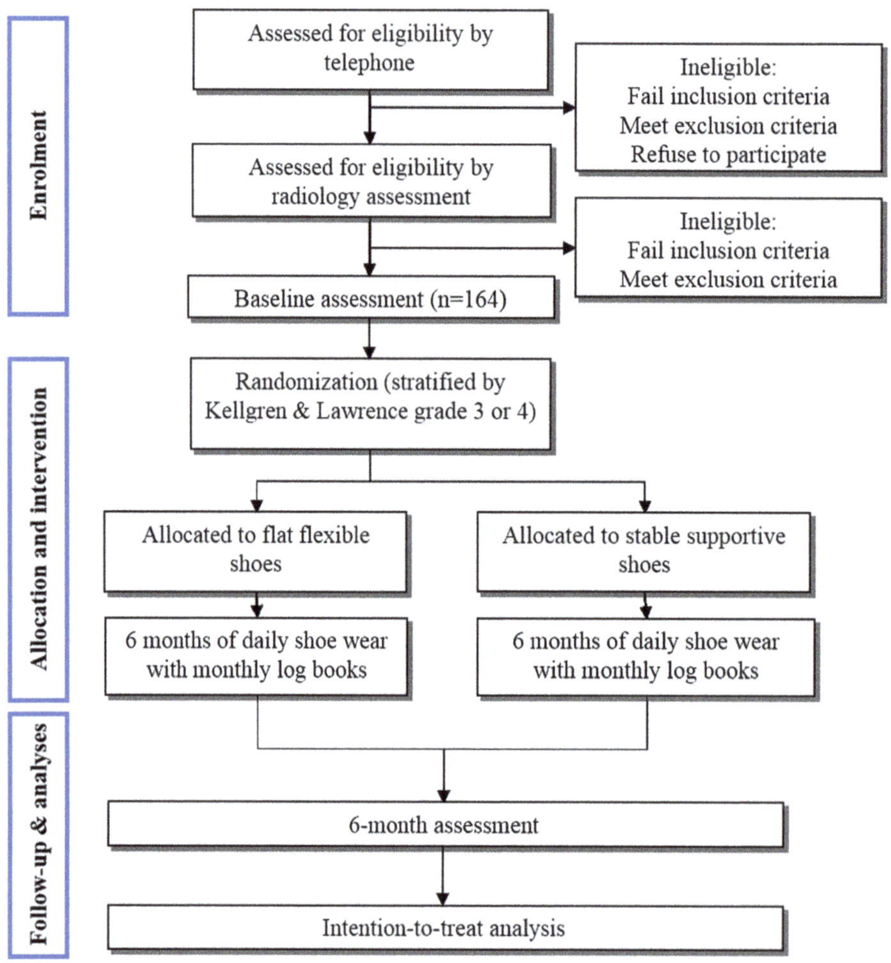

Fig. 1 Flow diagram of study phases

Procedure

Figure 1 outlines the trial phases and Table 1 describes the schedule for enrolment, intervention and assessments. Volunteers will be screened by an online form, then over the telephone by the Trial Coordinator. Potentially eligible participants will undergo standardised posteroanterior standing x-rays. Participants who have undergone standing x-ray in the prior 12 months, and can provide the images to research staff for screening, will not undergo new x-rays due to ethical concerns of exposing them to additional radiation. For participants with bilaterally eligible knees, the most symptomatic knee will be deemed the study knee with respect to outcome measurement.

Baseline assessments will be carried out at the Department of Physiotherapy, the University of Melbourne. At the 6-month follow-up, participants will complete questionnaires either on paper or electronically at home. Participants will also complete a short log book to record adherence with allocated footwear for one week of each month during the intervention period. If questionnaires or log books are not returned, the participant will be contacted by email and or phone to prompt their return, or as a last resort, to obtain primary outcome data. Ethical approval has been obtained from the University of Melbourne Human Research Ethics Committee (HREC No. 1748784). All participants will provide written informed consent.

Randomisation and allocation concealment

Eligible participants will be randomised to receive either flat flexible or stable supportive shoes following baseline data collection of primary and secondary outcomes. Randomisation (generated by the study biostatistician) will be by random permuted blocks (size 6 to 12) and stratified by radiographic disease severity (Kellgren & Lawrence grades 3 and 4 [27]). The schedule will be stored on a password-protected website (REDCap) maintained by a researcher not involved in either participant recruitment or administration of outcome measures. Group allocation will be revealed by this same researcher after baseline outcomes have been completed.

Participants will be blinded to group allocation by the process of limited disclosure. Participants will be

Table 1 Schedule of enrolment, interventions and assessments

	STUDY PERIOD							
	Enrolment	Allocation	Post-allocation					Close-out
TIMEPOINT	$-t_1$	0	1m	2m	3m	4m	5m	6m
ENROLMENT:								
Eligibility screen	X							
Informed consent	X							
Allocation		X						
INTERVENTIONS:								
Flat flexible shoes		◆—	—	—	—	—	—	—◆
Stable supportive shoes		◆—	—	—	—	—	—	—◆
ASSESSMENTS:								
Primary outcomes								
Knee pain on walking (11-point numerical scale)		X						X
Physical function (WOMAC physical function subscale)		X						X
Secondary outcomes								
Knee pain (KOOS pain subscale)		X						X
Sport and recreation activities (KOOS sport and recreation subscale)		X						X
Quality of life (KOOS quality of life subscale)		X						X
Patellofemoral pain and OA (KOOS PFJ pain and OA subscale)		X						X
Other joint pain (11-point numerical scale)		X						X
Health-related quality of life (AQoL-6D)		X						X
Physical activity (PASE)		X						X
Global improvement in pain								X
Global improvement in physical function								X
Other outcomes								
Co-interventions		X						X
Adverse events								X
Adherence to wearing shoes			X	X	X	X	X	X

informed that the trial is evaluating two different undisclosed "classes" of footwear to compare effects on knee OA symptoms. Participants will not be told about the classes of footwear under investigation, nor the specific shoe make/models that will be evaluated. Participants will not be informed about the study hypotheses, or which group they are allocated to until the study is completed, at which time they will be provided a lay summary of study purpose, hypotheses and findings. As the primary and secondary outcomes are participant-reported, and participants are blinded, this study is also considered assessor-blinded. Research staff administering and entering the participant-reported data will be blinded. Statistical analyses will be performed by a blinded biostatist ician. Descriptive baseline characteristics that are rese archer-measured using objective methods in the laboratory (e.g. height, weight, foot posture and pressure) will be measured before randomisation by the unblinded staff member who will allocate participants to footwear group, and fit participants to allocated shoes.

Interventions

We previously identified five criteria (Table 2) that distinguish flat flexible shoes from stable supportive shoes and showed that flat flexible shoes were associated with lower knee joint loads compared to stable supportive shoes [18]. Using our established criteria, we have selected a range of commercially-available shoes for each intervention arm. Once allocated to an intervention group, participants will choose two different pairs of shoes from the range of options in order to maximize adherence.

Consumers with chronic knee pain (68 women and 43 men) were consulted in the trial planning phase to help refine shoe selection for the study to ensure that the chosen shoes would be acceptable and likely to be worn as instructed (minimum of 6 h/day for 6 months). In a survey format, consumers were presented with a wide range of commercially available shoes (that fulfilled the criteria for each shoe class) in different styles and colours. Survey respondents mostly indicated that black was the preferred shoe colour, where black was an option. Where possible, the most popular shoe styles in each class were selected for the trial. These are shown in Fig. 2, and include:

Flat flexible shoes

Merrell Bare Access (Men and Women), Vivobarefoot Primus Lite (Men and Women), Vivobarefoot Mata Canvas (Men) and Converse Dainty Low (Women).

Stable supportive shoes

ASICS Kayano (Men and Women), Merrell Jungle Moc (Men), Nike Air Max 90 Ultra (Women), Rockport Edge Hill (Men) and New Balance 624 (Women).

As footwear manufacturers frequently change shoe models from season to season and year to year, we expect that shoes readily available at trial commencement may cease to be available during the course of the trial or may be rebranded with a different shoe name. In such instances, shoes will be replaced by another pair of commercially available shoes that fulfil the listed criteria in Table 2.

Participants will be instructed to wear either pair of their allocated shoes as much as possible every day for 6 months, and to avoid wearing their own usual footwear as much as possible. At a minimum, participants will be asked to wear the shoes for at least 6 h every day.

Outcome measures

Table 1 summarises the outcome measures that are being collected for this study. Our primary outcomes are validated measures of pain and physical function that have been recommended for use in knee OA clinical trials [28]. Conclusions regarding treatment efficacy will be based on the 6-month changes in our primary outcome measures. Our two primary outcomes, measured at baseline and 6 months, are:

- *Severity of knee pain during walking, scored on an 11-point NRS.* Average overall pain on walking in the last week will be self-reported using an 11-point NRS. Scores range from 0 to 10, where 0 = no pain and 10 = worst pain possible. This outcome measure has demonstrated reliability in OA [29].

Table 2 Criteria for selecting shoes

	Flat flexible shoes	Stable supportive shoes
Heel height/thickness	< 15 mm	> 30 mm
Shoe pitch	< 10 mm	> 10 mm
Arch support/motion control	Absent	Present
Sole flexibility	"Minimal" rigidity (Footwear Assessment Tool [45])	"Rigid" (Footwear Assessment Tool [45])
Weight[a]	≤200 g	> 300 g

Measurements are based on a size 9 US Men's and size 9 US Women's sized shoe
[a]A tolerance of +/− 10% was used for shoe weight

	Flat flexible shoes	Stable supportive shoes
Men's shoes	1) Merrell Bare Access 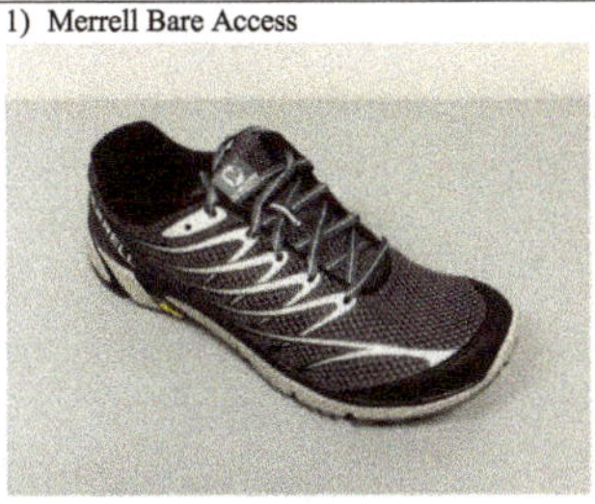	1) ASICS Kayano 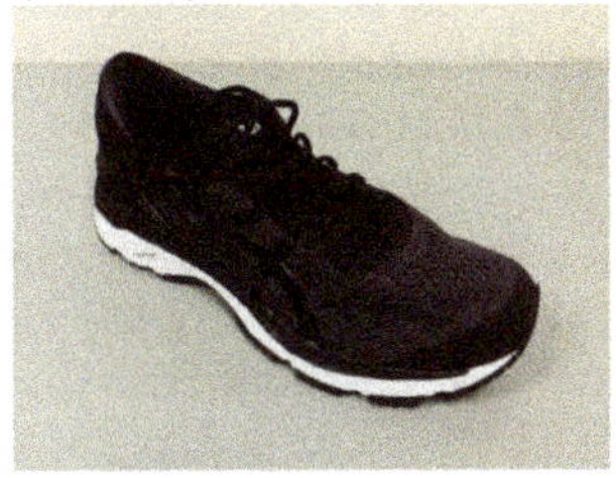
	2) Vivobarefoot Primus Lite 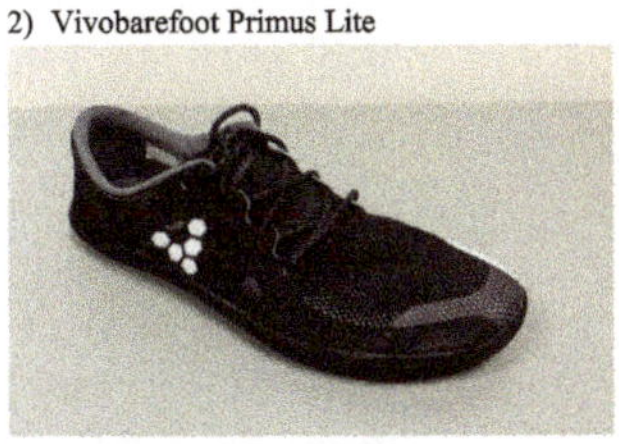	2) Merrell Jungle Moc 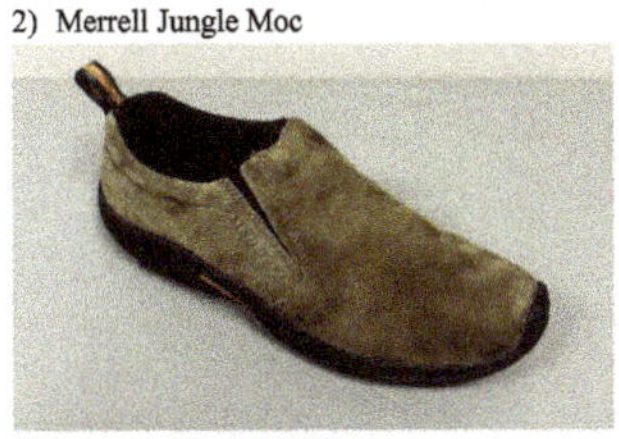
	3) Vivobarefoot Mata Canvas 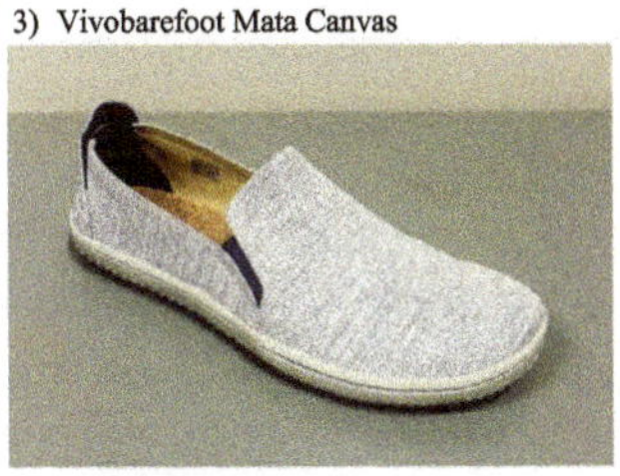	3) Rockport Edge Hill 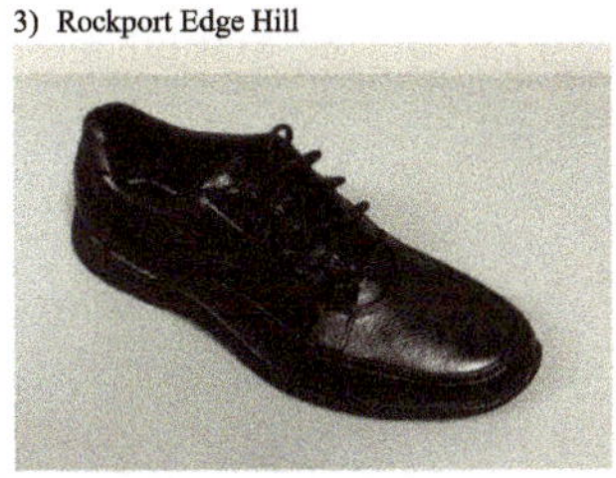
Women's shoes	1) Merrell Bare Access 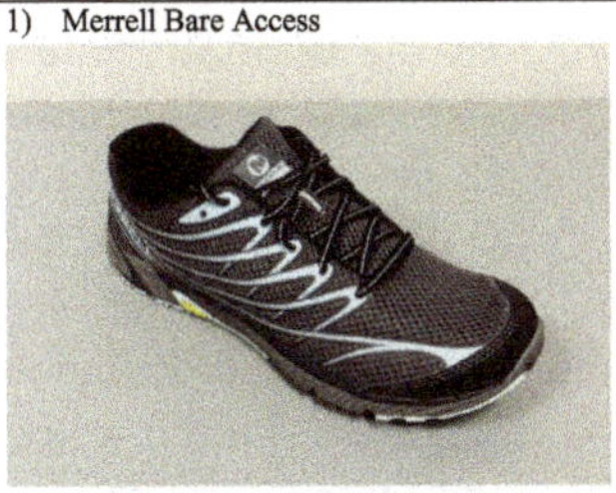	1) ASICS Kayano 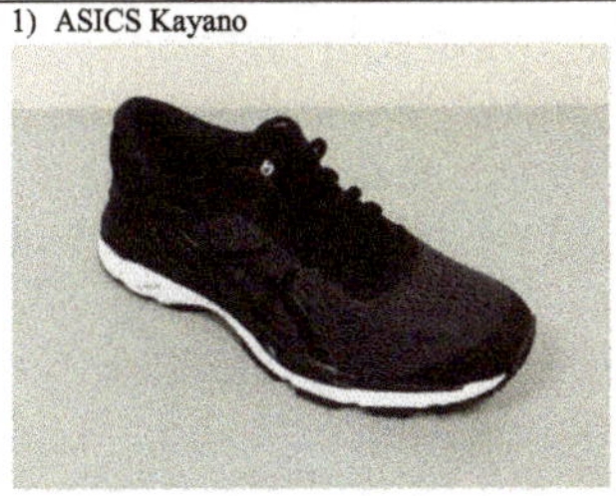
	2) Vivobarefoot Primus Lite 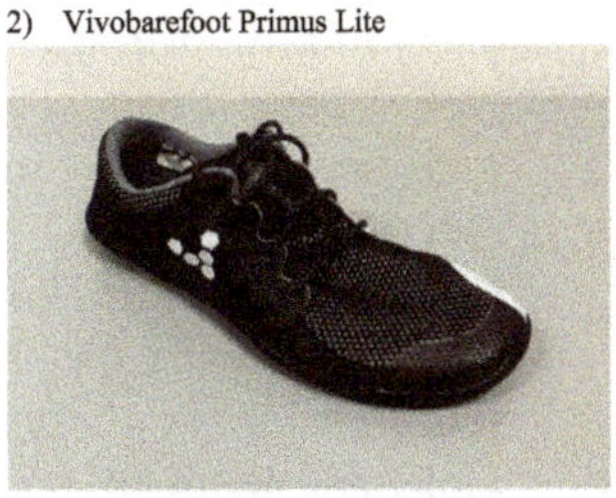	2) Nike Air Max 90 Ultra 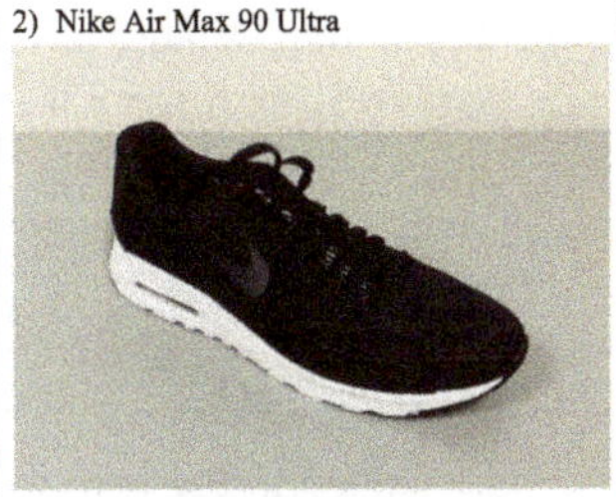
	3) Converse Dainty Low 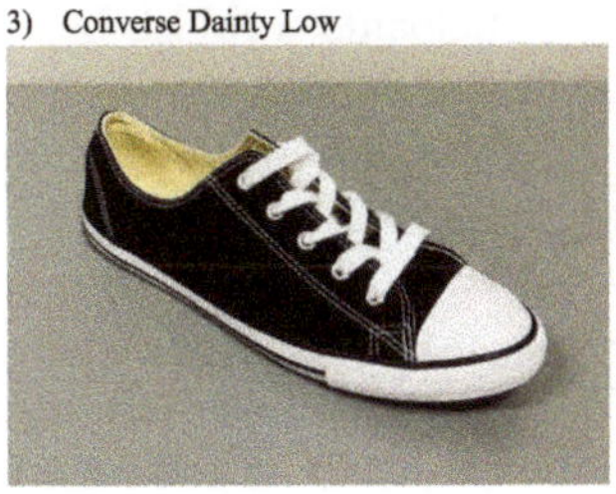	3) New Balance 624 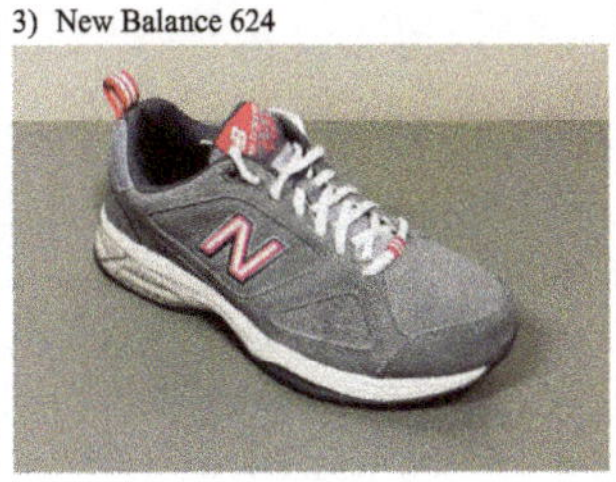

Fig. 2 Shoes selected at trial commencement

- *Physical function subscale of the WOMAC.* Limitations with physical functioning will be measured by the Western Ontario and McMaster Universities (WOMAC) Osteoarthritis Index (Likert version 3.1) [30]. The WOMAC is a self-report, disease-specific instrument which has established validity, reliability and responsiveness in an extensive range of OA studies [31]. The WOMAC physical function subscale contains 17 questions regarding knee function over the past week, with Likert response options ranging from 0 (no dysfunction) to 4 (extreme dysfunction). WOMAC scores will be extracted from the Knee Injury and Osteoarthritis Outcome Score (KOOS) [32] questionnaire, which contains the WOMAC questions. Total score ranges from 0 to 68, with higher scores indicating worse function.

Secondary outcome measures will be administered at baseline and at 6 months unless otherwise indicated. These include:

- *Pain subscale of the KOOS.* The subscale is scored using 9 questions about knee pain experienced in the last week, with Likert response options from None to Extreme. Scores range from 0 to 100, with lower scores indicating worse pain [32].
- *Sport and recreation subscale of the KOOS.* The subscale is scored using five questions regarding function with sport and recreational activities in the last week, with Likert response options ranging from None to Extreme [32]. Scores range from 0 to 100, with lower scores indicating worse function [32].
- *Quality of life subscale of the KOOS.* The subscale consists of four questions about knee-related quality of life experienced in the last week, with five Likert response options for each question. Scores range from 0 to 100, with lower scores indicating worse quality of life [32].
- *Patellofemoral pain and OA subscale of the KOOS.* The subscale is comprised of 11 questions about knee pain and function experienced in the last week, with five Likert response options for each question. Scores range from 0 to 100, with lower scores indicating worse patellofemoral symptoms [33].
- *Lower limb pain severity.* Average overall pain in the last week will be recorded using an 11-point NRS (0 = no pain and 10 = worst pain possible) at each of the following sites: (i) study knee, (ii) contralateral knee, (iii) ipsilateral hip, (iv) contralateral hip, (v) ipsilateral foot/ankle, (vi) contralateral foot/ankle, and (vii) back.
- *Participant-perceived global change.* At 6 months, participants will rate their overall global change in a) pain and b) physical function since enrolling in the study. Response to treatment will be scored using a 7-point global rating of change Likert scale, with terminal descriptors of 'much worse' to 'much better' [34]. Participants who report 'moderately better' or 'much better' will be classified as improved. All other respondents will be classified as not improved.
- *Health-related quality of life.* The Assessment of Quality of Life (AQoL) [35] (version AQoL-6D) will be used to measure health-related quality of life. It consists of 20 items that assess independent living, mental health, relationships, pain, coping and senses. Scores range from − 0.04 to 1.00 with higher scores indicating better quality of life.
- *Physical activity levels.* The Physical Activity Scale for the Elderly (PASE) will be used to measure physical activity over the previous week [36]. Scores range from 0 to over 400, with higher scores indicating greater physical activity.

Treatment adherence

Participants will rate their perceived overall level of adherence over the past 6 months with the instruction to wear their allocated shoes for a minimum of 6 h per day on an 11-point NRS (with terminal descriptors of 'shoes not worn all' and 'shoes worn completely as instructed'). At the 6-month follow up assessment, participants will also indicate whether they stopped wearing either pair of study shoes during the 6 months on a categorical scale (Yes or No). Participants who score Yes will describe when and why they ceased wearing their allocated shoes, and this will be reported descriptively. Finally, participants will record in log books how many hours each day they wear their allocated shoes, for 7 consecutive days every month, over the 6-month intervention period.

Adverse effects of treatment and co-interventions

Adverse events will be defined as any problem experienced in the study knee or elsewhere in the body because of wearing the study shoes. Adverse events will be self-reported by participants using a custom-developed table, and by open-ended questioning at 6 months. Participants will also be asked to contact the researchers at any time by telephone or email to report adverse events. Use of co-interventions (medications for knee pain and any other treatments for knee OA) will also be recorded at baseline and 6-months. Participants will complete a custom-developed table to indicate the frequency of use (over the past 6 months) of a range of pain and arthritis medications and co-interventions.

Descriptive measures

A range of other measures will be collected to describe demographic characteristics, treatment expectations, self-efficacy, foot biomechanics and current footwear characteristics. These measures will not be used to determine treatment efficacy but will be used for descriptive purposes. They include height, weight and body mass index; radiographic disease severity using the Kellgren & Lawrence scale [27]; current employment status; a rating of participant expectation of treatment outcome, measured on a 5-point ordinal scale; self-efficacy, determined using the Arthritis Self Efficacy Scale [37]; objective measures of foot posture, mobility and function including the Foot Posture Index (FPI [38]), Foot Mobility Magnitude [39], navicular drop [40] and in-shoe regional foot pressure patterns (Novel Pedar, Munich, Germany) during walking; and characteristics of each participant's three most commonly worn shoes, including shoe weight, heel height, pitch, motion control properties and flexibility [18].

Sample size calculations

We aim to detect the minimal clinically important difference (MCID) on primary outcomes between groups (1.8 (out of 10) [41] for NRS pain and 6 (out of 68) for WOMAC function) [42]. We assume between-participant standard deviations of 2.7 and 11.4, and baseline to 6-month correlations of 0.21 and 0.39 for pain and function respectively (data from our footwear trial in a similar sample) [43]. Using analysis of covariance adjusted for baseline score, we need 46 per arm to achieve 90% power to detect MCID in pain and 65 per arm for function. Allowing for 20% attrition, we will recruit 82 people per arm ($n = 164$).

Statistical analyses

A biostatistician will analyse data in a blinded manner, with p values less than 0.05 considered significant. Main comparative analyses between groups will be performed using intention-to-treat. If more than 5% of primary outcomes are missing, multiple imputation will be applied. For the primary hypothesis, differences in mean change in pain and function (baseline minus follow-up) will be compared between groups using linear regression modelling adjusted for baseline values and the stratifying variable of Kellgren & Lawrence grade. Similar analyses will be conducted for continuous secondary outcomes. Improvement based on global change will be compared across groups using risk differences, calculated from fitted logistic regression models. The effect of patient characteristics on outcomes will be explored by including relevant terms as covariates in models. Standard diagnostic plots will be used to check model assumptions.

To assess whether the effect of shoe class on the primary outcomes is moderated by any of Kellgren & Lawrence grade, Foot Posture Index score, body mass index or baseline score on the KOOS patellofemoral pain and OA subscale, appropriate interaction terms between randomised group and each of these variables will be included in regression models for the primary outcomes, and for each potential effect modifier separately. For the continuous moderators, a fractional polynomial approach will be applied [44].

Timelines

The application for project funding was successful in October 2016 and funding commenced in August 2017. Ethics approval was obtained from the Human Research Ethics Committee of the University of Melbourne in May 2017. Recruitment commenced in August 2017 and will be completed in December 2019. The trial is due for completion in July 2020 when all participants will have completed 6-month follow-up.

Discussion

This paper has outlined the theoretical foundation, and presented the protocol, for a two-arm pragmatic, comparative effectiveness RCT comparing flat flexible to stable supportive shoes for people with knee OA. Clinical OA guidelines recommend appropriate footwear for knee OA self-management [4, 8], with some guidelines specifying shoes with supportive features, based solely on expert opinion [8]. Stable supportive footwear are also recommended by clinicians for people with knee OA, and are typically worn by people with the disease [21]. Yet these styles increase knee loads compared to flat flexible shoes [18–20], while limited clinical data suggests flat flexible shoes may lead to symptomatic benefits [23]. Given the lack of high quality RCTs comparing footwear styles, leading international organisations [4, 8] have highlighted footwear clinical trials as an important OA research priority. Findings from the Footstep trial will assist clinicians and patients with knee OA in selecting the most appropriate footwear to help self-manage symptoms associated with the disease.

Abbreviations

AQoL: Assessment of Quality of Life; CONSORT: Consolidated Standards of Reporting Trials; HREC: Human Research Ethics Committee; KOOS: Knee Injury and Osteoarthritis Outcome Score; MCID: Minimal clinically important difference; NRS: Numerical rating scale; OA: Osteoarthritis; PASE: Physical Activity Scale for the Elderly; RCT: Randomised controlled trial; WOMAC: Western Ontario and McMaster Universities

Funding

This study is funded by the National Health and Medical Research Council (Project Grant #1124418). RSH is supported by an Australian Research Council Future Fellowship (FT130100175) and KLB by a National Health and Medical Research Council Principal Research Fellowship (APP1058440).

Authors' contributions
KLP, KLB, TVW and RSH conceived the idea for the study and RSH is leading the trial. KLP, TVW, JK and RSH obtained funding for the study. KLP, KLB, TVW and RSH designed the trial protocol with input from BRM, PKC and JK. KLP drafted the manuscript with input from KLB, TVW, BRM, PKC, JK and RSH. All authors read and approved the final manuscript.

Consent for publication
Not applicable.

Competing interests
KLP is a member of the Editorial Board of BMC Musculoskeletal Disorders. The other authors declare that they have no competing interests.

Author details
[1]Centre for Health, Exercise and Sports Medicine, Department of Physiotherapy, School of Health Sciences, Faculty of Medicine Dentistry & Health Sciences, The University of Melbourne, Melbourne, VIC, Australia. [2]Department of Epidemiology and Preventive Medicine, Monash University, Melbourne, Australia.

References
1. Cross M, Smith E, Hoy D, Nolte S, Ackerman I, Fransen M, Bridgett L, Williams S, Guillemin F, Hill CL, et al. The global burden of hip and knee osteoarthritis: estimates from the global burden of disease 2010 study. Ann Rheum Dis. 2014; 73:1323–30.
2. Arthritis & Osteoporosis Victoria. A Problem Worth Solving. The rising cost of musculoskeletal conditions in Australia. In: Arthritis & Osteoporosis Victoria; 2013.
3. Salmon JH, Rat AC, Sellam J, Michel M, Eschard JP, Guillemin F, Jolly D, Fautrel B. Economic impact of lower-limb osteoarthritis worldwide: a systematic review of cost-of-illness studies. Osteoarthr Cartil. 2016;24:1500–8.
4. National Clinical Guideline Centre: Osteoarthritis. Care and management in adults. In: Clinical guideline CG177. Methods, evidence and recommendations. London: National Institute for Health and Care Excellence; 2014.
5. McAlindon TE, Bannuru RR, Sullivan MC, Arden NK, Berenbaum F, Bierma-Zeinstra SM, Hawker GA, Henrotin Y, Hunter DJ, Kawaguchi H, et al. OARSI guidelines for the non-surgical management of knee osteoarthritis. Osteoarthr Cartil. 2014;22:363–88.
6. Andriacchi TP, Mundermann A. The role of ambulatory mechanics in the initiation and progression of knee osteoarthritis. Curr Opin Rheumatol. 2006;18:514–8.
7. Chehab EF, Favre J, Erhart-Hledik JC, Andriacchi TP. Baseline knee adduction and flexion moments during walking are both associated with 5 year cartilage changes in patients with medial knee osteoarthritis. Osteoarthr Cartil. 2014;22:1833–9.
8. Fernandes L, Hagen KB, Bijlsma JW, Andreassen O, Christensen P, Conaghan PG, Doherty M, Geenen R, Hammond A, Kjeken I, et al. EULAR recommendations for the non-pharmacological core management of hip and knee osteoarthritis. Ann Rheum Dis. 2013;72:1125–35.
9. Bennell KL, Creaby MW, Wrigley TV, Bowles KA, Hinman RS, Cicuttini F, Hunter DJ. Bone marrow lesions are related to dynamic knee loading in medial knee osteoarthritis. Ann Rheum Dis. 2010;69:1151–4.
10. Lo GH, McAlindon T, Niu J, Zhang Y, Beals C, Dabrowski C, Le Graverand MH, Hunter D. Bone marrow lesions and joint effusion are strongly and independently associated with weight-bearing pain in knee osteoarthritis: data from the osteoarthritis initiative. Osteoarthr Cartil. 2009;17:1562–9.
11. Creaby MW, Wang Y, Bennell KL, Hinman RS, Metcalf BR, Bowles KA, Cicuttini FM. Dynamic knee loading is related to cartilage defects and tibial plateau bone area in medial knee osteoarthritis. Osteoarthr Cartil. 2010;18:1380–5.
12. Bennell KL, Bowles KA, Wang Y, Cicuttini F, Davies-Tuck M, Hinman RS. Higher dynamic medial knee load predicts greater cartilage loss over 12 months in medial knee osteoarthritis. Ann Rheum Dis. 2011;70:1770–4.
13. Miyazaki T, Wada M, Kawahara H, Sato M, Baba H, Shimada S. Dynamic load at baseline can predict radiographic disease progression in medial compartment knee osteoarthritis. Ann Rheum Dis. 2002;61:617–22.
14. Chang AH, Moisio KC, Chmiel JS, Eckstein F, Guermazi A, Prasad PV, Zhang Y, Almagor O, Belisle L, Hayes K, et al. External knee adduction and flexion moments during gait and medial tibiofemoral disease progression in knee osteoarthritis. Osteoarthr Cartil. 2015;23:1099–106.
15. Kemp G, Crossley K, Wrigley T, Metcalf B, Hinman R. Reducing joint loading in medial knee osteoarthritis: shoes and canes. Arthritis Care Res. 2008;59:609–14.
16. Shakoor N, Block J. Walking barefoot decreases loading on the ower extremity joints in knee osteoarthritis. Arthritis Rheum. 2006;54:2923–7.
17. Radzimski AO, Mündermann A, Sole G. Effect of footwear on the external knee adduction moment — a systematic review. Knee. 2012;19:163–75.
18. Paterson KL, Bennell KL, Wrigley TV, Metcalf BR, Kasza J, Hinman RS. Effects of footwear on the knee adduction moment in medial knee osteoarthritis: classification criteria for flat flexible vs stable supportive shoes. Osteoarthr Cartil. 2017;25:234–41.
19. Shakoor N, Sengupta M, Foucher KC, Wimmer MA, Fogg LF, Block JA. Effects of common footwear on joint loading in osteoarthritis of the knee. Arthritis Care Res. 2010;62:917–23.
20. Shakoor N, Lidtke RH, Sengupta M, Fogg LF, Block JA. Effects of specialized footwear on joint loads in osteoarthritis of the knee. Arthritis Care Res. 2008; 59:1214–20.
21. Paterson KL, Wrigley TV, Bennell KL, Hinman RS. A survey of footwear advice, beliefs and wear habits in people with knee osteoarthritis. J Foot Ankle Res. 2014;7:43.
22. Shakoor N, Lidtke RH, Wimmer MA, Mikolaitis RA, Foucher KC, Thorp LE, Fogg LF, Block JA. Improvement in knee loading after use of specialized footwear for knee osteoarthritis: results of a six-month pilot investigation. Arthritis Rheum. 2013;65:1282–9.
23. Trombini-Souza F, Matias AB, Yokota M, Butugan MK, Goldenstein-Schainberg C, Fuller R, Sacco IC. Long-term use of minimal footwear on pain, self-reported function, analgesic intake, and joint loading in elderly women with knee osteoarthritis: a randomized controlled trial. Clin Biomech. 2015;30:1194–201.
24. Wood L, Egger M, Gluud LL, Schulz KF, Juni P, Altman DG, Gluud C, Martin RM, Wood AJ, Sterne JA. Empirical evidence of bias in treatment effect estimates in controlled trials with different interventions and outcomes: meta-epidemiological study. BMJ. 2008;336:601–5.
25. Chan A, Tetzlaff JM, Altman DG, et al. Spirit 2013 statement: defining standard protocol items for clinical trials. Ann Intern Med. 2013;158:200–7.
26. Altman R, Asch E, Bloch D, Bole G, Borenstein D, Brandt K, Christy W, Cooke TD, Greenwald R, Hochberg M, et al. Development of criteria for the classification and reporting of osteoarthritis. Classification of osteoarthritis of the knee. Arthritis Rheum. 1986;29:1039–49.
27. Kellgren JH, Jeffrey MR, Ball J. The epidemiology of chronic rheumatism: atlas of standard radiographs. Vol. volume 2. Oxford: Blackwell Scientific; 1963.
28. Bellamy N. Outcome measurement in osteoarthritis clinical trials. J Rheumatol. 1995;22:49–51.
29. Bellamy N. Osteoarthritis clinical trials: candidate variables and clinimetric properties. J Rheumatol. 1997;24:768–78.
30. Bellamy N, Buchanan WW, Goldsmith CH, Campbell J, Stitt LW. Validation study of WOMAC: a health status instrument for measuring clinically important patient relevant outcomes to antirheumatic drug therapy in patients with osteoarthritis of the hip or knee. J Rheumatol. 1988;15:1833–40.
31. McConnell S, Kolopack P, Davis AM. The western Ontario and McMaster universities osteoarthritis index (WOMAC): a review of its utility and measurement properties. Arthritis Rheum. 2001;45:453–61.
32. Roos EM, Roos HP, Lohmander LS, Ekdahl C, Beynnon BD. Knee injury and osteoarthritis outcome score (KOOS) - development of a self-administered outcome measure. J Orthop Sports Phys Ther. 1998;28:88–96.
33. Crossley KM, Macri EM, Cowan SM, et al. The patellofemoral pain and osteoarthritis subscale of the KOOS (KOOS-PF): development and validation using the COSMIN checklist. Br J Sports Med. 2017. doi: https://doi.org/10.1136/bjsports-2016-096776

34. ten Klooster PM, Drossaers-Bakker KW, Taal E, van de Laar MA. Patient-perceived satisfactory improvement (PPSI): interpreting meaningful change in pain from the patient's perspective. Pain. 2006;121:151–7.
35. Osborne RH, Hawthorne G, Lew EA, Gray LC. Quality of life assessment in the community-dwelling elderly: validation of the assessment of quality of life (AQoL) instrument and comparison with the SF-36. J Clin Epidemiol. 2003;56:138–47.
36. Martin K, Rejeski W, Miller M, James M, Ettinger W Jr, Messier S. Validation of the PASE in older adults with knee pain and physical disability. Med Sci Sport Exer. 1999;31:627–33.
37. Lorig K, Chastain RL, Ung E, Shoor S, Holman HR. Development and evaluation of a scale to measure perceived self-efficacy in people with arthritis. Arthritis Rheum. 1989;32:37–44.
38. Redmond AC, Crosbie J, Ouvrier RA. Development and validation of a novel rating system for scoring standing foot posture: the foot posture index. Clin Biomech. 2006;21:89–98.
39. McPoil T, Vicenzino B, Cornwall M, Collins N, Warren M. Reliability and normative values for the foot mobility magnitude: a composite measure of vertical and medial-lateral mobility of the midfoot. J Foot Ankle Res. 2009;2:6.
40. Brody DM. Techniques in the evaluation and treatment of the injured runner. Orthop Clin N Am. 1982;13:541.
41. Bellamy N, Carette S, Ford P, Kean W, le Riche N, Lussier A, Wells G, Campbell J. Osteoarthritis antirheumatic drug trials. III. Setting the delta for clinical trials- results of a consensus development (Delphi) exercise. J Rheumatol. 1992;19:451–7.
42. Tubach F, Ravaud P, Baron G, Falissard B, Logeart I, Bellamy N, Bombardier C, Felson D, Hochberg M, van der Heijde D, et al. Evaluation of clinically relevant changes in patient reported outcomes in knee and hip osteoarthritis: the minimal clinically important improvement. Ann Rheum Dis. 2005;64:29–33.
43. Hinman RS, Wrigley TV, Metcalf BR, Hunter DJ, Campbell P, Paterson K, Staples MP, Bennell KL. Unloading shoes for osteoarthritis of the knee: protocol for the SHARK randomised controlled trial. BMC Musculoskelet Disord. 2014;15:48.
44. Royston P, Sauerbrei W. Two techniques for investigating interactions between treatment and continuous covariates in clinical trials. Stata J. 2009;9:230.
45. Barton CJ, Bonanno D, Menz HB. Development and evaluation of a tool for the assessment of footwear characteristics. J Foot Ankle Res. 2009;2:10.

18

Objective assessment of physical activity and sedentary behaviour in knee osteoarthritis patients – beyond daily steps and total sedentary time

Maik Sliepen[1*], Elsa Mauricio[1], Matthijs Lipperts[2], Bernd Grimm[2] and Dieter Rosenbaum[1,3]

Abstract

Background: Knee osteoarthritis patients may become physically inactive due to pain and functional limitations. Whether physical activity exerts a protective or harmful effect depends on the frequency, intensity, time and type (F.I.T.T.). The F.I.T.T. dimensions should therefore be assessed during daily life, which so far has hardly been feasible. Furthermore, physical activity should be assessed within subgroups of patients, as they might experience different activity limitations. Therefore, this study aimed to objectively describe physical activity, by assessing the F.I.T.T. dimensions, and sedentary behaviour of knee osteoarthritis patients during daily life. An additional goal was to determine whether activity events, based on different types and durations of physical activity, were able to discriminate between subgroups of KOA patients based on risk factors.

Methods: Clinically diagnosed knee osteoarthritis patients (according to American College of Rheumatology criteria) were monitored for 1 week with a tri-axial accelerometer. Furthermore, they performed three functional tests and completed the Knee Osteoarthritis Outcome Score. Physical activity levels were described for knee osteoarthritis patients and compared between subgroups.

Results: Sixty-one patients performed 7303 mean level steps, 319 ascending and 312 descending steps and 601 bicycle crank revolutions per day. Most waking hours were spent sedentary (61%), with 4.6 bouts of long duration (> 30 min). Specific events, particularly ascending and descending stairs/slopes, brief walking and sedentary bouts and prolonged walking bouts, varied between subgroups.

Conclusions: From this sample of KOA patients, the most common form of activity was level walking, although cycling and stair climbing activities occurred frequently, highlighting the relevance of distinguishing between these types of PA. The total active time encompassed a small portion of their waking hours, as they spent most of their time sedentary, which was exacerbated by frequently occurring prolonged bouts.
In this study, event-based parameters, such as stair climbing or short bouts of walking or sedentary time, were found more capable of discriminating between subgroups of KOA patients compared to overall levels of PA and sedentary time. Thereby, subtle limitations in physical behaviour of KOA-subgroups were revealed, which might ultimately be targeted in rehabilitation programs.
(Continued on next page)

* Correspondence: mpl.sliepen@gmail.com
[1]Institut für Experimentelle Muskuloskelettale Medizin (IEMM), Universitätsklinikum Münster (UKM), Westfälische Wilhelms-Universität Münster (WWU), Albert-Schweitzer Campus 1, Gebäude D3, 48129 Münster, Germany
Full list of author information is available at the end of the article

(Continued from previous page)

Keywords: Knee osteoarthritis, Physical activity, Sedentary behaviour, Accelerometer, Body-worn sensors, F.I.T.T., Stair climbing, Objective assessment,

Background

Knee osteoarthritis (KOA) is a frequent cause of pain and disability, affecting over 250 million people worldwide [1, 2]. In part due to experienced pain and limitations, KOA patients generally spend most of their waking hours sedentary (i.e. sitting or lying as opposed to standing or in locomotion) and fail to adhere to physical activity recommendations [3, 4]. Such behaviour could ultimately lead to harmful co-morbidities such as cardiovascular diseases [5].

Physical activity (PA) is a multidimensional behaviour, which is suggested to consist of four dimensions (F.I.T.T.: frequency, intensity, time and type) according to the World Health Organization (WHO) [6]. Whether PA exerts a protective or harmful effect seems to depend primarily on the type, intensity and frequency of PA [7], which highlights the importance of assessing the four dimensions of PA during daily life. On one hand, PA could lead to the progression of KOA, as heavy, repetitive loading may detrimentally affect the articular cartilage of the knee [7]. On the contrary, PA has been shown to prevent functional impairment and maintain independence in KOA patients [7].

A multitude of methods exists to assess PA during daily life. Arguably, the most appropriate method is using accelerometer-based activity monitors, as these are able to implement an activity event-based approach and thus objectively capture the F.I.T.T. dimensions of PA [8]. Furthermore, these devices can objectively determine the time spent sedentary, which is known to detrimentally affect the general health and functional status of KOA patients [4].

So far, studies that have assessed the physical behaviour of KOA patients with activity monitors have generally not been able to describe the four individual dimensions of PA, particularly the type of activities that were performed by KOA patients. Therefore, potentially relevant knowledge regarding the effect of different types of PA on KOA might have been missed. Due to recent technological advancements, the objective assessment of stair/slope locomotion and bicycling, in addition to stepping behaviour, is now feasible [9]. Furthermore, the time patterns of activity and sedentary behaviour can now be determined objectively [9]. Stair locomotion might be a clinically relevant assessment outcome in KOA, as it is often reported as one of the most demanding or even painful activities and is essential for the independence of patients in daily life [10]. Similarly, objectively quantifying bicycling in a free-living environment is important, since the joint moments experienced during cycling are considered small compared to other activities [11]. Cycling is therefore perceived as less painful and commonly prescribed as rehabilitating exercise in KOA patients [12]. In addition, bicycling is a common mode of transportation and recreational activity in Europe [13]. Interrupting sedentary behaviour has been shown to improve physical function and general health of older adults [14, 15]. Consequently, assessing the distribution of sedentary bout durations and interruptions, in addition to overall levels of sedentary time, should be a valuable measurement outcome in a KOA population.

Physical behaviour of KOA patients should not only be assessed on a population-level, but also within subgroups, as they are suggested to engage in different types of PA and experience varying activity limitations [16, 17]. Thus, differentiating between subgroups, which can be characterized based on risk factors (e.g. gender, BMI and knee injury) [18], might reveal subgroup-specific PA limitations. For this purpose, an event-based approach (e.g. activity bouts of specific durations and types) has been suggested to be more discriminative compared to general outcome measures that describe overall levels of PA (e.g. total amount of daily steps) [19].

Therefore, this study aimed to comprehensively describe physical activity, by assessing F.I.T.T. dimensions, and sedentary behaviour of knee osteoarthritis patients during daily life. An additional goal was to determine whether activity events, based on different types and durations of PA, were able to discriminate between subgroups of KOA patients based on risk factors.

Methods

Study design

A cross-sectional, exploratory study was conducted to assess physical activity, sedentary behaviour and physical function in German knee osteoarthritis patients during daily life.

Participants

Eligible adults were required to present with clinical KOA (according to the guidelines of the American College of Rheumatology) and to report pain on most (≥4) days of the week for more than 3 months [20]. Individuals were excluded if they: (1) suffered from rheumatoid arthritis; (2) had a knee replacement, or were scheduled for replacement surgery within 3 months at the beginning of study participation; (3) suffered from medical conditions which could interfere with the activity and test performance, such as neurologic or severe cardiovascular conditions, (4) used an ambulatory aid for more than 50% of the ambulatory time. All participants were recruited at local hospitals and general practices.

Physical activity assessment

Physical activity was monitored using the AX3, a small tri--axial accelerometer (23 × 32.5 × 7.6 mm; sampling frequency: 50 Hz; Axivity Ltd., Newcastle, UK). Patients were instructed to wear the device for seven consecutive days during waking hours, except for water-based activities. The device was worn on the lateral side of the right thigh, halfway between femoral head and tibial plateau, attached by double-adhesive tape. To ensure consistency, the researcher marked the wear location.

Relevant parameters of the F.I.T.T. dimensions were extracted using custom-developed Matlab algorithms (detailed information has been described elsewhere [9]), which have shown highly accurate results in both healthy participants and orthopaedic lower-extremity patients [9]. In short, various types of activities were assessed (i.e. walking, sitting, standing, stair/slope climbing and bicycling). Furthermore, the frequency with which these activities were performed and the time spent within the activities was monitored. The intensity of walking (i.e. walking cadence) was also determined (Table 1). Participants filled in a daily log reporting on wear times, experienced pain through a numeric rating scale (NRS; 0 is no pain, 10 is worst conceivable pain) and physical activity events that could not be monitored with the algorithms (i.e. resistance exercise, swimming, gardening and household activities).

Table 1 Parameters extracted from AX3, categorized according to F.I.T.T. acronym

Dimension	Parameter
Frequency	Number of level steps Number of ascending steps Number of descending steps Number of bicycling crank revolutions Bouts of level steps Bouts of ascending steps Bouts of descending steps Number of walking bouts (0–5 s) Number of walking bouts (5–10 s) Number of walking bouts (300–600 s) Number of walking bouts (> 600 s) Number of sedentary bouts (0–10 s) Number of sedentary bouts (10–60 s) Number of sedentary bouts (1200–1800 s) Number of sedentary bouts (> 1800 s)
Intensity	Walking cadence
Time	Time spent walking (incl. Level, ascend and descend). Time spent bicycling Time spent sitting Time spent standing
Type	Walking Stair/slope ascending Stair/slope descending Bicycling Sitting Standing STS transfers

STS Sit-to-stand

Physical function scores

The participants performed three functional tests, rather than a single one, in order to represent different activities of daily life. They performed the 40 m (4 × 10 m) fast-paced Walk Test (WT), Timed Up and Go Test (TUGT) and 15-Stair Climb Test (SCT). The tests are proven to be valid, reliable and sensitive for knee OA patients [21]. Tests were conducted following the standard protocol instructing patients to perform as fast as possible while the time was recorded with a stopwatch [21]. Each test was performed three times and the average time was used for further analysis.

Questionnaire

Patients were asked to fill in the Knee Osteoarthritis Outcome Score (KOOS), a valid and responsive questionnaire covering several disease-related domains, ranging from 0 (most severely affected) to 100 (not affected) [22]. Furthermore, patients were asked about a previous knee injury ('Have you ever had a knee injury, which resulted in the inability to walk for over one week'), their job and employment status (i.e. employed, unemployed or retired) and whether they performed any sports on a regular basis (specifics regarding type of sports and frequency).

Statistical analysis

After the measurement, all participant data was pseudonymised. For the activity monitor data, a minimum of 4 valid wear days (i.e. at least 10 daily wear hours) was used as threshold, as these are minimally needed to obtain reliable PA estimates [23, 24]. Participants with insufficient valid wear days were excluded from further analysis.

All analyses were performed with SPSS (Version 23, SPSS Inc., USA), with the significance level set at $\alpha = 0.05$. First, descriptive statistics regarding socio-demographics, health-related factors and activity parameters were calculated for the total patient sample. Spearman's rank correlations were computed between activity parameters, the function test scores and KOOS outcomes.

Next, patients were grouped using their respective gender (male/female), BMI category (normal, BMI < 25; overweight, BMI 25–30; obese, BMI > 30) and history of knee injury (knee injury/no knee injury) as a variable. Data was tested for normality using the Shaphiro-Wilk Test and distribution histograms. In case of positively-skewed data (i.e. a violation of the normality-assumption), either a square-root or logarithmic transformation was used to generate a normal distribution [25]. One-way ANCOVA's were then used to examine the difference in PA parameters between subgroups of KOA patients, while adjusting for possible confounders (i.e. age, gender, BMI, pain and knee injury) [26]. A post-hoc Bonferroni correction was incorporated to adjust for multiple comparisons [25]. Afterwards, the transformed data was back-transformed to present meaningful values [25]. If the data was extremely skewed and a normal distribution could not be achieved (e.g. data that frequently contains '0'), non-parametric tests were used (e.g. Mann-Whitney U Test). Data regarding the socio-demographics, health factors and physical function of the complete sample were presented as mean ± standard deviation (SD). The differences between subgroups were presented as adjusted mean ± standard error (SE). Finally, transformed data was presented as adjusted mean (95% confidence interval (CI)) [25].

Results

Socio-demographics, health factors and physical function

In total, 61 of the included 64 participants provided valid activity data and were included for further analysis (56% female). The average age was 60 (±10) years. Of the included patients, 18, 30 and 13 were categorized as having a 'normal', 'overweight' and 'obese' BMI, respectively. They reported a mean pain score of 3.0 (NRS) or 57.4 ($KOOS_{pain}$). A slight majority of the patients (51%) had previously suffered a knee injury (Table 2). Most were still employed (57%) and 56% of the participants reported to perform some form of sports, twice per week. With respect to the functional tests, the patients needed a mean time of 26.1 (±4.7), 7.2 (±1.6) and 14.0 (±4.9) seconds to complete the WT, TUGT and SCT respectively (Table 2).

Physical activity and sedentary parameters

The AX3 was worn for a mean of 6.5 (±1.0) days, with an average wear time of 14.7 (±1.2) hours per day. Patients spent 11% of the waking hours walking (incl. Stair locomotion) and 1% bicycling, whereas most of the time was spent with non-locomotion behaviour (88%).

A mean amount of 7934 (±2326) steps were recorded per day, with an average cadence during walking bouts of 100 (±11) steps per minute. A quarter of the participants performed prolonged walking periods (lasting more than 10 min), twice per week. Ascending and descending stairs or slopes occurred 25 and 22 times on a daily basis, with a large variation ranging from 2 to 64 bouts (Table 3). The majority of participants (72%) cycled during the measurement period for a mean of 20 (±17) minutes per day. If crank revolutions were added as steps (since step-based PA recommendations do not discriminate between walking and cycling behaviour) 8535 steps would be counted on a daily basis. This way 25% of the participants would reach the commonly advocated threshold of 10,000 daily steps [3].

Table 2 Participant characteristics, physical function and knee osteoarthritis outcome scores (n = 61)

Characteristics	Mean (±SD)	Range
Sociodemographics		
Age (years)	60.7 (10.0)	37.0–79.0
Gender (male/female)	27/34	
Employment status (employed/retired)	35/26	
Regular sport participation (yes/no)	34/27	
Health factors		
BMI (kg/m^2)	27.3 (4.7)	19.7–42.8
Injury history (yes/no)	31/30	
Pain (NRS)	3.0 (1.5)	1.0–7.8
Physical function tests		
40 m Walk Test (s)	26.1 (4.7)	19.1–37.1
Timed Up and Go Test (s)	7.2 (1.6)	4.5–12.0
Stair Climb Test (s)	14.0 (4.9)	7.6–37.2
Knee Osteoarthritis Outcome Score		
Pain	57.4 (20.5)	5.6–96.4
Symptoms	55.0 (20.3)	14.3–96.4
Activities of daily living	64.1 (21.3)	0–100
Sports	36.1 (25.3)	0–100
Quality of life	31.0 (19.1)	0–81.3

BMI Body Mass Index, *NRS* Numeric Rating Scale

Non-locomotion time (mean: 12.9 h/day) primarily comprised of sedentary behaviour (69%) in comparison with standing (31%). On average, 52 sit-to-stand (STS) transfers were performed per day. Continuous sedentary periods lasting between 20 and 30 min and longer than 30 min occurred 2.6 (±0.9) and 4.6 (±1.7) times per day, resp. (Table 3).

The time spent within activities or sedentary behaviour was not associated with functional test outcomes (ρ < 0.21, p > 0.11). Furthermore, associations between the total amount of daily steps and functional test outcomes were insignificant or weak at best (ρ < 0.40, p ≥ 0.05). However, the amount of ascending/descending steps (ρ = – 0.55 to – 0.68), short activity periods (max. 5 s, ρ = – 0.61 to – 0.64) and short sedentary periods (max. 10 s, ρ = – 0.58 to – 0.62) were significantly associated with the time taken to complete the functional tests (p < 0.001).

Comparison of subgroups based on gender

No significant difference was found in the amount of daily steps between male and female participants (p = 0.89). However, the male participants performed 81% more ascending steps (adjusted mean (CI): 294 (250, 344) vs. 162 (141, 186), p < 0.01) and 84% more descending steps (adjusted mean (CI): 269 (229, 316) vs. 146 (127, 168), p < 0.01) during daily life. In addition, male participants completed the SCT significantly faster

Table 3 Physical activity outcomes, extracted from the AX3 ($n = 61$)

Parameter	Mean (±SD)	Range
Total wear time	14. 7 (1.2)	11.7–17.6
Time spent (h)		
Sitting	8.9 (1.8)	4.7–13.3
Standing	4.0 (1.4)	1.3–9.2
Walking	1.6 (0.4)	0.4–2.4
Bicycling	0.2 (0.3)	0.0–1.3
Bouts of steps (n)		
Level	232 (66)	48–379
Up	25 (15)	4–64
Down	22 (14)	2–55
Amount of steps (n)		
Total	7934 (2326)	1902–13,560
Level	7303 (2137)	1611–12,984
Up	319 (288)	15–1255
Down	312 (343)	18–2280
Cycling		
Crank revolutions	601 (754)	0–3959
Walking periods (n)		
0–5 s	4.4 (2.7)	0.0–10.7
5–10 s	61.2 (22.4)	10.2–123.2
300–600 s	0.5 (0.5)	0.0–1.9
> 600 s	0.1 (0.2)	0.0–0.8
Sedentary periods (n)		
0–10 s	3.6 (2.7)	0.38–12.0
10–60 s	15.4 (9.1)	3.3–37.7
1200–1800 s	2.6 (0.9)	0.6–4.6
> 1800 s	4.6 (1.7)	1.2–9.2
STS transfers (*n*)	52 (18)	26–105
Cadence (steps/min)	100.3 (10.6)	74.0–136.8

STS Sit-to-stand

compared to females (adjusted mean ± SE: 12.2 ± 0.8 vs. 15.5 ± 0.7, $p < 0.01$). Males spent a larger proportion of waking hours sedentary (adjusted mean ± SE: 64 ± 2% vs. 57 ± 2%, $p = 0.02$) compared to females. This difference was highlighted by more prolonged sedentary bouts lasting longer than 30 min (adjusted mean ± SE: 5.2 ± 0.3 vs. 4.2 ± 0.3 per day, $p = 0.03$). Females spent more time standing (adjusted mean ± SE: 30 ± 2% vs. 23 ± 2%, $p < 0.01$).

Comparison of subgroups based on BMI

Between the BMI categories, no significant differences were found in the time spent walking, cycling, standing or sitting ($p > 0.55$). Normal-weight KOA patients walked more steps on a daily basis than overweight KOA patients (adjusted mean ± SE: 8974 ± 558 vs. 7153 ± 420 steps/day, $p = 0.04$). However, no significant differences in daily steps were found between the other subgroups (normal vs. obese and overweight vs. obese, $p > 0.43$). Normal-weight participants performed 158% more ascending steps (adjusted mean (CI): 341 (281, 413) vs. 132 (106, 164), $p < 0.01$) and 175% more descending steps (adjusted mean (CI): 375 (326, 429) vs. 117 (152, 86), $p < 0.001$) compared to obese individuals. Furthermore, significant differences were found between the amount of brief walking bouts (up to 5 s) and short sedentary periods (max. 10 s) (Fig. 1). These differences were present between the normal vs. overweight and normal vs. obese group. During the functional tests, the obese participants needed more time to finish the WT and TUGT compared to the normal-weight participants. They also performed the WT significantly slower than the overweight individuals (Fig. 1).

Comparison of subgroups based on previously experienced knee injury

The majority of the activity and functional parameters was comparable between the participants with and without a knee injury history. Yet, the patients, who had previously suffered from a knee injury, performed fewer continuous walking bouts lasting more than 10 min (median (interquartile range): 0.00 (0.14) vs. 0.14 (0.34), $p < 0.01$), compared to the group with no injury history. They also tended to report lower scores on the KOOS-subscale related to symptoms (adjusted mean ± SE: 49.9 ± 3.3 vs. 60.7 ± 3.4, $p = 0.03$).

Discussion

Although PA and sedentary behaviour of KOA patients have been examined before, previous studies have not objectively investigated the four dimensions of PA, particularly the type of activities performed during daily life. The included KOA patients accumulated 7303 mean level steps, representing the majority of daily PA. In addition, most of the patients engaged in bicycling for which time and crank revolutions were measured. Mean steps for ascending and descending stairs or slopes, which comprised a significant part of the overall step count, were also assessed. The daily PA was executed during a small portion of the waking hours, since these were primarily spent sedentary, mainly through prolonged bouts (> 30 min). Furthermore, subgroups of KOA patients, based on risk factors (i.e. gender, BMI and history of knee injury), showed only few significant differences in general activity parameters. However, event-based parameters, such as the amount of ascending and descending steps and short bouts of walking or sedentary time (< 10 s), were significantly different in most of the subgroup-comparisons.

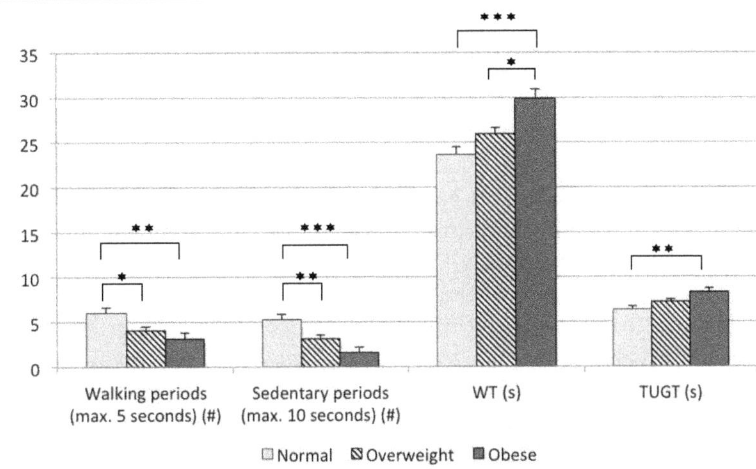

Fig. 1 The difference in activity parameters between healthy, overweight and obese KOA patients. Note: * = $p < 0.05$, ** = $p < 0.01$, *** = $p < 0.001$. Abbreviations: 40 m fast-paced Walk Test (WT) and Timed-Up-and-Go Test (TUGT)

Overall, KOA patients walked 7934 steps (including level, ascending and descending steps) on a daily basis. These findings compare well with the results of a recent systematic review, including over 3000 KOA patients that averaged 7750 daily steps [3]. The review included patients who varied extensively with respect to the severity of disease (including early-stage KOA up to pre-TKA patients) and country of origin (including countries from Europe, USA and Asia). Most of the participants (75%) did not perform prolonged walking activities (lasting over 10 min), which are suggested to be health-relevant [3]. The individuals that engaged in such continuous walking activity averaged only 2 bouts per week, whereas 3 daily bouts are recommended in PA guidelines [3]. KOA patients ascended and descended stairs or slopes regularly (25 and 22 times per day, resp.), even though it is regarded as one of the most demanding and potentially painful activities of daily life [10]. The large inter-participant variation might indicate that some individuals only engage in stair locomotion if necessary (e.g. within one's home), whereas others engage in it voluntarily and consciously, possibly for exercise purposes (e.g. during commuting or at work). In the latter example, stair climbing might have been avoided by taking the elevator, although this option is not always available. Furthermore, the majority of participants (72%) cycled during the measurement period for 20 min per day, which probably occurred as bicycling is a common mode of transportation and recreational activity in Europe [13]. Although level walking is the most common form of activity (85%), cycling (7%), ascending (4%) and descending stairs and slopes (4%) in addition occurred frequently in this sample of KOA patients, which underlines the importance of distinguishing between various types of PA.

Sedentary behaviour was commonly observed in the majority of the patients. To emphasize, 60% of the waking time was spent sedentary, which is slightly below the percentage reported by other studies (65–66%) [5, 27]. The sedentary time is accumulated to a large degree during long bouts (longer than 30 min), which are suggested to detrimentally affect general health [15]. The continuous bouts occurred more often in this population (4.6 times per day) compared to previous reports of pre- and post-total knee arthroplasty (TKA) patients (3.4 and 3.1, respectively) [5]. The variations in total sedentary time and amount of prolonged sitting bouts, however, might have occurred due to differences in applied activity monitors and methods [28]. When examining the sit-to-stand transfers, KOA patients performed 52 transitions per day, which compares well with the results of a recent review, reporting a range of 45 to 71 STS transfers [29]. Within the review, a large variety of participant groups were included, varying from healthy older adults to cancer patients. This suggests that KOA patients are still equally able to perform STS-transfers compared to other populations, which is important for maintaining independence during daily life [29].

This study also aimed to determine whether activity events, based on different types and durations of PA, were able to discriminate between subgroups of KOA patients. Such subgroups might engage in different types of PA during daily life and experience varying activity limitations [16, 17], which would be missed if the population were only analysed as a whole.

No gender differences were found in the number of daily steps. However, the male participants engaged in stair climbing more regularly during daily life compared to females. Males are known to ascend and descend stairs at higher speeds and are thus suggested to possess a superior physical capacity to climb stairs [30]. Stair climbing is known to be a challenging activity, especially for individuals with a poorly functioning lower-extremity [31]. Females, who generally have a poorer physical function than males, might therefore have tried to avoid stair climbing during daily life (e.g. by taking an elevator). Furthermore, the male individuals spent more waking hours sedentary, by engaging in prolonged sedentary bouts (> 30 min) more frequently, and less hours standing compared to females. This difference did not occur due to employment status, as the amount of employed males and females was comparable ($p = 0.80$). In addition to their occupation, females however engage in domestic activities more regularly [32]. Such activities (e.g. ironing and cooking) do not necessarily affect the amount of PA, but will reduce sedentary time. These findings show that male individuals climb more stairs and slopes and perform better on functional tests, but are also more sedentary compared to women, which confirms that PA and sedentary behaviour are two distinct dimensions that should be assessed separately [33].

Normal-weight patients walked more steps during daily life than overweight patients, which seems to confirm that BMI is negatively related to daily steps [34]. Unexpectedly, no differences in daily steps were found between the other subgroups. A possible explanation might be that the levels of PA were affected through factors that were not incorporated within this study. Psychological barriers, such as embarrassment, lack of motivation and the fear of experiencing pain upon being physically active, have been suggested to greatly affect the physical behaviour of KOA patients [35, 36].

Significant differences were also found in the amount of ascending and descending steps between the 'normal-weight' and 'obese' subgroup. During stair climbing, knee loading is more demanding in obese individuals [37]. As a result, they appear to minimize this kind of loading by engaging in fewer ascending and descending steps. Obese and overweight patients furthermore performed significantly less brief sedentary periods than normal-weight participants. STS transfers are suggested to be more challenging for these subgroups [38]. Consequently, they might attempt to avoid short sitting bouts (up to 10 s) and remain standing, thereby avoiding the need for sit-to-stand loading in a brief time period. Unexpectedly, the 27% difference in STS transfers was found to be insignificant, which could be due to the relative small subsamples (18 normal-weight, 30 overweight and 13 obese patients). In addition, normal-weight participants performed more brief walking bouts (up to 5 s) than the overweight and obese individuals. Perhaps, they should not be described as short-lasting walking bouts, yet more as an individual activity category. Household activities, such as cooking, gardening or cleaning, would probably include many of these short activity bouts. Normal-weight patients might be more likely to perform such activities, thereby explaining that a high amount of these walking bouts (which hardly affect the total step count) occurred more frequently in this subgroup. Examining activity events, based on different types and durations of PA seems to reveal differences between BMI categories that could not be revealed whilst assessing the total amount of daily steps or sedentary time.

A knee injury is strongly related to the progression of KOA and increases the risk of developing disease-related pain and symptoms [39]. In the current population, this seems to have resulted in a reduced amount of long-lasting activities (min. 10 min) in patients that have experienced a knee injury. Unexpectedly, both groups reported comparable pain levels. Pain scores, such as the NRS, might be inadequate to properly capture the complexity and fluctuations of pain in KOA, as they assess only average levels of pain and do not specify the experienced pain during such a particular activity (i.e. prolonged walking of at least 10 min) [40]. Patients with a history of knee injury also reported to suffer from more severe disease-related symptoms, as has been suggested previously [39]. The difference between the two groups was considered clinically relevant, since they exceed the difference of 8 to 10 points on the KOOS-scale [41].

In general, the total amount of daily steps or time spent within activities and postures (e.g. sedentary time) did not differ between subgroups of KOA patients. In addition, daily steps and time spent within activities were at best weakly associated with physical function. However, event-based parameters (e.g. stair climbing and brief periods of activity or sedentary behaviour) were shown to discriminate between subgroups of KOA patients more adequately. The significant association between the same parameters and physical function strengthened these findings. Thus, event-based parameters have an enhanced discriminatory capacity, not only between subgroups, but also with respect to physical function, compared to parameters of overall PA and sedentary behaviour. Furthermore, subtle limitations in physical behaviour of KOA-subgroups were revealed. To our knowledge, this has not been reported previously in this population. Although these findings need to be confirmed in future studies, these activity limitations might ultimately be targeted in rehabilitation programs to aid in maintaining the independence of KOA patients.

Several limitations should be acknowledged. First, radiographic imaging was not available for all participants, which resulted in the inability to grade the structural degeneration of the joint using common radiographic scales. Therefore, this study was unable to assess the physical behaviour of different grades of KOA. Although differences could be expected, a previous review reported comparable PA levels between patients with mild and severe KOA [3]. This however, might have occurred as only overall levels of PA were assessed and the included studies did not report specific types or durations of activities. Secondly, due to the design of the study, the same outcome measures have been compared and analysed multiple times, thereby possibly inducing family-wise errors [42]. Therefore, a Bonferroni correction was implemented in the ANCOVA's [25]. It should be noted that no consensus currently exists whether p-value adjustments are preferential, mainly because a reduction in the chance of type-I errors will lead to an increased probability of type-II errors [42, 43]. Thirdly, we were able to control for confounding parameters in the majority of analysed activity parameters. However, two activity parameters (walking bouts lasting between 5 to 10 min and walking bouts lasting more than 10 min) generally did not occur amongst the majority of the patients. Therefore, their distribution was extremely positively-skewed and could not be transformed to achieve a normal distribution. As a result, ANCOVA's could not be performed with these two parameters, so that we were not able to control for confounding variables.

This study included a relatively small patient sample, which might have reduced the odds of detecting a true effect [44]. For example, obese patients were found to perform less brief sedentary periods compared to normal-weight individuals. Surprisingly, there was no significant difference between the amounts of STS transfers performed by these subgroups ($p > 0.25$), although the difference between group means was 27%. This lack of significance might have occurred due to the small subgroup samples. It should be noted that the included participants were similar with respect to BMI, age and gender ratio compared to the average values of a recent systematic review, including 3266 KOA patients from 21 different studies [3]. Therefore this sample was considered comparable to other KOA studies. Nonetheless, this study's findings cannot be generalized towards every other KOA population. For example, non-European KOA patients might cycle significantly less, as bicycling is less common in other continents [13].

Due to the wording of the injury question, mild knee injuries (e.g. small meniscal tears) might have been missed. Yet, more severe knee injuries, which are known to increase the risk of developing KOA [45], have most probably been captured. Finally, some limitations that can occur while examining PA with accelerometers should be recognized. Not all types of physical activity (i.e. water-based activities and strengthening exercises) can correctly be captured [46]. In addition, patients might adjust their habitual behaviour as a response to wearing an accelerometer (e.g. due to social desirability), although this effect is suggested to last only briefly in general [46]. Nonetheless, accelerometry is considered an objective and accurate method for monitoring PA during daily life [46].

Future studies with larger samples are needed to confirm the specific PA limitations that seemed to be present in this population. In addition, radiographic data should be included to comprehensively assess the differences in physical behaviour between patients with different KOA severities.

Conclusions

In this sample of German KOA patients, the most common form of activity was level walking, although cycling and stair climbing activities occurred frequently, highlighting the relevance of distinguishing between these types of PA. The total active time encompassed only a small portion of their waking hours, as they spent most of their time sedentary, which was exacerbated by frequently occurring prolonged sedentary bouts.

In this study, event-based parameters, such as stair climbing or short bouts of walking or sedentary time, were found more capable of discriminating between subgroups of KOA patients compared to overall levels of PA and sedentary time. Thereby, subtle limitations in physical behaviour of KOA-subgroups were revealed, which might ultimately be targeted in rehabilitation programs to aid in maintaining the independence of KOA patients.

Abbreviations

BMI: Body-mass index; CI: Confidence Interval; F.I.T.T: Frequency, intensity, time and type; KOA: Knee osteoarthritis; KOOS: Knee osteoarthritis outcome score; NRS: Numeric rating scale; PA: Physical activity (PA); SCT: 15-Stair Climb Test; SD: Standard deviation; SE: Standard error; STS: Sit-to-stand; TKA: Total Knee Arthroplasty; TUGT: Timed up and Go Test; WHO: World Health Organization; WT: 40 m (4 × 10 m) fast-paced Walk Test

Acknowledgements

The authors would like to thank Joyce van Tunen and Alessio Bricca for their valuable feedback on the manuscript.

Funding

This research received funding from the European Union Seventh Framework Programme (FP7/2007–2013) under grant agreement n° 607510. The funding body had no role in the design, collection, analysis and interpretation of data.

Authors' contributions

Conception and design of study: MS, DR. Acquisition of data: MS, EM. Analysis and interpretation of data: MS, ML, BG, DR. Involved in drafting the manuscript or revising it for important intellectual content: MS, EM, ML, BG, DR. Gave final approval of the version to be published: MS, EM, ML, BG, DR. Agreed to be accountable for all aspects of the work: MS, EM, ML, BG, DR. All authors read and approved the final manuscript.

Consent for publication

Not applicable.

Competing interests

Dieter Rosenbaum is a member of the editorial board of BMC Musculoskeletal Disorders. The remaining authors declare that they have no competing interests.

Author details

[1]Institut für Experimentelle Muskuloskelettale Medizin (IEMM), Universitätsklinikum Münster (UKM), Westfälische Wilhelms-Universität Münster (WWU), Albert-Schweitzer Campus 1, Gebäude D3, 48129 Münster, Germany. [2]AHORSE, Department of Orthopaedics, Zuyderland Medical Centre, Henri Dunantstraat 5, 6419, PC, Heerlen, the Netherlands. [3]Otto Bock Healthcare GmbH, Hermann-Rein-Str. 2a, 37075 Göttingen, Germany.

References

1. Vos T, Flaxman AD, Naghavi M, Lozano R, Michaud C, Ezzati M, Shibuya K, Salomon JA, Abdalla S, Aboyans V, et al. Years lived with disability (YLDs) for 1160 sequelae of 289 diseases and injuries 1990-2010: a systematic analysis for the global burden of disease study 2010. Lancet. 2012;380(9859):2163–96.
2. Winter CC, Brandes M, Muller C, Schubert T, Ringling M, Hillmann A, Rosenbaum D, Schulte TL. Walking ability during daily life in patients with osteoarthritis of the knee or the hip and lumbar spinal stenosis: a cross sectional study. BMC Musculoskelet Disord. 2010;11:233.
3. Wallis JA, Webster KE, Levinger P, Taylor NF. What proportion of people with hip and knee osteoarthritis meet physical activity guidelines? A systematic review and meta-analysis. Osteoarthr Cartil. 2013;21(11):1648–59.
4. Lee J, Chang RW, Ehrlich-Jones L, Kwoh CK, Nevitt M, Semanik PA, Sharma L, Sohn MW, Song J, Dunlop DD. Sedentary behavior and physical function: objective evidence from the osteoarthritis initiative. Arthritis Care Res. 2015; 67(3):366–73.
5. Webber SC, Strachan SM, Pachu NS. Sedentary behavior, cadence, and physical activity outcomes after knee arthroplasty. Med Sci Sports Exerc. 2017;
6. Cavill N, Kahlmeier S, Racioppi S. Physical activity and health in Europe: evidence for action. WHO Regional Office for Europe: Copenhagen, Denmark; 2006.
7. Terwee CB, Bouwmeester W, van Elsland SL, de Vet HC, Dekker J. Instruments to assess physical activity in patients with osteoarthritis of the hip or knee: a systematic review of measurement properties. Osteoarthr Cartil. 2011;19(6):620–33.
8. Verlaan L, Bolink SA, Van Laarhoven SN, Lipperts M, Heyligers IC, Grimm B, Senden R. Accelerometer-based physical activity monitoring in patients with knee osteoarthritis: objective and ambulatory assessment of actual physical activity during daily life circumstances. Open Biomed Eng J. 2015;9:157–63.
9. Lipperts M, Van Laarhoven SN, Senden R, Heyligers IC, Grimm B. Clinical validation of a body-fixed 3D accelerometer and algorithm for activity monitoring in orthopaedic patients. J Orthop Translat. 2017;11:19–29.
10. Hensor EM, Dube B, Kingsbury SR, Tennant A, Conaghan PG. Toward a clinical definition of early osteoarthritis: onset of patient-reported knee pain begins on stairs. Data from the osteoarthritis initiative. Arthritis Care Res. 2015;67(1):40–7.
11. Ericson MO, Bratt A, Nisell R, Nemeth G, Ekholm J. Load moments about the hip and knee joints during ergometer cycling. Scand J Rehabil Med. 1986; 18(4):165–72.
12. Westby MD. A health professional's guide to exercise prescription for people with arthritis: a review of aerobic fitness activities. Arthritis Rheum. 2001;45(6):501–11.
13. Bassett DR Jr, Pucher J, Buehler R, Thompson DL, Crouter SE. Walking, cycling, and obesity rates in Europe, North America, and Australia. J Phys Act Health. 2008;5(6):795–814.
14. Sardinha LB, Santos DA, Silva AM, Baptista F, Owen N. Breaking-up sedentary time is associated with physical function in older adults. J Gerontol A Biol Sci Med Sci. 2015;70(1):119–24.
15. Thorp AA, Healy GN, Winkler E, Clark BK, Gardiner PA, Owen N, Dunstan DW. Prolonged sedentary time and physical activity in workplace and non-work contexts: a cross-sectional study of office, customer service and call centre employees. International J Behav Nutrition Physical Activity. 2012;9:128.
16. Knoop J, van der Leeden M, Thorstensson CA, Roorda LD, Lems WF, Knol DL, Steultjens MP, Dekker J. Identification of phenotypes with different clinical outcomes in knee osteoarthritis: data from the osteoarthritis initiative. Arthritis Care Res. 2011;63(11):1535–42.
17. Waarsing JH, Bierma-Zeinstra SM, Weinans H. Distinct subtypes of knee osteoarthritis: data from the osteoarthritis initiative. Rheumatology (Oxford). 2015;54(9):1650–8.
18. Dell'Isola A, Allan R, Smith SL, Marreiros SS, Steultjens M. Identification of clinical phenotypes in knee osteoarthritis: a systematic review of the literature. BMC Musculoskelet Disord. 2016;17(1):425.
19. Grimm B, Bolink SA. Evaluating physical function and activity in the elderly patient using wearable motion sensors. EFORT Open Rev. 2016;1:112–20.
20. Altman R, Asch E, Bloch D, Bole G, Borenstein D, Brandt K, Christy W, Cooke TD, Greenwald R, Hochberg M, et al. Development of criteria for the classification and reporting of osteoarthritis. Classification of osteoarthritis of the knee. Diagnostic and therapeutic criteria Committee of the American Rheumatism Association. Arthritis Rheum. 1986;29(8):1039–49.
21. Dobson F, Hinman RS, Roos EM, Abbott JH, Stratford P, Davis AM, Buchbinder R, Snyder-Mackler L, Henrotin Y, Thumboo J, et al. OARSI recommended performance-based tests to assess physical function in people diagnosed with hip or knee osteoarthritis. Osteoarthr Cartil. 2013;21(8):1042–52.
22. Roos EM, Toksvig-Larsen S. Knee injury and osteoarthritis outcome score (KOOS) - validation and comparison to the WOMAC in total knee replacement. Health Qual Life Outcomes. 2003;1:17.
23. Dunlop DD, Song J, Lee J, Gilbert AL, Semanik PA, Ehrlich-Jones L, Pellegrini CA, Pinto D, Ainsworth B, Chang RW. Physical activity minimum threshold predicting improved function in adults with lower-extremity symptoms. Arthritis Care Res. 2017;69(4):475–83.
24. Troiano RP, Berrigan D, Dodd KW, Masse LC, Tilert T, McDowell M. Physical activity in the United States measured by accelerometer. Med Sci Sports Exerc. 2008;40(1):181–8.
25. McDonald JH: Handbook of biological statistics, 3rd edn: sparky house publishing; 2014.
26. Pourhoseingholi MA, Baghestani AR, Vahedi M. How to control confounding effects by statistical analysis. Gastroenterol Hepatol Bed Bench. 2012;5(2):79–83.
27. Semanik PA, Lee J, Song J, Chang RW, Sohn MW, Ehrlich-Jones LS, Ainsworth BE, Nevitt MM, Kwoh CK, Dunlop DD. Accelerometer-monitored sedentary behavior and observed physical function loss. Am J Public Health. 2015;105(3):560–6.
28. Judice PB, Santos DA, Hamilton MT, Sardinha LB, Silva AM. Validity of GT3X and Actiheart to estimate sedentary time and breaks using ActivPAL as the reference in free-living conditions. Gait Posture. 2015;41(4):917–22.
29. Bohannon RW. Daily sit-to-stands performed by adults: a systematic review. J Phys Ther Sci. 2015;27(3):939–42.
30. Tiedemann AC, Sherrington C, Lord SR. Physical and psychological factors associated with stair negotiation performance in older people. J Gerontol A Biol Sci Med Sci. 2007;62(11):1259–65.
31. Nadeau S, McFadyen BJ, Malouin F. Frontal and sagittal plane analyses of the stair climbing task in healthy adults aged over 40 years: what are the challenges compared to level walking? Clin Biomech (Bristol, Avon). 2003;18(10):950–9.
32. Van Domelen DR, Koster A, Caserotti P, Brychta RJ, Chen KY, McClain JJ, Troiano RP, Berrigan D, Harris TB. Employment and physical activity in the U. S. Am J Prev Med. 2011;41(2):136–45.
33. Owen N, Healy GN, Matthews CE, Dunstan DW. Too much sitting: the population health science of sedentary behavior. Exerc Sport Sci Rev. 2010; 38(3):105–13.
34. White DK, Neogi T, Zhang Y, Felson D, Lavalley M, Niu J, Nevitt M, Lewis CE, Torner J, Douglas Gross K. The association of obesity with walking independent of knee pain: the multicenter osteoarthritis study. J Obes. 2012;2012:261974.
35. Somers TJ, Keefe FJ, Pells JJ, Dixon KE, Waters SJ, Riordan PA, Blumenthal JA, McKee DC, LaCaille L, Tucker JM, et al. Pain catastrophizing and pain-related fear in osteoarthritis patients: relationships to pain and disability. J Pain Symptom Manag. 2009;37(5):863–72.
36. Stevenson JD, Roach R. The benefits and barriers to physical activity and lifestyle interventions for osteoarthritis affecting the adult knee. J Orthop Surg Res. 2012;7:15.
37. Aaboe J, Bliddal H, Messier SP, Alkjaer T, Henriksen M. Effects of an intensive weight loss program on knee joint loading in obese adults with knee osteoarthritis. Osteoarthr Cartil. 2011;19(7):822–8.
38. Galli M, Crivellini M, Sibella F, Montesano A, Bertocco P, Parisio C. Sit-to-stand movement analysis in obese subjects. Int J Obes Relat Metab Disord. 2000;24(11): 1488–92.
39. Zhang Y, Jordan JM. Epidemiology of osteoarthritis. Clin Geriatr Med. 2010; 26(3):355–69.

40. Hawker GA, Mian S, Kendzerska T, French M. Measures of adult pain: visual analog scale for pain (VAS pain), numeric rating scale for pain (NRS pain), McGill pain questionnaire (MPQ), short-form McGill pain questionnaire (SF-MPQ), chronic pain grade scale (CPGS), short Form-36 bodily pain scale (SF-36 BPS), and measure of intermittent and constant osteoarthritis pain (ICOAP). Arthritis Care Res. 2011;63(Suppl 11):S240–52.
41. Roos EM, Lohmander LS. The knee injury and osteoarthritis outcome score (KOOS): from joint injury to osteoarthritis. Health Qual Life Outcomes. 2003;1:64.
42. Feise RJ. Do multiple outcome measures require p-value adjustment? BMC Med Res Methodol. 2002;2:8.
43. Rothman KJ. No adjustments are needed for multiple comparisons. Epidemiology. 1990;1(1):43–6.
44. Button KS, Ioannidis JP, Mokrysz C, Nosek BA, Flint J, Robinson ES, Munafò MR. Power failure: why small sample size undermines the reliability of neuroscience. Nat Rev Neurosci. 2013;14(5):365–76.
45. Chaganti RK, Lane NE. Risk factors for incident osteoarthritis of the hip and knee. Curr Rev Musculoskelet Med. 2011;4(3):99–104.
46. Hills AP, Mokhtar N, Byrne NM. Assessment of physical activity and energy expenditure: an overview of objective measures. Front Nutr. 2014;1:5.

A randomized, controlled study to evaluate the efficacy of intra-articular, autologous adipose tissue injections for the treatment of mild-to-moderate knee osteoarthritis compared to hyaluronic acid

Ian A. Jones[1], Melissa Wilson[2], Ryan Togashi[1], Bo Han[3], Austin K. Mircheff[4] and C. Thomas Vangsness JR[1*]

Abstract

Background: Osteoarthritis (OA) is a highly debilitating joint disease that causes progressive, irreversible damage to articular cartilage. OA takes a massive toll on society that has grown in recent decades, but no therapy has been shown to halt or reverse the progression of the disease. The critical need for better treatments and increased interest cellular therapies has spawned a new generation of "minimally manipulated" cell treatments. Autologous adipose tissue injections are among the most controversial of these new treatments. Despite a lack of clinical evidence, adipose tissue injections are often marketed as "stem cell" injections with wide-ranging regenerative benefits. The purpose of this study is to estimate the effect size of the treatment by comparing the efficacy of autologous fat to hyaluronic acid (HA). As a secondary aim, we will test for preliminary evidence of efficacy of autologous fat vs. HA.

Methods: This is a prospective, single-center, parallel-group, randomized, controlled trial. Participants ($n = 54$) will receive either a single intra-articular, ultrasound-guided injection of autologous adipose tissue or a single intra-articular, ultrasound-guided injection of HA (1:1 ratio). Outcome data will be obtained at baseline, week-6 and month-6. The Western Ontario and McMaster Universities Osteoarthritis Index (WOMAC) pain domain (WOMAC-A) will be used as the primary outcome measure. Secondary clinical outcome measures include WOMAC (full), clinical anchors (pain, function, and stiffness), and the 29-point Patient-Reported Outcomes Measurement Information System (PROMIS®) profile. We will also take synovial fluid samples and assess sway velocity using a force plate, as well as analyze excess/discard adipose tissue to gain a better understanding of how intra-articular adipose tissue injections influence the biochemical environment of the joint.

Discussion: Given the widespread use of intra-articular fat injections in the United States, it is critical that randomized, controlled human studies evaluating efficacy and biological activity be performed. This study is the first step in addressing this unmet need, but it is not without limitations. The most notable limitations of this study are its small size and lack of blinding, which predisposes the study to both investigator and participant bias.

Keywords: Lipogems, Stem cell, Knee, Osteoarthritis, Intra-articular injection, Adipose tissue, Fat MSC, ADSC

* Correspondence: vangsness@usc.edu
[1]Department of Orthopaedic Surgery, Keck School of Medicine of USC, HCT 1520 San Pablo Street, suite 2000, Los Angeles, CA 90033, USA
Full list of author information is available at the end of the article

Background

Introduction

Osteoarthritis (OA) is a debilitating "whole joint disease" that causes progressive, irreversible damage to articular cartilage that results in debilitating joint pain and stiffness [1]. OA places a massive financial burden ln society [2] that has grown in recent decades [3–5]. There are no approved disease modification therapies for OA, and the only non-invasive pharmacologic therapies recommended for OA symptom management are analgesics and non-steroidal anti-inflammatory drugs (NSAIDs) [6, 7]. Intra-articular therapies, including corticosteroids and hyaluronic acid (HA) are frequently used to treat knee OA, but both treatments have limitations. The American Academy of Orthopaedic Surgeons (AAOS) determined that there was inconclusive evidence to support the use of intra-articular corticosteroids of OA [8] and several recent studies have suggested that corticosteroids may have detrimental catabolic effects on cartilage [9–11]. While generally assumed to be safe, the AAOS concluded that the apparent effectiveness of HA compared to saline placebo is clinically negligible, and strongly recommended against its use [12]. The recommendation has been met by push back [12, 13], and meta-analysis published since have both confirmed [14] and contradicted [15] the appropriateness of the AAOS recommendation. Nevertheless, even if assumed to be effective, HA provides (at best) modest, short-term, symptomatic relief compared to placebo control.

OA is frequently referred to as a "wear and tear" disease. However, OA pathophysiology is multifactorial, and complex interactions between genetic, metabolic, biochemical, and biomechanical factors are also likely to play an important role in the progression of the disease [16, 17]. In recent years, studies have suggested that inflammatory mechanisms contribute to OA pathogenesis, particularly synovitis, which has been correlated with the structural progression of OA, cartilage degeneration and osteophyte formation [18]. Indeed, an emerging body of evidence indicates that OA is a whole-organ disease that involves the production of cytokines by a variety of different tissues [1, 19] and a number of cytokines have been implicated in OA pathogenesis [20–24].

There is considerable interest in exploiting the anti-inflammatory activities of cellular treatments to treat OA [25]; however, adipose tissue-derived cell therapies require enzymatic processing and isolation techniques that may impact safety and efficacy [26]. These concerns have prompted the United States Food and Drug Administration (US FDA) to regulate autologous cell therapies that have been cultured and/or enzymatically processed as drugs. The promise of cellular therapies, particularly those containing so called mesenchymal "stem" or stromal cells (collectively referred to as MSCs), combined with regulatory barriers and the critical need for new therapies, has spawned a new generation of "minimally manipulated" cell treatments for OA. Among these new "minimally manipulated" cell treatments are autologous adipose tissue injections, which are often marketed as "stem" cell injections and are currently available at orthopaedic clinics across the United States [27].

In the US, the rules governing the clinical use of treatments claiming to be "minimally manipulated", particularly intra-articular adipose tissue injections, are ambiguous. This ambiguity can be attributed to special regulatory exemptions for blood-derived cell products [28], as well as Section 361 of the US Public Health Service Act, which exempts certain human cells, tissues, and cellular and tissue-based products (HCT/Ps) from the regulations that require regulatory submissions for the conduct of clinical trials and marketing [29]. Orthopaedic surgeons administering these treatments claim that they are being administered for reconstruction, repair, and replacement, and that the mechanical processing of the fat does not alter the original relevant characteristics of the transferred tissue [30]. Opponents argue that, despite the presence and importance of fat in the knee joint [31], subcutaneous fat is very different than the adipose tissue of the knee joint, and so the injection of adipose tissue into the intra-articular space should not be considered homologous use. Despite regulatory ambiguity and little evidence demonstrate their effectiveness [32], "minimally manipulated" adipose tissue injections are widely available at clinics throughout the US. To date, there have been no randomized, controlled clinical studies performed to evaluate the efficacy intra-articular adipose tissue injections for the treatment of OA.

Basic science for clinical study aspects

The principle difference between cell therapies and "minimally manipulated" fat injections is that fat injections are not enzymatically digested. As a result, autologous fat treatments contain both autologous cells, including MSCs [33], and extra-cellular matrix (ECM). Therapies containing ECM are thought to have the following advantages over treatments prepared using enzymatic digestion: (1) preservation of the stromal vascular niche, which allows time-release of the regenerative factors [34]; (2) release of bioactive molecules by exosomes, which have been demonstrated to be significantly greater in mechanically processed fat than enzymatically processed fat [35]; and (3) maintenance of the structural and morphologic unit, which is thought to increase efficacy by making the cells more resilient to the harsh, inflamed conditions in the recipient environment [36]. Enzymatic digestion, which is used to remove the cells from ECM, may remove critical elements involved in tissue repair and may damage the cells, affecting their function and viability. In vitro studies have suggested that cell-containing lipoaspirate obtained without enzymatic digestion may act as a scaffold when administered via intra-articular injection, allowing for the formation of fibrous tissue that provides mechanical support [37]. While non-enzymatic processing produces a lower progenitor cell yield [38, 39], the preserved ECM and growth factors are thought to contribute to the treatments' overall therapeutic effectiveness.

Preclinical [37] and clinical [40, 41] studies investigating the use of "minimally manipulated" adipose tissue injections have demonstrated preliminary safety, but a number of questions remain unanswered. While ECM has been shown to be beneficial for tissue repair [42] and is commonly used to as a bridging material between new and old tissues [43], these advantages are less applicable to intra-articular fat injections because there are no tissue fragments for the ECM to bridge [44] and because agents injected into the joint tend to be quickly cleared from the body [45]. Most importantly, ECM itself has the potential to produce inflammatory signals [46]. In fact, collagen fragments are known to induce arthritis in animals [47].

Feasibility justification for clinical aspects of the study

Adipose tissue will be obtained and administered in a single point-of-care procedure. The rapid processing (approx. 20 min) within a closed system reduces the possibility of contamination. However, this also means that the specific composition of the adipose tissue therapy cannot be determined prior to injection. As a result, there will be inherent, unavoidable variability between the treatments that participants receive. In order to help minimize this variability, each patient will receive exactly 6 ml of processed adipose tissue. The decision to inject 6 ml is based on anatomic considerations and the principal investigator's clinical experience. A 6 ml injection is conservative, as the synovial fluid volume has been estimated to be 6.7 +/− 2.3 ml [48], with the average volume of the knee joint itself being 131 ± 53 ml [49]. The 6 ml "dose" is also in line with published case studies, where fat processed with the Lipogems® device has been injected into the knee [40]. Lastly, a 6 ml volume improves comparability because the comparator treatment is also a 6 ml intra-articular injection.

The entire fat transfer procedure will be completed in under an hour. Adipose tissue will be harvested from the abdomen using lipoaspiration, which does not require general anesthesia [50]. The tissue will be mechanically broken down using the Lipogems® device. While a number of other similar fat processing systems are available [51], the differences between the products produced by different systems and their implications for osteoarthritis are unclear [32].

Our study will use Hyaluronic acid (HA) as an active control. In accordance with the requirements for the administrations for HA, only patients that fail to respond to the standard conservative treatment options (exercise, analgesics, NSAIDS [7]) will be recruited. The use of HA as an active control for autologous cell-based therapies is well-established [52, 53]. We have chosen to use Synvic One® because it has been included in more than 300 publications and has been used to treat more than 13 million knees worldwide. Synvic One® is also an ideal comparator treatment for this study because it has been shown to have an effect that last for up to 6 months [54].

Study overview

This is a prospective, single-center, parallel-group, randomized, controlled study. The aim of this study is to estimate statistical power and gather preliminary efficacy data. Qualified participants will receive either a single, intra-articular injection of autologous adipose tissue or a single, intra-articular injection of HA. We hypothesize that participants treated with autologous adipose tissue will show a greater improvement in pain (as determined using the pain items of the Western Ontario and McMaster Universities Osteoarthritis Index, or WOMAC-A) than participants treated with HA. WOMAC (full questionnaire), the 29-point Patient-Reported Outcomes Measurement Information System (PROMIS®) profile, and clinical anchors will be used as secondary clinical outcome measures. Synovial fluid samples and excess adipose tissue (treatment group) will also be analyzed to gain a better understanding of how adipose tissue affects the biochemical environment of the joint.

Methods

Participants, interventions, and outcomes

All study-related activities will be performed at the USC Department of Orthopaedic Surgery Outpatient Clinic, including subject identification, screening, treatment, and outcome assessments. Patients between the ages of 45 and 75 with Kellgren-Lawrence grades 2–3 OA (inclusive) that are interested in participating in the study will be screened for eligibility by the principal investigator using pre-defined criteria (Fig. 1). Those who meet inclusion/exclusion criteria and decide to participate will sign an informed consent before randomization (see Assignment of Interventions). Because the fat treatment requires the removal of adipose tissue from the abdomen, participants will not be blinded to their assigned group.

Male and/or female patients will be randomized to either the HA (Synvic One®) treatment group ($n = 27$) or autologous fat (Lipogems®) treatment group (n = 27). To

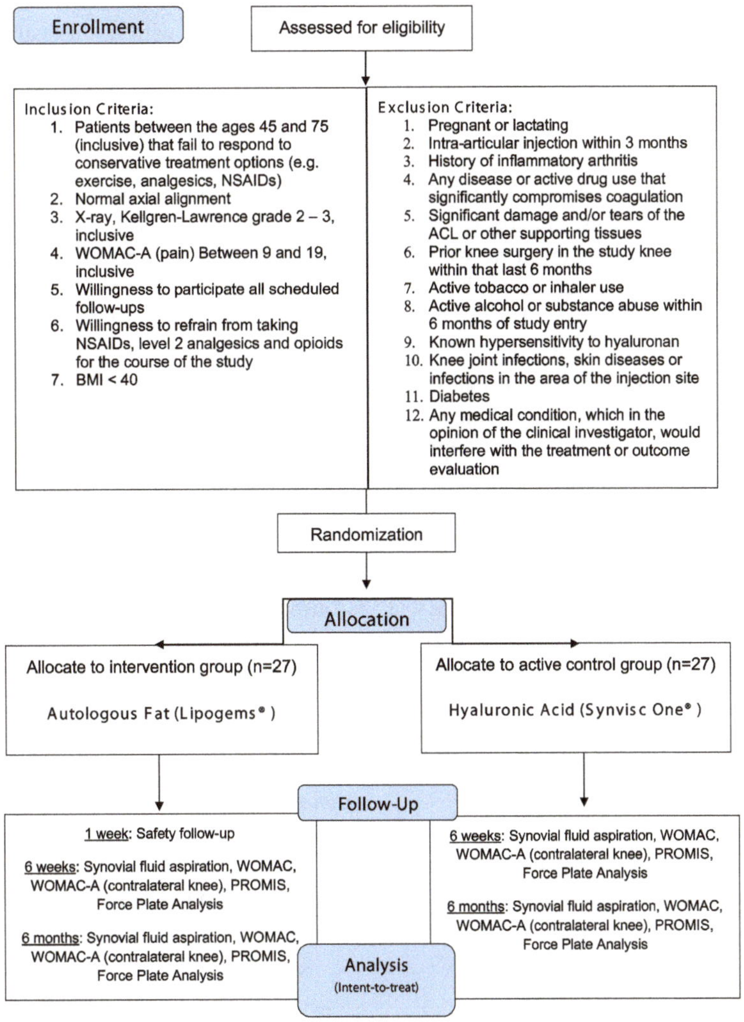

Fig. 1 Study design flow chart

ensure enrollment goals are met, the investigator will draw from a waitlist of current patients that have expressed interest in participating in clinical trials. We also have IRB-approved flyers/brochures that will be shared with patients and nearby orthopaedic clinics (Additional file 1). Additionally, to improve adherence to the intervention protocol, participant who are allocated to the control group that complete all scheduled follow-up visits will be offered the adipose tissue treatment at the end of their final visit at no cost.

Since our primary aim is to estimate the effect size for future well-powered studies, we estimate the precision around which we can measure the effect. Based on a prior study using similar methods, but comparing WOMAC-A scores among patients receiving placebo to Hylan G-F (a joint lubricant) [54], we assumed standard deviations in the control and treatment groups of 0.66 and 0.67, respectively. With a sample size of 54 (27 per group), we will be able to estimate a two-sided 95% confidence interval within ±0.36 distance from the mean difference. For our secondary aim, we estimated the mean difference we would be able to detect, assuming a similar effect size for HA as was observed for Hylan G-F ($\mu = -0.84$, $\sigma = 0.67$) and found that we would have 80% power to detect a mean difference of – 1.4 in the autologous adipose group with a two-sided Type I error rate of 0.05.

Power was calculated using Pass 14 (Kaysville, UT).

At the treatment visit (day 0), patients will be randomly assigned to receive either a single intra-articular, ultrasound-guided injection autologous adipose tissue (6 ml) or a single intra-articular, ultrasound-guided injection of hyaluronic acid (6 ml). Patients with bilateral OA will be allowed to participate in this study, but only their more painful eligible knee will be treated (as determined by WOMAC-A). To control for possible responder differences between bilateral and unilateral symptomatic patients [55, 56], WOMAC-A for the contralateral knee will be obtained at baseline, 6 weeks, and 6 months (Table 1). If a participant has bilateral OA of equal pain intensity in both knees, the treatment knee will be selected randomly.

Lipoaspiration procedure

For patients receiving the adipose tissue injection, fat tissue will be harvested under semi-sterile conditions (sterile draping and gloves, gown, face masks, and head cover). The participant will be positioned supine on an examination bench. Local anesthesia (2% lidocaine) will be applied to the area to be harvested (approx. 8 cm × 20 cm just below the umbilicus) and a small incision (6-8 mm) will be made. Approximately 500 mL of normal saline containing 50 mL of 2% lidocaine and 1amp epinephrine will be infused to reduce bleeding and trauma. Approximately 15 min will be allowed for infiltration. Then, a thin cannula will be inserted through the incision and a controlled back and forth motion will be used to loosen excess fat. Using a 13-gauge cannula connected to a VacLok® syringe, 20 ml to 40 ml of subcutaneous adipose tissue will be harvested. Following the harvest procedure, a pressure dressing will be applied. Participants will be told to remove the dressing 24–48 h after the procedure and return approximately 1 week after receiving the treatment so that the harvest site can be evaluated.

Injection procedure

The same injection procedure will be used for both treatments. With the patient in the supine position, the affected knee will be extended, and the femoral condyle will be marked with a surgical marker. The area will be cleaned, and local anesthesia will be applied to the injection site (2 cc, 1% lido). A 21-gauge needle will be inserted into the suprapatellar pouch under ultrasound guidance. Synovial fluid will be aspirated from the knee and autologous fat or HA will be administered through the same needle used to aspirate the synovial fluid. The synovial fluid aspiration portion of the procedure will also be performed at the 6-week and 6-month follow-up visits. A detailed summary of study procedures is provided in Table 1.

The mean change in WOMAC-A score over time will be used as the primary outcome measure. The PROMIS-29 profile, clinical anchors and WOMAC will be used as secondary clinical outcome measures. WOMAC is multidimensional, self-administered health status instrument for patients with OA of the hip and/or knee and been shown to fulfill conventional criteria for content and construct validity, reliability, responsiveness and relative efficiency [57]. The PROMIS-29 questionnaire is set of person-centered measures that encompasses domains that OA is likely to affect, including functional limitations, pain interference/intensity, ability to fulfill desired social roles, anxiety/depression, sleep disturbance and fatigue [58]. PROMIS-29 has been shown to correlate with scales measuring similar constructs for patients with OA [59] and is frequently used for research purposes [58]. Three clinical anchors (pain,

Table 1 Study Calendar

Timepoint**	Study period				
	Screening	Allocation	Follow-up visits		Close-out
	Day – 21 to 0	day 0	Safety follow-up visit Day 2–7 (inclusive)	Week 6 ± 7 days	Month 6 ± 30 days
Enrolment:					
Eligibility screen	X				
Informed consent	X				
Focused physical exam		X	X	X	X
Randomization / Allocation		X			
Interventions:					
Autologous Adipose Tissue Injection		X			
Hyaluronic Acid Injection		X			
Assessments:					
WOMAC	X	X		X	X
WOMAC-A (contralateral knee)	X	X		X	X
PROMIS-29		X		X	X
Force Plate Analysis (bilateral)		X		X	X
Clinical anchors		X		X	X
Synovial fluid aspiration		X		X	X

The *eligibility screen* includes a detailed physical exam/medical history and pregnancy testing (if applicable). The *focused physical exam* includes Height/weight/vitals, concomitant medications, knee exam, and wound evaluation (if applicable). Only patients that receive the fat treatment will be asked to come in for the safety follow-up. All assessments pertain only to the study knee, unless otherwise indicated

function and stiffness; 7-point Leichhardt scale) will be used to determine the patient's global impression of change, as described previously [60, 61].

We will assess participants using a proprietary system that includes a force plate (1000 Hz (9260AA6, Kistler Instruments, Winterthur, Switzerland), dedicated computer, and software (SpartaMARS, Sparta Performance Science, Menlo Park, USA). Participants will be assessed at baseline, 6 weeks and 6 months. The non-invasive standing assessment will take approximately 3 min to complete. Assessments will be performed after clinical outcome data has been obtained, but before synovial fluid has been aspirated. Participants will be instructed to stand on the scale with their hands on their hips and eyes closed to establish baseline force. The test consists of four, 20 s balance trials on each leg. A 10 s rest period will be provided between trials, and trials will be conducted on alternating legs. Displacement and sway velocity will be measured as described previously [62]. The results of the force plate assessment will be associated with clinical outcome data and synovial fluid biomarker profiles. Results of the force plate sub-set analysis will be reported separately.

Excess adipose tissue will be transferred to sterilized vials filled with phosphate buffered saline. Adipose tissue samples will be kept at 4 °C. Samples will be divided into two parts in the biosafety hood using sterile scalpel. One part of each sample will be processed for cell culture, and another part will be cryopreserved. For cell culture, samples will be transferred to a tube containing RPMI serum free medium, supplemented with 1% penicillin-streptomycin-fungizone. Tissue samples will be washed 3 times with the same medium, then finely minced for cell isolation using a standard collagenase digestion protocol.

Synovial fluid samples will be transferred to EDTA tubes, gently inverted 8–10 times, and then immediately transported to the lab on wet ice in accordance with university policies. Samples will be centrifuged within 1 h at 1500 x g for 10 min at 4 °C. The supernatant will then be aliquoted to cryovials containing protease inhibitor and stored at -80C until use.

Synovial fluid samples and excess adipose tissue will be analyzed to characterize the treatment and gain a better understanding of how adipose tissue affects the biochemical environment of the knee. To better monitor the disease progression and treatment efficacy, chemokines, cytokines, growth factors, and matrix metalloproteinases in the synovial fluid will be analyzed, including IL-1β, IL-6, IL-8, TNFα, C-terminal telopeptides of Type I collagen, and C-telopeptide of Type II collagen. The results will be made available for principle component analysis, which will be used to determine if pre-treatment synovial fluid inflammatory mediator and selected OA biomarker profiles that define different OA phenotypes predict the responses to autologous adipose tissue injections. The pro- and anti-inflammatory capabilities and cell viability of the autologous fat product will be evaluated and may also be compared to unprocessed preparations.

The use of NSAIDs may negatively impact healing [32, 63] and their prolonged half-life in synovial fluid allows them to accumulate in the joint [64], which is likely to impact synovial fluid biomarker profiles. To ensure that clinical outcomes, tissue healing and the biochemical profile of the synovial fluid are not influenced by the use of NSAIDs, participants will be asked not to take NSAIDs for at least 1 week prior to treatment and throughout the duration of the study.

Patients will be instructed to contact the study doctor before taking analgesic medications. Acetaminophen (250-500 mg) will be recommended if appropriate. The total number of days each patient takes acetaminophen will be logged and reported with published results. However, extended acetaminophen used will not be used as grounds for termination, as it has it is generally thought to have a clinically negligible effect on OA-related knee pain [65–67].

Assignment of interventions

A random number sequence was generated using the Stata 14.0 uniform distribution. Blocks of four were used to ensure equal numbers of subjects in each group. To carry out the randomization of study subjects, we will utilize sequentially numbered, opaque, sealed envelopes. The statistician will prepare the envelopes for the Principal Investigator in order to maintain the concealment of the sequence prior to randomization. Upon enrolment in the trial, the next sequentially numbered envelope will be selected by the investigator and the subject will be offered the assigned treatment.

Data collection, management, and analysis

Demographics and survey data will be stored using a REDcap database created specifically for the purpose of this study. REDcap has several security features, including off-site backups, an audit trail, secure logins, de-identified data exports, and built-in filtering methods to ensure data quality. Additionally, survey answers (clinical outcome data) will be directly entered into the database by the participants via iPad before they interact with the examining physician. Documentation not included in the quantitative analysis of clinical outcomes will be recorded using traditional source documents (Additional files 2 and 3). These documents will be kept in the participant's binder and locked in a secure location. All data collection will take place in the clinic.

Only those who require access to the database will be given access. Coding of the variables will be done within the database. A completed data file will be stored by the statistician in the shared folder for the Clinical Translational Science Institute Biostatistics core at USC and will be backed up regularly. The statistician's access to the database will be limited to de-identified data. Data quality will be assured by range checks for unusual or impossible data values. Data management will include a thorough data cleaning (checking ranges, evaluating distributions) and deriving of variables needed for analysis.

All protocol deviations will be recorded. The same outcome data will be obtained from all participants, regardless of protocol adherence. In order to promote retention and compliance, participants that receive the HA treatment and complete all schedule follow-up visits will be offered the fat treatment at the 6-month (final) follow-up visit at no charge. Imputation will be used if loss to follow-up is uncommon.

Preliminary analyses will include descriptive statistics of basic demographic and clinical characteristics to assess the degree to which randomization was effective in balancing treatment groups. If any factors are found to have clinically significant differences, they will be considered and evaluated as possible confounders. The analysis will be by intent-to-treat. That is, all subjects will be analyzed according to randomization status, regardless of actual treatment received, compliance with therapy, or adherence to the study protocol. We will compare the outcome, difference in WOMAC-A score from baseline to 6 months, between the treated and untreated groups using generalized linear models (GLM) with a Gaussian family specified, assuming the data are normally distributed. If the data are not normally distributed, we will specify a more appropriate distribution based on an evaluation of the data via histogram. We will also use GLM to examine the relationship between the treatment and outcome at each time point at which the WOMAC was measured. Last, we will model the effect across all time points using a multi-level mixed effects model to account for repeated measures. Confounders will be defined as those variables that were found to differ between groups either at baseline or post-randomization and which, when added to the model, alter the effect estimate by > 15%. Potential a priori confounders include BMI, Bilateral vs contralateral OA, gender, ethnicity, and race. Potential interactions between treatment and visit will be evaluated. A *p*-value of <.05 will be considered statistically significant. The 29-point PROMIS® questionnaire will be evaluated using GLM at each measured time point and across time points using a multi-level mixed effects model, as described above. Missing data, if ≤5%, will be imputed using multiple imputation methods. Any covariate missing > 5% will not be included in the analysis.

A per-protocol analysis will also be conducted including only those participants who were protocol-adherent. Protocol adherence is defined as: (1) Receiving the assigned study treatment and (2) completing all follow-up visits. Lastly, sensitivity analyses will be conducted to assess the impact of using multiple imputation methods, if such methods are employed in the analysis.

Monitoring

This is a small-scale, single-site, investigator-initiated clinical trial, so a data monitoring committee will not be utilized. The principle investigator will regularly review study data for the occurrence of adverse events (AEs), including moderate to severe effusion, synovitis, local infection, systemic infection, and toxicities. The study will be suspended if more than 1 out of the first 10 patients enrolled in the study group experiences a significant adverse event (SAEs) attributable to the investigational treatment. SAEs are defined (per US FDA) as those that are life threatening, require hospitalization, or result in death, disability or long-term damage. All adverse events (AEs and SAEs) will be recorded in study source documents and will be reported to the University IRB in accordance with federal, state and institutional requirements. Additionally, all AEs and SAEs will be reported with published results.

Ethics and dissemination of information

Ethics approval was received from the University of Southern California Health Science IRB (10/9/2017), USC Institutional Biosafety Committee (May 2017) and USC Radiation Safety Committee (September 2017). Continuing reviews and all protocol modifications will be submitted to the USC Health Science IRB through the University iStar System. Because the IRB has determined that this study involves 'greater than minimal risk', only the Principal Investigator will be allowed to obtain informed consent. All participants provided written informed consent to participate. Participants will be given a copy of the consent to take home, and an informed consent comprehension assessment will be performed before randomization.

To protect participant confidentiality, samples will not be labeled with information that can be used to directly identify participants. Samples will be labeled with subject identification numbers and only the investigator and IRB-approved study personnel will have access to information linking subject identification numbers to identifiable information. The link between study participants and their study ID numbers will be destroyed (shredded/purged) in accordance with federal regulations when study activities are complete. The final trial dataset will not contain identifiable data and will be available to all investigators listed in the IRB protocol.

There are no additional provisions for ancillary or post-trial care, or for compensation to those who suffer harm from trial participation. However, participants will be informed prior to enrollment that they are responsible for unscheduled visits/interventions and that they are not giving up any legal rights by agreeing to participate in the study (Additional file 4). Once study activities have been completed, results will be published and posted to clinicaltrials.gov.

Personal information will be collected using REDcap, which maintains a secure login and will only be accessible to appropriately delegated study staff, as indicated on the IRB protocol. De-identified data exports will be performed so that statisticians and collaborators may receive data sets without knowledge of personal health information. A de-identified dataset will be stored with the statistician indefinitely. The results of the study, whether positive or negative, will be published. An abstract based on the results may be submitted to an orthopaedics meeting prior to publication. Should the results prove impactful, we may contact the Keck Media Relations Team at USC to assist in developing a press release.

Discussion

In view of the already widespread use of intra-articular fat injections in the United States, it is critical that randomized, controlled studies aimed at evaluating the clinical efficacy of intra-articular autologous adipose tissue injections for osteoarthritis be performed [68]. This study is the first step towards addressing this unmet need, but it is not without limitations. The most notable limitation of this study is its small size, which is fixed due to funding constraints. However, in order to consider adopting autologous adipose tissue injections as a new therapy for OA, the clinical impact of the treatment would have to be substantial, as autologous fat injects are more costly, carry additional risks, and are more invasive than HA injections. Thus, detecting a small, statistically significant but clinically negligible difference would not advance the treatment of OA.

Another major limitation is the lack of blinding, which predisposes the study to both investigator and subject bias. However, the trauma associated with the removal of adipose tissue from the abdomen is not justified in patients receiving the control (hyaluronic acid). To minimize investigator bias, which is particularly noteworthy given that the study isn't multi-site, clinical outcomes will be assessed using self-reported measurement tools and responses will be directly entered into a REDcap database by the participants before they interact with the examining physician. Additionally, other response indictors (synovial fluid analysis, fat characterization) will be blinded for analysis.

The removal of synovial fluid presents minimal risk to patients and may help us better understand how autologous fat injections impact the biological environment of the joint. However, puncturing the joint cavity may have clinically important implications. To mitigate this potential limitation, the joint cavity will only be punctured once at the treatment visit. Additionally, outcome assessments will be performed before removing joint fluid and all synovial aspirations will be performed under ultrasound guidance. The number of successful/failed aspirations in each group will be logged and reported in the final published results. While synovial fluid can be challenging to obtain, prior studies conducted by the investigator and others have demonstrated feasibility [69, 70]. Based on the experience of the investigator, > 50% of aspirations are expected to yield analyzable synovial fluid samples.

This study has several strengths. While imperfect, prospective, randomized controlled trials are the gold standard for evaluating treatment effects because they mitigate selection and information bias, as well as confounding variables. Additionally, this study will use WOMAC, which is generally thought to be the gold standard for assessing patient-relevant treatment effects in osteoarthritis [71, 72]. Moreover, WOMAC has been shown to be more responsive than other outcome measures in short-term, small-scale studies [73]. Finally, we will characterize both the treatment (though analysis of discarded adipose) and the biologic response (though the analysis of synovial fluid), which is critical for understanding the treatment bioactivity [74].

Several aspects of this study were changed based on reviewer recommendations. No patients were recruited prior to the implementation and IRB approval of these changes.

Abbreviations

AE: Adverse event; ECM: Extra-cellular matrix; GLM: Generalized linear models\; HA: Hyaluronic acid; NSAID: Non-steroidal anti-inflammatory Drug; OA: Osteoarthritis; PROMIS: Patient-Reported Outcomes Measurement Information System; SAE: Severe adverse event; WOMAC: Western Ontario and McMaster Universities Osteoarthritis index

Funding

This research study is sponsored in part by a grant from the L.K. Whittier Foundation. Additional funding is provided by the investigator's discretional research account. This work was also supported by grants UL1TR001855 and UL1TR000130 from the National Center for Advancing Translational Science (NCATS) of the U.S. National Institutes of Health. The content is solely the responsibility of the authors and does not necessarily represent the official views of the National Institutes of Health. Lipogems kits for fat processing have been provided by the device manufacturer.

Authors' contributions

IAJ drafted Whittier grant application that was used to help fund this study and prepared and submitted both the IRB and published versions of the study protocol, as well as all other study documents, under the oversight CTV. MW developed the statistical analysis plan and reviewed and commented on all study materials/protocols. RT, BH, and AKM contributed to study design and preparation of the manuscript. All authors approved the final version of the manuscript.

Consent for publication

N/A.

Competing interests

Ian A Jones has nothing to disclose.
Melissa Wilson has nothing to disclose.
Ryan Togashi has nothing to disclose.
Bo Han has nothing to disclose.
Austin K. Mircheff, has nothing to disclose.
C. Thomas Vangsness, Jr., is a shareholder and board member of CarthroniX.

Author details

[1]Department of Orthopaedic Surgery, Keck School of Medicine of USC, HCT 1520 San Pablo Street, suite 2000, Los Angeles, CA 90033, USA. [2]Department of Preventive Medicine, Keck School of Medicine of USC, 2001 Soto Street, SSB1 318A, Los Angeles, CA 90033, USA. [3]Departments of Surgery and Biomedical Engineering, Keck School of Medicine of USC, 1333 San Pablo St. BMT-302, Los Angeles, CA 90033, USA. [4]Department of Physiology & Neuroscience, Keck School of Medicine of USC, 1333 San Pablo St. BMT B-11A, Los Angeles, CA 90033, USA.

References

1. Lories RJ, Luyten FP. The bone-cartilage unit in osteoarthritis. Nat Rev Rheumatol. Nature Publishing Group. 2011;7:43–9.
2. Murphy L, Helmick CG. The impact of osteoarthritis in the United States: a population-health perspective: a population-based review of the fourth most common cause of hospitalization in U.S. adults. Orthop Nurs. 2012;31:85–91.
3. Ethgen O, Kahler KH, Kong SX, Reginster J-Y, Wolfe F. The effect of health related quality of life on reported use of health care resources in patients with osteoarthritis and rheumatoid arthritis: a longitudinal analysis. J Rheumatol. 2002;29:1147–55.
4. Kotlarz H, Gunnarsson CL, Fang H, Rizzo JA. Insurer and out-of-pocket costs of osteoarthritis in the US: evidence from national survey data. Arthritis Rheum. Wiley subscription services, Inc., A Wiley Company. 2009;60:3546 53.
5. Losina E, Paltiel AD, Weinstein AM, Yelin E, Hunter DJ, Chen SP, et al. Lifetime medical costs of knee osteoarthritis management in the United States: impact of extending indications for total knee arthroplasty. Arthritis Care Res. 2015;67:203–15.
6. Brown GA. AAOS clinical practice guideline: treatment of osteoarthritis of the knee: evidence-based guideline, 2nd edition. J Am Acad Orthop Surg. 2013;21:577–9.
7. Maniar KH, Jones IA, Gopalakrishna R, Vangsness CT Jr. Lowering side effects of NSAID usage in osteoarthritis: recent attempts at minimizing dosage. Expert Opin Pharmacother. 2018;19(2):93–102.
8. Jevsevar DS. Treatment of osteoarthritis of the knee: evidence-based guideline, 2nd edition. J Am Acad Orthop Surg. 2013;21:571–6.
9. McAlindon TE, LaValley MP, Harvey WF, Price LL, Driban JB, Zhang M, et al. Effect of intra-articular triamcinolone vs saline on knee cartilage volume and pain in patients with knee osteoarthritis: a randomized clinical trial. JAMA Am Med Assoc. 2017;317:1967–75.
10. Bedard NA, Pugely AJ, Elkins JM, Duchman KR, Westermann RW, Liu SS, et al. The John N. Insall award: do intraarticular injections increase the risk of infection after TKA? Clin Orthop Relat Res. Springer US. 2017;475:45–52.
11. Wernecke C, Braun HJ, Dragoo JL. The Effect of Intra-articular Corticosteroids on Articular Cartilage: A Systematic Review. Orthop J Sports Med. SAGE PublicationsSage CA: Los Angeles, CA. 2015;3:2325967115581163.
12. McIntyre LF, Bannuru RR, Vaysbrot EE. Authors' reply. Arthroscopy. 2014;30: 658–9.
13. Bannuru RR, Vaysbrot EE, McIntyre LF. Did the American Academy of Orthopaedic surgeons osteoarthritis guidelines miss the mark? Arthroscopy. 2014;30:86–9.
14. Jevsevar D, Donnelly P, Brown GA, Cummins DS. Viscosupplementation for osteoarthritis of the knee: a systematic review of the evidence. J Bone Joint Surg Am. 2015;97:2047–60.
15. Vannabouathong C, Bhandari M, Bedi A, Khanna V, Yung P, Shetty V, et al. Nonoperative treatments for knee osteoarthritis: an evaluation of treatment characteristics and the intra-articular placebo effect: a systematic review. JBJS Rev. 2018;6:e5.
16. Liu-Bryan R. Synovium and the innate inflammatory network in osteoarthritis progression. Curr Rheumatol Rep. Current Science Inc. 2013;15:323.
17. Haseeb A, Haqqi TM. Immunopathogenesis of osteoarthritis. Clin Immunol. 2013;146:185–96.
18. Sellam J, Berenbaum F. The role of synovitis in pathophysiology and clinical symptoms of osteoarthritis. Nat Rev Rheumatol. Nature Publishing Group. 2010;6:625–35.
19. Chevalier X, Eymard F, Richette P. Biologic agents in osteoarthritis: hopes and disappointments. Nat Rev Rheumatol Nature Publishing Group. 2013;9:400–10.
20. Lambert C, Dubuc J-E, Montell E, Vergés J, Munaut C, Noël A, et al. Gene expression pattern of cells from inflamed and normal areas of osteoarthritis synovial membrane. Arthritis Rheumatol. 2014;66:960–8.
21. Kapoor M, Martel-Pelletier J, Lajeunesse D, Pelletier J-P, Fahmi H. Role of proinflammatory cytokines in the pathophysiology of osteoarthritis. Nat Rev Rheumatol. 2011;7:33–42.
22. Ashraf S, Cha B-H, Kim J-S, Ahn J, Han I, Park H, et al. Regulation of senescence associated signaling mechanisms in chondrocytes for cartilage tissue regeneration. Osteoarthr Cartil. 2016;24:196–205.
23. Lotz M, Martel-Pelletier J, Christiansen C, Brandi M-L, Bruyère O, Chapurlat R, et al. Value of biomarkers in osteoarthritis: current status and perspectives. Ann. Rheum. Dis. BMJ Publishing Group Ltd and European League Against Rheumatism. 2013;72:1756–63.
24. Tsuchida AI, Beekhuizen M, t Hart MC, TRDJ R, WJA D, DBF S, et al. Cytokine profiles in the joint depend on pathology, but are different between synovial fluid, cartilage tissue and cultured chondrocytes. Arthritis Res. Ther. BioMed Central. 2014;16:441.
25. McIntyre JA, Jones IA, Danilkovich A, Vangsness CT. The placenta: applications in Orthopaedic sports medicine. Am J Sports Med. 2017;122:363546517697682.
26. Bourin P, Bunnell BA, Casteilla L, Dominici M, Katz AJ, March KL, et al. Stromal cells from the adipose tissue-derived stromal vascular fraction and culture expanded adipose tissue-derived stromal/stem cells: a joint statement of the International Federation for Adipose Therapeutics and Science (IFATS) and the International Society for Cellular Therapy (ISCT). Cytotherapy. 2013;15:641–8.
27. Turner L, Knoepfler P. Selling stem cells in the USA: assessing the direct-to-consumer industry. Cell Stem Cell. 2016;19:154–7.
28. Jones IA, Togashi RC, Thomas VC. The economics and regulation of PRP in the evolving field of orthopedic biologics. Curr Rev Musculoskelet Med Springer US. 2018;17:602–8.
29. Marks P, Gottlieb S. Balancing safety and innovation for cell-based regenerative medicine. N Engl J Med. 2018;378:954–9.
30. Tremolada C, Ricordi C, Caplan AI, Ventura C. Mesenchymal stem cells in Lipogems, a reverse story: from clinical practice to basic science. Methods Mol. Biol. New York, NY: Springer New York. 2016;1416:109–22.
31. Clockaerts S, Bastiaansen-Jenniskens YM, Runhaar J, Van Osch GJVM, Van Offel JF, Verhaar JAN, et al. The infrapatellar fat pad should be considered as an active osteoarthritic joint tissue: a narrative review. Osteoarthr Cartil. 2010;18:876–82.
32. Bowen JE. Technical issues in harvesting and concentrating stem cells (bone marrow and adipose). PM R. 2015;7:S8–18.
33. Vangsness CT, Sternberg H, Harris L. Umbilical cord tissue offers the greatest number of harvestable mesenchymal stem cells for research and clinical application: a literature review of different harvest sites. Arthroscopy. 2015; 31:1836–43.
34. Bianchi F, Maioli M, Leonardi E, Olivi E, Pasquinelli G, Valente S, et al. A new nonenzymatic method and device to obtain a fat tissue derivative highly enriched in pericyte-like elements by mild mechanical forces from human lipoaspirates. Cell Transplant. 2013;22:2063 77.

35. Carelli S, Messaggio F, Canazza A, Hebda DM, Caremoli F, Latorre E, et al. Characteristics and properties of mesenchymal stem cells derived from microfragmented adipose tissue. Cell Transplant Cognizant Communication Corporation. 2015;24:1233–52.
36. Tonnard P, Verpaele A, Peeters G, Hamdi M, Cornelissen M, Declercq H. Nanofat grafting: basic research and clinical applications. Plast Reconstr Surg. 2013;132:1017–26.
37. Bosetti M, Borrone A, Follenzi A, Messaggio F, Tremolada C, Cannas M. Human Lipoaspirate as autologous injectable active scaffold for one-step repair of cartilage defects. Cell Transplant. Cognizant Communication Corporation. 2016;25:1043–56.
38. Aronowitz JA, Lockhart RA, Hakakian CS. Mechanical versus enzymatic isolation of stromal vascular fraction cells from adipose tissue. Springerplus. Springer International Publishing. 2015;4:713.
39. Shah FS, Wu X, Dietrich M, Rood J, Gimble JM. A non-enzymatic method for isolating human adipose tissue-derived stromal stem cells. Cytotherapy. 2013;15:979–85.
40. Striano RD, Chen H, Bilbool N, Azatullah K, Hilado J. Non-responsive knee pain with osteoarthritis and concurrent meniscal disease treated with autologous micro-fragmented adipose tissue under continuous. CellR4. 2015;3(5):e1690.
41. Franceschini M, Castellaneta C, Mineo G. Injection of autologous micro-fragmented adipose tissue for the treatment of post traumatic degenerative lesion of knee cartilage: a case report. CellR4. 2016;1768:4.
42. Badylak SF. The extracellular matrix as a biologic scaffold material. Biomaterials. 2007;28:3587–93.
43. Badylak SF. The extracellular matrix as a scaffold for tissue reconstruction. Semin Cell Dev Biol. 2002;13:377–83.
44. Filardo G, Kon E, Buda R, Timoncini A, Di Martino A, Cenacchi A, et al. Platelet-rich plasma intra-articular knee injections for the treatment of degenerative cartilage lesions and osteoarthritis. Knee Surg Sports Traumatol Arthrosc Springer-Verlag. 2011;19:528–35.
45. Altman RD, Akermark C, Beaulieu AD, Schnitzer T. Durolane International Study Group. Efficacy and safety of a single intra-articular injection of non-animal stabilized hyaluronic acid (NASHA) in patients with osteoarthritis of the knee. Osteoarthr. Cartil. 2004;12:642–9.
46. Lukashev ME, Werb Z. ECM signalling: orchestrating cell behaviour and misbehaviour. Trends Cell Biol. 1998;8:437–41.
47. Trentham DE, Townes AS, Kang AH. Autoimmunity to type II collagen an experimental model of arthritis. J Exp Med The Rockefeller University Press. 1977;146:857–68.
48. Heilmann HH, Lindenhayn K, Walther HU. [synovial volume of healthy and arthrotic human knee joints]. Z Orthop Ihre Grenzgeb. © 1996 F. Enke Verlag Stuttgart. 1996;134:144–8.
49. Matziolis G, Roehner E, Windisch C, Wagner A. The volume of the human knee joint. Arch Orthop Trauma Surg. Springer Berlin Heidelberg. 2015; 135:1401–3.
50. Tremolada C, Colombo V, Ventura C. Adipose tissue and mesenchymal stem cells: state of the art and Lipogems® technology development. Current stem cell reports. 2016;2:304–12.
51. Alexander RW. Autologous fat grafts as mesenchymal stromal stem cell source for use in prolotherapy: a simple technique to acquire lipoaspirants. J Prolotherapy. 2011;3:680–8.
52. Vangsness Jr CT, Jack Farr I, Boyd J, Dellaero DT, Mills CR, LeRoux-Williams M. Adult human mesenchymal stem cells delivered via intra-articular injection to the knee following partial medial meniscectomy: a randomized, Double-Blind, Controlled Study. J Bone Joint Surg Am. 2014;96(2):90–8.
53. Sánchez M, Fiz N, Azofra J, Usabiaga J, Aduriz Recalde E, Garcia Gutierrez A, et al. A randomized clinical trial evaluating plasma rich in growth factors (PRGF-Endoret) versus hyaluronic acid in the short-term treatment of symptomatic knee osteoarthritis. Arthroscopy. 2012;28:1070–8.
54. Chevalier X, Jerosch J, Goupille P, van Dijk N, Luyten FP, Scott DL, et al. Single, intra-articular treatment with 6 ml hylan G-F 20 in patients with symptomatic primary osteoarthritis of the knee: a randomised, multicentre, double-blind, placebo controlled trial. Ann. Rheum. Dis. BMJ Publishing Group Ltd. 2010;69:113–9.
55. Riddle DL, Stratford PW. Unilateral vs bilateral symptomatic knee osteoarthritis: associations between pain intensity and function. Rheumatology (Oxford). 2013;52:2229–37.
56. Kahn TL, Soheili AC, Schwarzkopf R. Poor WOMAC scores in contralateral knee negatively impact TKA outcomes: data from the osteoarthritis initiative. J Arthroplast. 2014;29:1580 5.
57. Bellamy N, Buchanan WW, Goldsmith CH, Campbell J, Stitt LW. Validation study of WOMAC: a health status instrument for measuring clinically important patient relevant outcomes to antirheumatic drug therapy in patients with osteoarthritis of the hip or knee. J Rheumatol. 1988;15(12):1833–40.
58. Losina E, Ranstam J, Collins JE, Schnitzer TJ, Katz JN. OARSI clinical trials recommendations: key analytic considerations in design, analysis, and reporting of randomized controlled trials in osteoarthritis. Osteoarthr Cartil. 2015;23:677–85.
59. Katz P, Pedro S, Michaud K. Performance of the Patient-Reported Outcomes Measurement Information System 29-Item Profile in Rheumatoid Arthritis, Osteoarthritis, Fibromyalgia, and Systemic Lupus Erythematosus. Arthritis Care Res. 2017;69(9):1312–21.
60. Jaeschke R, Singer J, Guyatt GH. Measurement of health status: ascertaining the minimal clinically important difference. Control Clin Trials Elsevier. 1989; 10:407–15.
61. Lundquist CB, Døssing K, Christiansen DH. Responsiveness of a Danish version of the disabilities of the arm, shoulder and hand (DASH) questionnaire. Dan Med J. 2014;61:A4813.
62. Prieto TE, Myklebust JB, Hoffmann RG, Lovett EG, Myklebust BM. Measures of postural steadiness: differences between healthy young and elderly adults. IEEE Trans Biomed Eng. 1996;43:956–66.
63. van Esch RW, Kool MM, van As S. NSAIDs can have adverse effects on bone healing. Med Hypotheses. 2013;81:343–6.
64. Crofford LJ. Use of NSAIDs in treating patients with arthritis. Arthritis Res. Ther. 2013;15(Suppl 3):S2.
65. McAlindon TE, Bannuru RR, Sullivan MC, Arden NK, Berenbaum F, Bierma-Zeinstra SM, et al. OARSI guidelines for the non-surgical management of knee osteoarthritis. Osteoarthr. Cartil. 2014;22:363–88.
66. da Costa BR, Reichenbach S, Keller N, Nartey L, Wandel S, Jüni P, et al. Effectiveness of non-steroidal anti-inflammatory drugs for the treatment of pain in knee and hip osteoarthritis: a network meta-analysis. Lancet. 2017; 390:e21–33.
67. Machado GC, Maher CG, Ferreira PH, Pinheiro MB, Lin C-WC, Day RO, et al. Efficacy and safety of paracetamol for spinal pain and osteoarthritis: systematic review and meta-analysis of randomised placebo controlled trials. BMJ. 2015;350:h1225.
68. Marks PW, Witten CM, Califf RM. Clarifying stem-cell Therapy's benefits and risks. N Engl J Med. 2017;376:1007–9.
69. Kraus VB, Conaghan PG, Aazami HA, Mehra P, Kivitz AJ, Lufkin J, et al. Synovial and systemic pharmacokinetics (PK) of triamcinolone acetonide (TA) following intra-articular (IA) injection of an extended-release microsphere-based formulation (FX006) or standard crystalline suspension in patients with knee osteoarthritis (OA). Osteoarthr Cartil. 2018;26:34–42.
70. Vangsness CT, Burke WS, Narvy SJ, MacPhee RD, Fedenko AN. Human knee synovial fluid cytokines correlated with grade of knee osteoarthritis--a pilot study. Bull NYU Hosp Jt Dis. 2011;69:122–7.
71. Brazier JE, Harper R, Munro J, Walters SJ, Snaith ML. Generic and condition-specific outcome measures for people with osteoarthritis of the knee. Rheumatology (Oxford). 1999;38:870–7.
72. Roos EM, Toksvig-Larsen S. Knee injury and Osteoarthritis Outcome Score (KOOS) - validation and comparison to the WOMAC in total knee replacement. Health Qual Life Outcomes. BioMed Central. 2003;1:17.
73. Bachmeier CJ, March LM, Cross MJ, Lapsley HM, Tribe KL, Courtenay BG, et al. A comparison of outcomes in osteoarthritis patients undergoing total hip and knee replacement surgery. Osteoarthr Cartil. 2001;9:137–46.
74. Mendicino M, Bailey AM, Wonnacott K, Puri RK, Bauer SR. MSC-based product characterization for clinical trials: an FDA perspective. Cell Stem Cell. 2014;14:141–5.

Vascular endothelial growth factor expression and their action in the synovial membranes of patients with painful knee osteoarthritis

Shotaro Takano[1], Kentaro Uchida[1*], Gen Inoue[1], Toshihide Matsumoto[2], Jun Aikawa[1], Dai Iwase[1], Manabu Mukai[1], Masayuki Miyagi[1] and Masashi Takaso[1]

Abstract

Background: Research suggests that vascular endothelial growth factor (VEGF) levels in the synovial fluid of knee osteoarthritis (KOA) patients are positively correlated with KOA severity. The relationship between synovial VEGF levels and pain in human KOA patients is not fully understood, and the role of VEGF in the pain pathway remains unclear.

Methods: We harvested synovial membrane (SM) from 102 patients with radiographic evidence of KOA (unilateral Kellgren/Lawrence [K/L] grade 2–4) during total knee arthroplasty. Patients scored their pain on a 0 to 10 cm visual analog scale (VAS). VEGF levels in the SM of KOA patients with strong/severe (VAS ≥ 6) and mild/moderate pain (VAS < 6) were compared. Correlations between VAS and VEGF mRNA expression were investigated. To investigate a possible mechanism for VEGF-induced pain, the distribution of VEGF and the neuropeptide apelin was determined by immunohistochemical analyses. To investigate the role of VEGF in regulating apelin expression, SM cells were exposed to VEGF.

Results: VEGF expression in the VAS ≥ 6 group was significantly greater than expression in the VAS < 6 group. Expression levels of VEGF were also positively correlated with VAS. VEGF-positive cells were identified in the lining of the SM. Expression of apelin mRNA and protein were significantly elevated in SM cells treated with exogenous VEGF compared to those treated with vehicle.

Conclusion: Synovial VEGF may be involved in pain pathways in KOA and its action may be mediated by apelin.

Keywords: Vascular endothelial growth factor, Synovial membrane, Pain, Osteoarthritis, Neuropeptides

Background

Osteoarthritis (OA) is the most common form of arthritis and a leading cause of disability worldwide. This disability is largely due to pain, a major symptom of the condition. Pain contributes to functional limitations and reduces quality of life [1–4]. Largely because of pain, lower extremity OA is well recognized as the leading cause of mobility impairment in older adults [5]. Pharmacologic treatment options for OA are centered around the relief of pain and support for functional improvement in patients. Nevertheless, the efficacy of treatments such as nonsteroidal anti-inflammatory drugs (NSAIDs) can be limited, and can cause significant adverse effects such as cardiorenal and gastrointestinal toxicity [6, 7]. It is therefore important to establish the mechanisms underlying OA pain to aid in drug development for OA treatment.

Vascular endothelial growth factor (VEGF) is a potent stimulator of angiogenesis, and also a contributor to inflammation. VEGF in OA patients has been found to be elevated in the synovial membrane (SM) [8–11], subchondral bone [12–14], synovial fluid (SF) [15–18], serum [16–19], and articular cartilage [20–28]. In particular, VEGF is strongly expressed in synovial lining cells in OA patients [29]. Intraarticular injection of anti-VEGF antibody reduced

* Correspondence: kuchida@med.kitasato-u.ac.jp
[1]Department of Orthopedic Surgery, Kitasato University School of Medicine, 1-15-1 Minami-ku Kitasato, Sagamihara City 252-0374, Japan
Full list of author information is available at the end of the article

synovial inflammation in a rabbit OA model [30]. Several studies have suggested that SF and plasma VEGF concentrations in OA patients correlate with OA severity [16, 17]. In addition, recent studies have reported that VEGF contributes to pain in a rodent neuropathic pain model [31–34] and cancer pain model [35]. The exact relationship between VEGF expression in SM and pain in human KOA patients is not fully understood.

Recent studies have suggested that several neuropeptides, such as calcitonin gene-related peptide (CGRP) and nerve growth factor (NGF), in the SM are involved in the OA pain pathway [36–39]. Apelin is a recognized member of the adipose-secreted cytokine family and is initially secreted as a pre-propeptide of 77 amino acid residues, which is then cleaved into a number of active forms [40]. The apelin signaling pathway was shown to play a major role in the development of the functional vascular network [41] and apelin expression was elevated in endothelial cell culture following VEGF stimulation [42]. Several studies also showed that apelin can regulate peripheral pain sensitivity mediated by apelin receptors (APJ) and GABAA receptors [21, 43]. Hu et al. reported that apelin concentration in SF is increased in OA patients [44]. These observations led us to investigate the role of VEGF in regulating apelin in SM and its contribution to the OA pain pathway.

We investigated the relationship between VEGF expression in SM and pain in knee osteoarthritis (KOA) patients. In addition, we investigated whether VEGF regulates apelin expression in the SM.

Methods

Patients

This study was approved by the Institutional Review Board for Clinical Research and Treatment in Kitasato University (approval No. B13–113). Sample size was determined with a power analysis for an alpha of 0.05 and power of 0.80 using G*POWER3. Patients scored their pain on a 0 to 10 cm visual analog scale (VAS). Power analysis showed that 44 SM samples of patients with VAS < 6 and 58 SM samples of patients with VAS ≥ 6 were required to identify a difference in VEGF expression between the two groups. SM samples were harvested from 102 patients undergoing total knee arthroplasty. The study enrolled 22 men and 80 women (age 46–89 years, mean ± standard error (SE) = 73.2 ± 0.8 years; body mass index (BMI) range 18.4–36.7, mean ± SE = 26.0 ± 0.4 kg/m^2) with radiographic evidence of KOA (unilateral Kellgren/Lawrence [K/L] grades 2 (3/102, 2.9%), 3 (36/102, 35.3%) and 4 (63/102, 61.8%)). All patients provided informed consent for participation in this study 1 day before surgery. SM samples were harvested intraoperatively from the suprapatellar pouch of each operated knee and immediately stored frozen in liquid nitrogen at − 80 °C until required for extraction of RNA. SM samples obtained from six patients were used for cell culture. The remaining samples were fixed in 4% paraformaldehyde phosphate-buffered solution (Nacalai Tesque, Kyoto, Japan) for 72 h for use in histological analysis.

Quantitative polymerase chain reaction (qPCR) analysis

Extraction of total RNA from SM and cultured SM cells and cDNA synthesis was conducted as reported previously [45]. PCR primer pair sequences for use in qPCR analysis were: VEGF-Forward (5′- TTGCCTTGCTGCTCTACCT C-3′) and VEGF-Reverse (5′- AGCTGCGCTGATAG ACATCC-3′) for VEGF amplification (product size: 117 bp); apelin-Forward (5′- GAATCTGCGGCTCT GCGT-3′) and apelin-Reverse (5′- CATCAGGGACCCTC CACACA-3′) for apelin amplification (product size: 76 bp); and GAPDH-Forward (5′-TGTTGCCATCAATGACCCC TT-3′) and GAPDH-Reverse (5′-CTCCACGACGTACT CAGCG-3′) for GAPDH amplification (product size: 223 bp). Specificity of the qPCR products was evaluated using melting curve analysis. Relative mRNA expression levels of VEGF and apelin were evaluated using qPCR (CFX-96®, Bio-Rad, Richmond CA, USA). Expression levels of VEGF and apelin mRNA were normalized to the expression of the housekeeping gene, GAPDH.

Expression levels of VEGF mRNA were compared between the strong/severe (VAS ≥ 6) and mild/moderate pain (VAS < 6) groups (Table 1), using VAS = 6 as a cutoff based on previous reports [39, 46, 47]. The correlation between VAS levels and VEGF mRNA expression was also determined. Relative VEGF expression was calculated based on the mean of all samples of the VAS < 6 group.

Table 1 Characteristics of patients in VAS < 6 and VAS ≥ 6 groups

Characteristic	VAS < 6 (*n* = 44)	VAS ≥ 6 (*n* = 58)
Age (y)	74.2 ± 1.1	72.3 ± 1.2
Male/Female, n	12/32	10/48
BMI (kg/m^2)	25.5 ± 0.6	26.3 ± 0.6
Number of patients with Kellgren/Lawrence grade 2, 3, 4	3, 14, 27	0, 22, 36
VAS (cm)	3.7 ± 0.2	8.4 ± 0.2

Data are mean ± standard error unless otherwise indicated
BMI body mass index, *VAS* visual analogue pain scale

To investigate the relationship between VEGF and K/L grades, the 102 knee OA patients were divided into three groups based on their K/L grade (2, 3, or 4). The clinical characteristics of patients in each of these groups are shown in Table 2. Relative VEGF expression was calculated based on the mean of all samples of the K/L2 group.

Immunohistochemistry

Following fixation, SM samples were embedded in paraffin, sectioned at 3 μm thickness, then deparaffinized (Clear Plus®, FALMA, Tokyo, Japan) and pretreated with sodium citrate buffer (pH 6.0) containing 0.1% polyoxyethylene sorbitan monolaurate (Nacalai Tesque, Kyoto, Japan) at 98 °C for 20 min for antigen retrieval. The sections were subsequently washed three times with phosphate-buffered saline for 5 min and incubated with rabbit polyclonal anti-VEGF antibody (1:100 dilution; Santa Cruz Biotechnology Inc., Santa Cruz CA, USA) and mouse monoclonal anti-apelin antibody (1:100 dilution; Santa Cruz Biotechnology) for 4 h at 4 °C. The sections were additionally incubated with Alexa 488 Fluor®-conjugated goat anti-rabbit IgG antibody (1:100 dilution; Thermo Fisher Scientific, Waltham MA, USA) and Alexa 594 Fluor®-conjugated goat anti-mouse IgG antibody (1:100 dilution; Thermo Fisher Scientific) for 1 h at room temperature. The distribution of fluorescence in SM sections was analyzed using a fluorescence microscope (Axiovert 200®, Zeiss, Jena, Germany).

Synovial membrane cell culture

Synovial membrane cells (SMCs) were isolated from 500 mg SM using 40 mL of a 1 mg/mL collagenase solution. The SMCs were incubated in α-minimal essential media (α-MEM; Nacalai Tesque) containing 10% fetal bovine serum in six-well plates. After 1 week, the SMCs were incubated with vehicle (serum free α-MEM) or 10 or 100 ng/mL human recombinant VGEF (Biolegend, San Diego CA, USA) for 24 h. Subsequently, total mRNA and protein were extracted and used in western blotting and qPCR analysis. Relative expression was calculated based on the mean of all samples of the vehicle-treated group.

Western blotting for apelin

To investigate the regulation of apelin by VEGF, SMCs harvested from six patients were stimulated with 1 ng/mL or 10 ng/mL VEGF for 24 h. Using methodology described elsewhere [48], SMCs were lysed in radioimmunoprecipitation buffer (Thermo Fisher Scientific) containing a protease inhibitor cocktail (Sigma-Aldrich, St. Louis MO, USA). Protein concentration was determined for each cell extract using a bicinchoninic acid (BCA) assay (Thermo Fisher Scientific). A total of 30 μg of each protein was separated by sodium dodecyl sulfate-polyacrylamide gel electrophoresis and electrophoretically transferred to polyvinyl difluoride membranes. These membranes were then blocked with polyvinylidene fluoride (PVDF) blocking reagent (DS Pharma Biomedical, Suita, Japan) for 1 h and incubated overnight at 4 °C with mouse monoclonal primary antibody against apelin (1:200 dilution; Santa Cruz Biotechnology Inc.). The membranes were washed with Tris-buffered saline containing 0.05% Tween and then incubated with horseradish peroxidase-conjugated anti mouse IgG (1:1000 dilution; GE Healthcare, Piscataway NJ, USA). Apelin proteins were visualized by chemiluminescence using an enhanced chemiluminescence detection system (GE Healthcare) and exposure of the membranes to x-ray film. Bands were quantified by densitometric scanning using ImageJ software (NIH, Bethesda MD, USA). Densitometry levels of apelin proteins were normalized against that of β-actin.

Table 2 Clinical characteristics of patients (K/L 2, 3 and 4)

Characteristic	K/L2 (n = 3)	K/L3 (n = 36)	K/L4 (n = 63)
Age (y)	72.0 ± 2.6	72.0 ± 4.2	73.9 ± 8.4
Male/Female, n	1/2	9/27	12/51
BMI (kg/m^2)	25.8 ± 3.4	26.4 ± 4.3	25.7 ± 4.1
VAS (cm)	3.7 ± 2.5	6.9 ± 2.6	6.2 ± 2.6

Data are mean ± standard error unless otherwise indicated
BMI body mass index, *VAS* visual analogue pain scale, *K/L* Kellgren/Lawrence grade

Statistical analysis

Differences in VEGF expression between the VAS < 6 and VAS ≥ 6 groups were compared using the Mann-Whitney *U*-test. Differences in VEGF expression among K/L2, 3 and 4 subjects were compared using the Kruskal-Wallis test. Tukey's multiple comparisons test was used to compare vehicle control and VEGF-treated cells. The relationship between VEGF expression and VAS was evaluated using Spearman's correlation coefficient. All statistical analyses were conducted using SPSS software (v. 19.0; SPSS, Chicago IL, USA), with a P value < 0.05 considered statistically significant for all analyses.

Results

Relationship between VEGF expression and VAS

The VAS ≥ 6 and VAS < 6 groups did not differ with regard to patient age, male/female ratio, BMI, or KL 2/3/4 ratio (Table 1). qPCR analysis showed that VEGF expression in the SM was significantly higher in the VAS ≥ 6 group than the VAS < 6 group (Fig. 1a, $P < 0.05$). VEGF levels were also positively correlated with VAS (Fig. 1b, $\rho = 0.346$, $P < 0.05$).

Relationship between VEGF expression and K/L grades

The three K/L grade groups did not differ with regard to patient age, male/female ratio, BMI, or VAS (Table 2). There was no difference in synovial VEGF expression among the K/L2, 3 and 4 groups (Fig. 2).

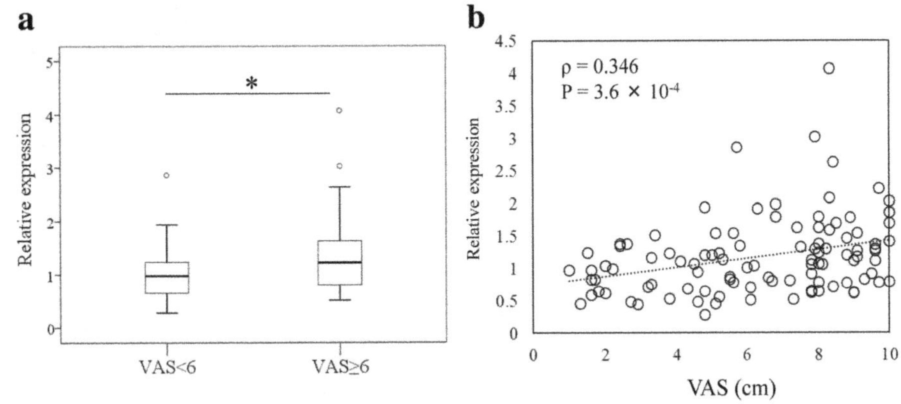

Fig. 1 qPCR analysis of VEGF expression in the synovial membranes (SMs) of knee osteoarthritis (KOA) patients according to their VAS score. **a** "Box and whisker" plot of VEGF expression in the SMs of KOA patients with mild/moderate (VAS < 6) ($n = 44$) and strong/severe pain (VAS ≥ 6) ($n = 58$). The plot shows the median values (bold horizontal line), interquartile range (IQR) (box), and range. Outliers beyond 1.5-fold of the IQR from the box are plotted. * $P = 0.008$. VAS, visual analog scale. **b** Scatter plot showing the correlation between VAS scores and VEGF levels. Relative expression was calculated based on the mean of all samples of the VAS < 6 group

Distribution of VEGF and apelin in the SMs of KOA patients

Immunohistochemical analysis was conducted to investigate the distribution of VEGF and apelin in the SMs of KOA patients (Fig. 3). Immunostaining showed that VEGF and apelin protein were both expressed in the synovial lining layers (Fig. 3).

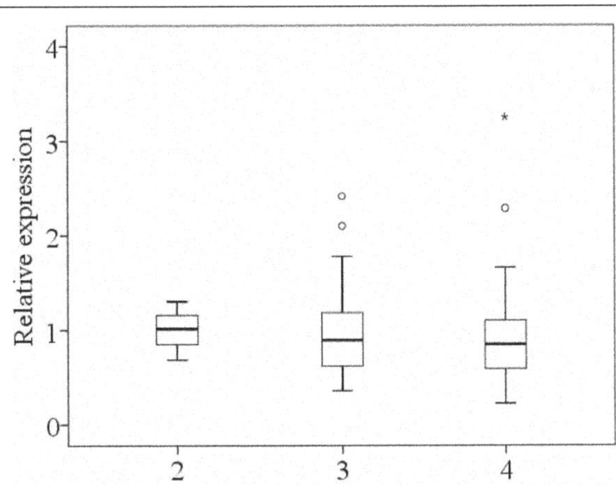

Fig. 2 Relationship between VEGF mRNA expression level and Kellgren/Lawrence (K/L) grade. To investigate the relationship between VEGF and K/L grades, 102 knee OA patients were divided into three groups according to their K/L grade (2, 3, or 4). The three groups did not differ by patient age, male/female ratio, body mass index, or pain score based on the visual analog scale. Relative expression was calculated based on the mean of all samples of the KL2 group. The plot indicates median (bold horizontal line), interquartile range (IQR) (box), and range. Outliers beyond 1.5-fold of the IQR from the box are plotted

Effects of VEGF on apelin expression in SMCs

qPCR analysis showed that the expression of apelin mRNA increased significantly in SMCs following 10 and 100 ng/mL VEGF stimulation (1.73-fold and 1.69-fold, respectively, $P < 0.05$; Fig. 4). Western blotting analysis showed that the expression of apelin was significantly increased in SMCs in the presence of exogenously added 10 and 100 ng/mL VEGF (1.85-fold and 1.56-fold, respectively, $P < 0.05$; Fig. 5a and b).

Discussion

In the SM of KOA patients, VEGF mRNA expression in the VAS ≥ 6 group was significantly higher than that in the VAS < 6 group. VEGF and apelin were both expressed in the synovial lining layers and VEGF stimulated apelin mRNA and protein expression in SM cell culture. Together, these findings indicate that VEGF expression in SM may be involved in knee pain via apelin in KOA patients.

Several studies have reported that VEGF may contribute to chronic pain conditions [31, 32, 49]. Injection of VEGF in spinal cord-injured rats causes mechanical allodynia [49]. VEGF neutralization in rat chronic constriction injury (CCI) models attenuates chronic pain behavior by reducing the VEGF receptor expression level in dorsal root ganglia to inhibit neuropathic pain signaling [32]. Perineural injection of a VEGF inhibitor inhibited tactile allodynia and thermal hyperalgesia caused by partial sciatic nerve ligation [31]. Here, KOA patients who experienced severe/strong pain showed increased VEGF expression levels in SM. These findings suggest that synovial VEGF seems to play an important role in the pain pathway associated with KOA.

Several studies have reported that VEGF regulates apelin expression in vitro and in vivo [42, 50, 51]. VEGF

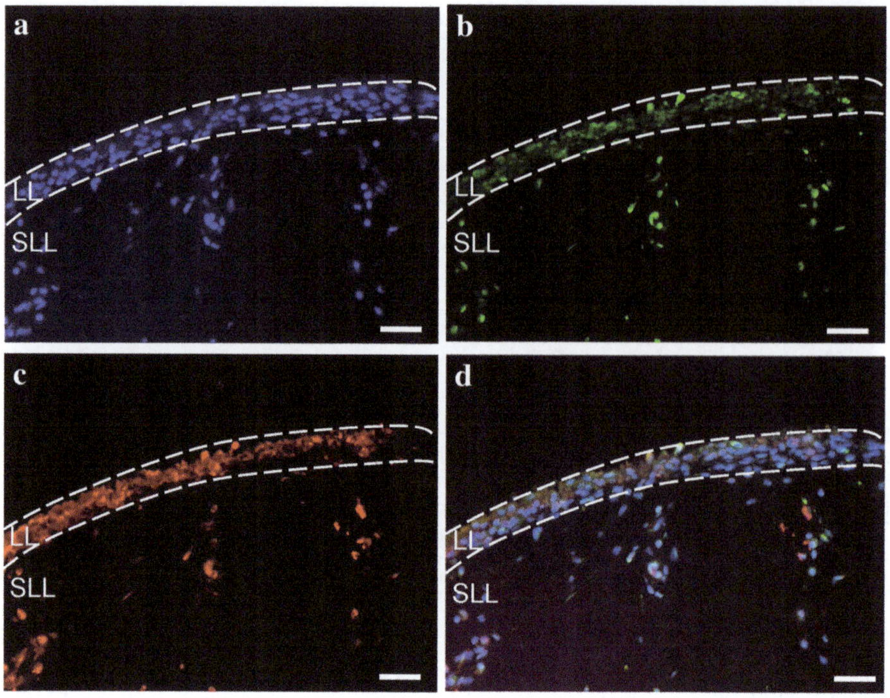

Fig. 3 Immunostaining of VEGF and apelin in the synovial membranes of knee OA patients. Synovial membranes stained with **a** DAPI (nuclei), **b** VEGF, or **c** apelin. **d** The merged images. Region enclosed by dotted lines indicates the lining layer (LL), which is above the sublining layer (SLL) in the synovial membrane. Scale bar = 100 μm

stimulates apelin mRNA in human umbilical venous endothelial cells in vitro [50]. Local injection of bevacizumab, an anti-VEGF antibody, inhibits apelin expression in monkeys with occlusion of the central retinal vein [51]. Apelin-APJ systems are located in the central and peripheral nervous systems [52, 53]. In the central nervous system, apelin and its receptors have been detected in pain-associated regions. Previous studies have reported that intrathecal injection of apelin-13 (the isoform that binds most strongly to the APJ) induces hyperalgesia [21], and when "intrathecal administration of ML221, an APJ blocker, was used, this transiently reduced CCI-induced pain hypersensitivity" [43]. In addition, higher apelin concentrations in serum and SF were found in OA patients compared to non-OA patients [44]. Here, VEGF stimulated apelin mRNA and protein expression in SMCs, suggesting that further investigation of a direct link between apelin and pain may explain the mechanism underlying VEGF-induced OA pain.

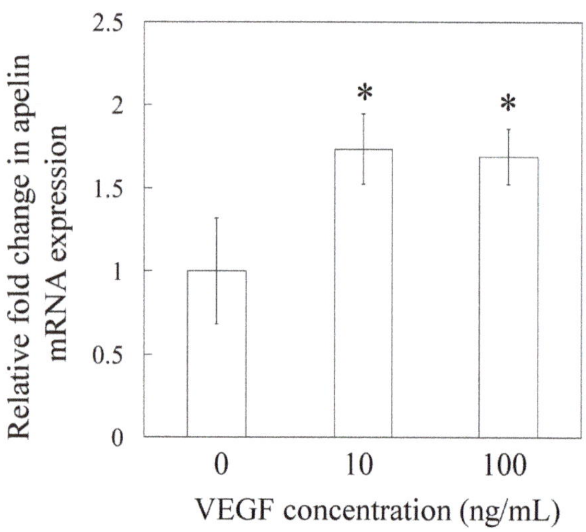

Fig. 4 Effect of VEGF on apelin mRNA expression. qPCR analysis for apelin. Synovial membrane cells were stimulated with 10 or 100 ng/mL human recombinant VGEF or vehicle for 24 h preceding the extraction and analysis of apelin mRNA. All data are shown as the mean ± standard error ($n = 6$). *$P < 0.05$

A number of limitations of this study warrant mention. First, the absence of a non-KOA control patient population reduces the certainty of our results. Additional evaluations aimed at confirming whether VEGF levels are raised in the SMs of KOA patients compared to non-KOA patients are needed. Second, whether SMCs extracted from OA knees will behave the same as SMCs from healthy knees when treated with VEGF remains to be determined. Third, although our findings support the idea that altered VEGF levels in SMs are associated with KOA pain, whether a direct causative link exists between VEGF and apelin remains to be clarified.

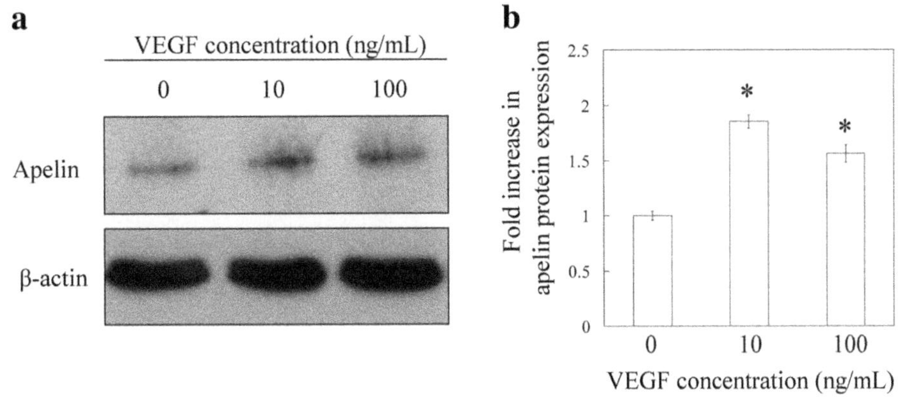

Fig. 5 Effect of VEGF on apelin protein expression. Western blotting analysis for apelin. Synovial membrane cells were stimulated with 10 or 100 ng/mL human recombinant VGEF or vehicle for 24 h preceding protein extraction and analysis of apelin protein. **a** Western blot of apelin and β-actin. **b** Densitometric analysis of apelin bands. All data are shown as the mean ± standard error ($n = 6$). $*P < 0.05$ compared with the vehicle control

Finally, the relationship between apelin and pain in SMs was not determined.

Conclusions

Elevated VEGF expression in SMs was associated with an increase in pain in KOA patients with severe/strong pain. VEGF may regulate apelin expression in SMCs. The present findings suggest that altering the regulation of VEGF and apelin expression in SMs may represent a promising and suitable pharmaceutical strategy for the management of KOA pain.

Abbreviations

BCA: Bicinchoninic acid; BMI: Body mass index; CGRP: Calcitonin gene-related peptide; K/L: Kellgren/Lawrence; KOA: Knee osteoarthritis; NGF: Nerve growth factor; NSAIDs: Nonsteroidal anti-inflammatory drugs; OA: Osteoarthritis; PVDF: Polyvinylidene fluoride; SE: Standard error; SF: Synovial fluid; SM: Synovial membrane; SMCs: Synovial membrane cells; VAS: Visual analog scale; VEGF: Vascular endothelial growth factor

Acknowledgements

We thank Ms. Yuko Onuki for her assistance with real time PCR analysis. We thank Libby Cone, MD, MA, and Heidi Tran, PhD, from DMC Corp. (dmed.co.jp) for editing drafts of this manuscript.

Funding

This investigation was supported in part by a Kitasato University Research Grant for Young Researchers, Grant of Japan Orthopaedics and Traumatology Research Foundation, Inc. No. 373, JSPS KAKENHI Grant No. 18K09119, and research grants from the Parents' Association of Kitasato University School of Medicine.

Authors' contributions

ST, KU and MT designed the study and performed the analysis of the data. ST and KU wrote the manuscript. ST, GI, TM, JA, DI, MM (Mukai), and MM (Miyagi) participated in the data collection, analysis, and interpretation. All authors read and approved the final manuscript.

Consent for publication

Not applicable

Competing interests

The authors declare that they have no competing interests.

Author details

[1]Department of Orthopedic Surgery, Kitasato University School of Medicine, 1-15-1 Minami-ku Kitasato, Sagamihara City 252-0374, Japan. [2]Department of Pathology, Kitasato University School of Medicine, 1-15-1 Minami-ku Kitasato, Sagamihara City 252-0374, Japan.

References

1. Ayis S, Dieppe P. The natural history of disability and its determinants in adults with lower limb musculoskeletal pain. J Rheumatol. 2009;36(3):583–91.
2. Dominick KL, Ahern FM, Gold CH, Heller DA. Health-related quality of life and health service use among older adults with osteoarthritis. Arthritis Rheum. 2004;51(3):326–31.
3. Hadler NM. Knee pain is the malady–not osteoarthritis. Ann Intern Med. 1992;116(7):598–9.
4. McAlindon TE, Cooper C, Kirwan JR, Dieppe PA. Determinants of disability in osteoarthritis of the knee. Ann Rheum Dis. 1993;52(4):258–62.
5. Guccione AA, Felson DT, Anderson JJ, Anthony JM, Zhang Y, Wilson PW, Kelly-Hayes M, Wolf PA, Kreger BE, Kannel WB. The effects of specific medical conditions on the functional limitations of elders in the Framingham study. Am J Public Health. 1994;84(3):351–8.
6. Johnsen SP, Larsson H, Tarone RE, McLaughlin JK, Norgard B, Friis S, Sorensen HT. Risk of hospitalization for myocardial infarction among users of rofecoxib, celecoxib, and other NSAIDs: a population-based case-control study. Arch Intern Med. 2005;165(9):978–84.
7. Whelton A. Renal and related cardiovascular effects of conventional and COX-2-specific NSAIDs and non-NSAID analgesics. Am J Ther. 2000;7(2):63–74.
8. Giatromanolaki A, Sivridis E, Maltezos E, Athanassou N, Papazoglou D, Gatter KC, Harris AL, Koukourakis MI. Upregulated hypoxia inducible factor-1alpha and -2alpha pathway in rheumatoid arthritis and osteoarthritis. Arthritis Res Ther. 2003;5(4):R193–201.
9. Haywood L, McWilliams DF, Pearson CI, Gill SE, Ganesan A, Wilson D, Walsh DA. Inflammation and angiogenesis in osteoarthritis. Arthritis Rheum. 2003;48(8):2173–7.

10. Jackson JR, Minton JA, Ho ML, Wei N, Winkler JD. Expression of vascular endothelial growth factor in synovial fibroblasts is induced by hypoxia and interleukin 1beta. J Rheumatol. 1997;24(7):1253–9.
11. Lambert C, Mathy-Hartert M, Dubuc JE, Montell E, Verges J, Munaut C, Noel A, Henrotin Y. Characterization of synovial angiogenesis in osteoarthritis patients and its modulation by chondroitin sulfate. Arthritis Res Ther. 2012;14(2):R58.
12. Corrado A, Neve A, Cantatore FP. Expression of vascular endothelial growth factor in normal, osteoarthritic and osteoporotic osteoblasts. Clin Exp Med. 2013;13(1):81–4.
13. Huh JE, Seo DM, Baek YH, Choi DY, Park DS, Lee JD. Biphasic positive effect of formononetin on metabolic activity of human normal and osteoarthritic subchondral osteoblasts. Int Immunopharmacol. 2010;10(4):500–7.
14. Neve A, Cantatore FP, Corrado A, Gaudio A, Ruggieri S, Ribatti D. In vitro and in vivo angiogenic activity of osteoarthritic and osteoporotic osteoblasts is modulated by VEGF and vitamin D3 treatment. Regul Pept. 2013;184:81–4.
15. Fay J, Varoga D, Wruck CJ, Kurz B, Goldring MB, Pufe T. Reactive oxygen species induce expression of vascular endothelial growth factor in chondrocytes and human articular cartilage explants. Arthritis Res Ther. 2006;8(6):R189.
16. Mabey T, Honsawek S, Saetan N, Poovorawan Y, Tanavalee A, Yuktanandana P. Angiogenic cytokine expression profiles in plasma and synovial fluid of primary knee osteoarthritis. Int Orthop. 2014;38(9):1885–92.
17. Saetan N, Honsawek S, Tanavalee A, Yuktanandana P, Meknavin S, Ngarmukos S, Tanpowpong T, Parkpian V. Relationship of plasma and synovial fluid vascular endothelial growth factor with radiographic severity in primary knee osteoarthritis. Int Orthop. 2014;38(5):1099–104.
18. Sohn DH, Sokolove J, Sharpe O, Erhart JC, Chandra PE, Lahey LJ, Lindstrom TM, Hwang I, Boyer KA, Andriacchi TP, Robinson WH. Plasma proteins present in osteoarthritic synovial fluid can stimulate cytokine production via toll-like receptor 4. Arthritis Res Ther. 2012;14(1):R7.
19. Ballara S, Taylor PC, Reusch P, Marme D, Feldmann M, Maini RN, Paleolog EM. Raised serum vascular endothelial growth factor levels are associated with destructive change in inflammatory arthritis. Arthritis Rheum. 2001;44(9):2055–64.
20. Cui RR, Mao DA, Yi L, Wang C, Zhang XX, Xie H, Wu XP, Liao XB, Zhou H, Meng JC, Yuan LQ, Liao EY. Apelin suppresses apoptosis of human vascular smooth muscle cells via APJ/PI3-K/Akt signaling pathways. Amino Acids. 2010;39(5):1193–200.
21. Lv S, Yang YJ, Hong S, Wang N, Qin Y, Li W, Chen Q. Intrathecal apelin-13 produced different actions in formalin test and tail-flick test in mice. Protein Pept Lett. 2013;20(8):926–31.
22. Lv SY, Qin YJ, Wang NB, Yang YJ, Chen Q. Supraspinal antinociceptive effect of apelin-13 in a mouse visceral pain model. Peptides. 2012;37(1):165–70.
23. Perjes A, Skoumal R, Tenhunen O, Konyi A, Simon M, Horvath IG, Kerkela R, Ruskoaho H, Szokodi I. Apelin increases cardiac contractility via protein kinase Cepsilon- and extracellular signal-regulated kinase-dependent mechanisms. PLoS One. 2014;9(4):e93473.
24. Reaux A, Gallatz K, Palkovits M, Llorens-Cortes C. Distribution of apelin-synthesizing neurons in the adult rat brain. Neuroscience. 2002;113(3):653–62.
25. Reaux A, De MN, Skultetyova I, Lenkei Z, El MS, Gallatz K, Corvol P, Palkovits M, Llorens-Cortes C. Physiological role of a novel neuropeptide, apelin, and its receptor in the rat brain. J Neurochem. 2001;77(4):1085–96.
26. Smith TP, Schlenz AM, Schatz JC, Maitra R, Sweitzer SM. Modulation of pain in pediatric sickle cell disease: understanding the balance between endothelin mediated vasoconstriction and apelin mediated vasodilation. Blood Cells Mol Dis. 2015;54(2):155–9.
27. Than A, Cheng Y, Foh LC, Leow MK, Lim SC, Chuah YJ, Kang Y, Chen P. Apelin inhibits adipogenesis and lipolysis through distinct molecular pathways. Mol Cell Endocrinol. 2012;362(1–2):227–41.
28. Xu N, Wang H, Fan L, Chen Q. Supraspinal administration of apelin-13 induces antinociception via the opioid receptor in mice. Peptides. 2009;30(6):1153–7.
29. Giatromanolaki A, Sivridis E, Athanassou N, Zois E, Thorpe PE, Brekken RA, Gatter KC, Harris AL, Koukourakis IM, Koukourakis MI. The angiogenic pathway "vascular endothelial growth factor/flk-1(KDR)-receptor" in rheumatoid arthritis and osteoarthritis. J Pathol. 2001;194(1):101–8.
30. Nagai T, Sato M, Kobayashi M, Yokoyama M, Tani Y, Mochida J. Bevacizumab, an anti-vascular endothelial growth factor antibody, inhibits osteoarthritis. Arthritis Res Ther. 2014;16(5):427.
31. Kiguchi N, Kobayashi Y, Kadowaki Y, Fukazawa Y, Saika F, Kishioka S. Vascular endothelial growth factor signaling in injured nerves underlies peripheral sensitization in neuropathic pain. J Neurochem. 2014;129(1):169–78.
32. Lin J, Li G, Den X, Xu C, Liu S, Gao Y, Liu H, Zhang J, Li X, Liang S. VEGF and its receptor-2 involved in neuropathic pain transmission mediated by P2X(2)(/)(3) receptor of primary sensory neurons. Brain Res Bull. 2010;83(5):284–91.
33. Liu S, Xu C, Li G, Liu H, Xie J, Tu G, Peng H, Qiu S, Liang S. Vatalanib decrease the positive interaction of VEGF receptor-2 and P2X2/3 receptor in chronic constriction injury rats. Neurochem Int. 2012;60(6):565–72.
34. Malykhina AP, Lei Q, Erickson CS, Epstein ML, Saban MR, Davis CA, Saban R. VEGF induces sensory and motor peripheral plasticity, alters bladder function, and promotes visceral sensitivity. BMC Physiol. 2012;12:15.
35. Selvaraj D, Gangadharan V, Michalski CW, Kurejova M, Stosser S, Srivastava K, Schweizerhof M, Waltenberger J, Ferrara N, Heppenstall P, Shibuya M, Augustin HG, Kuner R. A functional role for VEGFR1 expressed in peripheral sensory neurons in Cancer pain. Cancer Cell. 2015;27(6):780–96.
36. Takano S, Uchida K, Miyagi M, Inoue G, Fujimaki H, Aikawa J, Iwase D, Minatani A, Iwabuchi K, Takaso M. Nerve growth factor regulation by TNF-alpha and IL-1beta in synovial macrophages and fibroblasts in osteoarthritic mice. J Immunol Res. 2016;2016:5706359.
37. Takano S, Uchida K, Miyagi M, Inoue G, Aikawa J, Fujimaki H, Minatani A, Sato M, Iwabuchi K, Takaso M. Synovial macrophage-derived IL-1beta regulates the calcitonin receptor in osteoarthritic mice. Clin Exp Immunol. 2016;183(1):143–9.
38. Takano S, Uchida K, Inoue G, Miyagi M, Aikawa J, Iwase D, Iwabuchi K, Matsumoto T, Satoh M, Mukai M, Minatani A, Takaso M. Nerve growth factor regulation and production by macrophages in osteoarthritic synovium. Clin Exp Immunol. 2017;190:235–43.
39. Takano S, Uchida K, Inoue G, Minatani A, Miyagi M, Aikawa J, Iwase D, Onuma K, Mukai M, Takaso M. Increase and regulation of synovial calcitonin gene-related peptide expression in patients with painful knee osteoarthritis. J Pain Res. 2017;10:1099–104.
40. Tatemoto K, Hosoya M, Habata Y, Fujii R, Kakegawa T, Zou MX, Kawamata Y, Fukusumi S, Hinuma S, Kitada C, Kurokawa T, Onda H, Fujino M. Isolation and characterization of a novel endogenous peptide ligand for the human APJ receptor. Biochem Biophys Res Commun. 1998;251(2):471–6.
41. Kunduzova O, Alet N, esque-Touchard N, Millet L, Castan-Laurell I, Muller C, Dray C, Schaeffer P, Herault JP, Savi P, Bono F, Valet P. Apelin/APJ signaling system: a potential link between adipose tissue and endothelial angiogenic processes. FASEB J. 2008;22(12):4146–53.
42. Kojima Y, Quertermous T. Apelin-APJ signaling in retinal angiogenesis. Arterioscler Thromb Vasc Biol. 2008;28(10):1687–8.
43. Xiong Q, He W, Wang H, Zhou J, Zhang Y, He J, Yang C, Zhang B. Effect of the spinal apelinAPJ system on the pathogenesis of chronic constriction injuryinduced neuropathic pain in rats. Mol Med Rep. 2017;16:1223–31.
44. Hu PF, Tang JL, Chen WP, Bao JP, Wu LD. Increased apelin serum levels and expression in human chondrocytes in osteoarthritic patients. Int Orthop. 2011;35(9):1421–6.
45. Minatani A, Uchida K, Inoue G, Takano S, Aikawa J, Miyagi M, Fujimaki H, Iwase D, Onuma K, Matsumoto T, Takaso M. Activation of calcitonin gene-related peptide signaling through the prostaglandin E2-EP1/EP2/EP4 receptor pathway in synovium of knee osteoarthritis patients. J Orthop Surg Res. 2016;11(1):117.
46. Collins SL, Moore RA, McQuay HJ. The visual analogue pain intensity scale: what is moderate pain in millimetres? Pain. 1997;72(1–2):95–7.
47. rendt-Nielsen L, Nie H, Laursen MB, Laursen BS, Madeleine P, Simonsen OH, Graven-Nielsen T. Sensitization in patients with painful knee osteoarthritis. Pain. 2010;149(3):573–81.
48. Uchida K, Takano S, Matsumoto T, Nagura N, Inoue G, Itakura M, Miyagi M, Aikawa J, Iwase D, Minatani A, Fujimaki H, Takaso M. Transforming growth factor activating kinase 1 regulates extracellular matrix degrading enzymes and pain-related molecule expression following tumor necrosis factor-alpha stimulation of synovial cells: an in vitro study. BMC Musculoskelet Disord. 2017;18(1):283.
49. Nesic O, Sundberg LM, Herrera JJ, Mokkapati VU, Lee J, Narayana PA. Vascular endothelial growth factor and spinal cord injury pain. J Neurotrauma. 2010;27(10):1793–803.

50. Kasai A, Shintani N, Oda M, Kakuda M, Hashimoto H, Matsuda T, Hinuma S, Baba A. Apelin is a novel angiogenic factor in retinal endothelial cells. Biochem Biophys Res Commun. 2004;325(2):395–400.
51. Zhao T, Lu Q, Tao Y, Liang XY, Wang K, Jiang YR. Effects of apelin and vascular endothelial growth factor on central retinal vein occlusion in monkey eyes intravitreally injected with bevacizumab: a preliminary study. Mol Vis. 2011;17:1044–55.
52. Kawamata Y, Habata Y, Fukusumi S, Hosoya M, Fujii R, Hinuma S, Nishizawa N, Kitada C, Onda H, Nishimura O, Fujino M. Molecular properties of apelin: tissue distribution and receptor binding. Biochim Biophys Acta. 2001; 1538(2–3):162–71.
53. Medhurst AD, Jennings CA, Robbins MJ, Davis RP, Ellis C, Winborn KY, Lawrie KW, Hervieu G, Riley G, Bolaky JE, Herrity NC, Murdock P, Darker JG. Pharmacological and immunohistochemical characterization of the APJ receptor and its endogenous ligand apelin. J Neurochem. 2003; 84(5):1162–72.

21

Analysis of DNA methylation in chondrocytes in rats with knee osteoarthritis

Xinxin Wang[1,2], Dezhi Tang[2*], Peng Shen[1,2], Hao Xu[2], Hongfu Qiu[1], Tao Wu[1] and Xiang Gao[1*]

Abstract

Background: Knee osteoarthritis (KOA) is a degenerative knee disease commonly found in the ageing population. DNA methylation works with histone acetylation to participate in aging. Alterations of DNA methylation may involve the joint chondrocyte degeneration in KOA. The aim of this study is to detect DNA methylation changes in chondrocytes of rats with KOA.

Methods: The rat KOA model was established with the Hulth method (n = 10), while rats receiving sham operation served as the control (n = 10). At 16 weeks after modeling, the knee joint tissue was collected from half of the rats in each group for Micro-CT scanning, Haematoxylin& Eosin (HE) staining, ABH/OG staining, immunohistochemistry for Bax, Bcl-2 and Fas, and TUNNEL staining. Meanwhile, the articular cartilage was collected from the other half to detect promoter methylation in target genes with the MethylTarget approach.

Results: Micro-CT scanning, HE staining, ABH/OG staining, immunohistochemistry, and TUNNEL staining all showed more severe cartilage injury in the KOA group than in the control group, indicating successful establishment of KOA model. The methylation rate in the KOA group was significantly decreased for C/ebpα-2 (within a CpG island -452 bp to the initiation codon on chromosome 1 91,363,511), Cdk2 (within a CpG island -55 bp to the initiation codon on chromosome 7 3,132,362), Bak1 (within a CpG island 6452 bp to the initiation codon on chromosome 20 5,622,277), and Fas (within a CpG island on the entire chromosome 1 gene), compared with the sham group (P = 0.005, 0.008, 0.022 and 0.027, respectively).

Conclusion: The chondrocyte apoptosis and significantly reduced methylation levels of C/ebpα-2, Cdk2, Bak1, and Fas may participate in the pathogenesis of KOA. However, the exact mechanisms remain to be determined.

Keywords: Knee osteoarthritis, C/ebpα, Cdk2, Fas, Bak, Methylation

Background

Knee osteoarthritis (KOA) is a degenerative knee disease commonly found in the ageing population. It is usually derived from pathology of the cartilage, subchondral bone and synovial membrane of the knee joint. KOA is clinically characterized as progressive knee pain, swelling, stiffness, and restricted joint range of motion, and even joint deformity in serious conditions, resulting in loss-of-function of the joint, largely affecting the life quality of patients and posing a great economic burden [1]. Currently, there is no well treatment for KOA. All therapeutic approaches are aimed at ameliorating symptoms and improving joint functions. KOA is a multifactorial disease. Apart from living style and healthy conditions, other factors like genetic aberrations and environmental factors also contribute to its occurrence. Changes in genetic modulation in cartilage have been implicated in the pathogenesis and progression of KOA. DNA methylation is one such player that has been receiving more and more attention. DNA methylation is a typical epigenetic modification of DNA to modify gene expression, which involves a process of transference of a methyl group on S-adenosyl methionine to the 5th atom of the cytosine ring under the catalysis effect of DNA methyltransferase, forming 5-methylcytosine. DNA methylation plays critical roles in embryo development, X chromosome inactivation, regulation of gene expression, gene imprinting and silencing, and tumorigenesis [2]. In addition, it works with histone acetylation to participate in aging. Alterations of DNA methylation

* Correspondence: dztang702@126.com; gaoxiang19710312@sina.com
[2]Spine Research Institute, Shanghai University of Traditional Chinese Medicine, Shanghai 200032, China
[1]Department of Surgery, Huadong Hospital Affiliated to Fudan University, Shanghai 200040, China

may involve the joint chondrocyte degeneration in the elderly KOA patients. In this study, methylation was analyzed in KOA rats for 31 genes (C/ebpa, Cdk, Bak, Bax, Fas, Bcl, Tnfaip3, Tnfsf11, Il6r, Rel, Ikzf3, Irf5, Kdm4b, Aire, Nr3c1, Ptpn2, Mlh1, Irf8, Ifngr2, Nfkbie, Irak1, and Kdm6b, etc.) selected by searching the literatures [3–19]. These genes are directly or indirectly related to the metabolism of bone or cartilage through a common mechanism. By detecting the changes in methylation level of these genes, we hope to clarify the relationship between methylation alterations and KOA pathogenesis.

Methods

Animals

Twenty SPF-grade male SD rats (8 weeks, 180–200 g, Charles River Laboratories, Beijing, China) were randomly assigned into sham-operation and KOA model groups (n = 10 in each group). The rats were housed in groups of 5 in cages under room temperature of 21–22 °C with a 12 h light/dark cycle and free access to food and water. KOA modeling was performed after 1-week habituation. After fasting for 12 h, KOA model was established in the rats with the Hulth method [20]. Briefly, after anesthesia with intraperitoneal injection of 10% chloral hydrate, a longitudinal incision of 10 cm was made on skin at the inner side of the right hind knee of rat placed in a supine position. The medial collateral ligament was cut to open up the joint cavity, and medial meniscus was resected, then the anterior and posterior cruciate ligaments were cut. The anteriordrawer test was used to confirm rupture of the ligaments. Efforts were made to avoid artificial injury to articular cartilage. Sutures were made layer-by-layer. Rats in the sham group received only the same operation of skin incision. After surgery, chlortetracycline ointment was applied to the incision site and the surroundings to prevent infection.

Sample preparation

At 16 weeks after modeling, rats in each group were sacrificed by injection with pentobarbital sodium at a dose of 0.2 ml/100 g. The articular cartilage was collected from 5 rats in each group and stored in formalin until use for methylation analysis. Meanwhile, the knee joint of the right hind limb was collected from the left rats, fixed in formalin for 48 h, and stored in 75% ethanol at room temperature until Micro-CT scanning, Haematoxylin& Eosin (HE) staining, orange G (ABH/OG) staining, immunohistochemistry and TUNNEL staining.

Sample processing

After Micro-CT scanning (Scanco, vivaCT80), the knee joint tissue was decalcified in 14% EDTA (pH 7.40 ± 0.05) for 4 weeks with replacement of the decalcification medium every 2–3 days, followed by dehydration, wax immersing and embedding. Then the tissue was cut at 5 μm, and subsequently HE and ABH/OG staining, immunohistochemistry, and TUNNEL staining were conducted.

The articular cartilage underwent MethylTarget analysis of methylation of CpGIsland in the promoter region of 31 genes including C/ebpa, Cdk, Bak, Bax, Fas, Bcl, Tnfaip3, Tnfsf11, Il6r, Rel, Ikzf3, Irf5, Kdm4b, Aire, Nr3c1, Ptpn2, Mlh1, Irf8, Ifngr2, Nfkbie, Irak1, Kdm6b, etc. The MethylTarget test is an approach for DNA methylation level mapping following bisulfite treatment and bioinformatics data analysis, based on the second-generation high throughput sequencing platform [21, 22].

Bisulfite conversion and multiplex amplification

DNA methylation level was analyzed by MethylTargetTM, an NGS-based multiple TargetedCpG methylation analysis method.Specifically, the genomic regions of interest were analyzed and transformed to bisulfite-converted sequences by geneCpG software. PCR primers (Table 1) were designed using the Methylation Primer software based on the bisulfate converted DNA.

Genomic DNA (400 ng) was treated with sodium bisulfite using an EZ DNA Methylation™-GOLD Kit (Zymo Research) according to the manufacturer's protocols. Multiplex PCR was performed with an optimized combination of primers. A 20 μl PCR reaction mixture was prepared for each reaction, which included 1× reaction buffer (Takara), 3 mM Mg2+, 0.2 mMdNTP, 0.1 μM of each primer, 1 U HotStarTaq polymerase (Takara) and 2 μl template DNA.The PCR program included 95 °C for 2 min; 11 cycles of 94 °C for 20 s, 63 °C for 40s with a decreasing temperature step of 0.5 °C per cycle, 72 °C for 1 min; then 24 cycles of 94 °C for 20 s, 65 °C for 30 s, 72 °C for 1 min; and finally 72 °C for 2 min.

Index PCR

PCR amplicons were diluted and amplified using indexed primers. Specifically, a 20 μl mixture was prepared for each reaction, including 1× reaction buffer (NEB Q5TM), 0.3 mMdNTP, 0.3 μM F primer, 0.3 μM index primer, 1 U Q5TM DNA polymerase (NEB) and 1 μL diluted template. The PCR program was 98 °C for 30 s; 11 cycles of 98 °C for 10 s, 65 °C for 30 s, 72 °C for 30 s; and 72 °C for 5 min. PCR products (170 bp–270 bp) were separated by agarose electrophoresis and purified using QIAquick Gel Extraction kit (QIAGEN).

Table 1 Primers of target genes

NO	Primer Name	sequence
1	Aire_F	ATAGTATTTAGATATTTAAGGGAGAAGGGAA
	Aire_R	ACCTAAAACTTATCCTCAAAAACCAC
2	Atm_F	GGTTTTATTGGYGGTGTTGAAT
	Atm_R	CACTCRCTCCCCTCAAAACATT
3	Bak1_1F	GTGGAYGAGAGTAGTTTTAAGTGGTG
	Bak1_1R	CATTTCTTCCCTAAACCATTAACC
	Bak1_2F	GGAGTTGATTTTTGTYGGGAGTT
	Bak1_2R	AACTCCTAACTACTCCCRAAACCAA
4	Bax_1F	GTATGYGTGAATTTAATGGTAGAGGTTT
	Bax_1R	TAATTCTCCRCCTCCCRCCTC
5	Bcl2_1F	GTTTTAGATTTTTAGGGGAGAGATATGTT
	Bcl2_1R	ACACAATACRCRAACTACTCCTTAAACAC
	Bcl2_2F	GGGYGTTAGGTGTAGTTGATTGGATA
	Bcl2_2R	CCTAACATCTTCTCCTTCCAACCT
6	Cdk2_2F	AAATTGTTAAGAGTTGAGTTTTGTTTG
	Cdk2_2R	TACCCTCTCCAATCTTCTCCAC
7	Cebpa_22F	GGATAGAAGGGGTTTGGTGAG
	Cebpa_22R	AACCATTACACTAAAAAATCTTAACCTTAC
	Cebpa_2F	TGGAAAGTTATAAGAGAAGGTAGGTTT
	Cebpa_2R	CCACCCAATACCCCAACTC
	Cebpa_3F	GTAAGGTTAAGAAGTYGGTGGATAAGA
	Cebpa_3R	CCTTAACCAAAAAACTCTCAAACAAC
	Cebpa_F	GGTTTTTTAGAGTAGTAGGGYGTTAGGA
	Cebpa_R	CCRAAACATTTAACTAAAAACTCCAC
8	Cflar_F	GGTTTTTTGAGATTTTTAGGGTTTATTAG
	Cflar_R	CTCCATTTTATAAACCCCAAAACA
9	Esr1_F	AAGATGTTTATGGAGAGGGTTTTG
	Esr1_R	AAAACCCCCAAACTATTAACACC
10	Fas_1F	GAGTTGTGTGGGTGTTAGTTTGTG
	Fas_1R	AACTACATATAAACATCTCTCATCACCAA
11	Icam1_F	TGGGGAGTTATTAAGAYGTTTTAGTAGTTA
	Icam1_R	CATTCAAAAATATCCCTCTCCCTA
12	ICOSLG_F	AGAGTGGAGAGTTGTAGTTGTTGG
	ICOSLG_R	CCCTACCCAACATCAAACTAAAC
13	Ifngr2_F	GTGGGTGTYGTTGGGAGTTT
	Ifngr2_R	CCTTCAACAAATCTCCCTAACA
14	Ikzf3_F	GGGTTGTAGTTGTTGTTTAGGTTT
	Ikzf3_R	CAAAATTCCTCAAACTTAACATTCAA
15	Il6r_F	GATTTAGGATGTAGTTGAGTAAGATTTGT
	Il6r_R	ACCAACCTAAAACTAACCCACCTATACT
16	Irak1_F	TGGATTTAGGTTTTTGGAGTTGA
	Irak1_R	CCCATCCCTAAAATCCCTAAAA
17	Irf5_F	GGAGTAGGGAGGATGTTTATTGG
	Irf5_R	AACTACTACCAAACCACCRCTCC
	Irf8_F	TAGTTGGGTTTTTTGGGAAAGTAA
	Irf8_R	ACCCCRCCCTATCTATAAAAACAAA
18	Kdm4b_2F	GGGTTGGTTGTGTGTATTTTGA
	Kdm4b_2R	CTCCCCTCATCAACACCTAAC
	Kdm4b_4F	AAGGGTGGAGTTYGGAGTATATAAGA
	Kdm4b_4R	TCAAAATACACACAACCAACCC
19	Kdm6b_2F	GAGTATATTTTAGGTTTTGGTAGGTAGGG
	Kdm6b_2R	CRCCAAAAACCCTTCTACCTTTAT
	Kdm6b_F	GGGAAGGTTAGGGAAGGGA
	Kdm6b_R	ACACRCATTTAACCAACACCCAC
20	Mlh1_1F	GTTGGGAAGGTGGTTTAGGA
	Mlh1_1R	CCAATTTTCAATCATCTCTTTAATAACA
	Mlh1_2F	GGTGTATTTTGTTYGGGTGATTTG
	Mlh1_2R	CRCAAACTCCACCACCAAATAAC
21	Nfkbie_F	GGGATTTAGGGTTTAGTGGGATT
	Nfkbie_R	AAAACCCTTCAACTACCCAAAA
22	Nr3c1_23F	GGTAGTTAGAGTTTTTGAGGGGATAGTT
	Nr3c1_23R	CTAACCCTCTCCTCTACRCTCCC
	Nr3c1_24F	AAGTTTGGGTTGTAGGTTGTGAG
	Nr3c1_24R	CRCCACCATCCCTAACCC
23	Nr3c1_F	GATTTTTAAGAGGTTAGGTAGAGGAGAT
	Nr3c1_R	CCCTCTACCTCATACCATAAACTAAA
24	Ppara_2F	GGTGTTAGGGTGGGTGTGG
	Ppara_2R	TACCCCCTACRCTATCAATTAACAA
	Ppara_F	TGAGGTGGGTGGATAGGG
	Ppara_R	CTCCAACCCACAAAACAACTAC
25	Ptpn2_F	GGAGGTTGTTGGTTTTGAAGG
	Ptpn2_R	CTAACCCCATCAAAAAACTCTCTC
26	Rel_F	GAATAGGTGTTTATTAGTAAGGGAAGG
	Rel_R	CAACCTTATTTTCCCTCTATATCTACATT
27	Tnfaip3_F	GGATGTGAYGTGGAAGGTAGTTTT
	Tnfaip3_R	AAAACTACAAACTAAACAATTCCCTTT
28	Tnfsf11_F	AGGAGATGGGTAGTTGTTTTGG
	Tnfsf11_R	AATCCTAAAACCAAACTCAATTTCC
29	Traf6_F	GGAGATATTTGATTTYGGAGTGTTG
	Traf6_R	CAACRACACRTCCTTATCCCTT
30	Tyk2_F	GATGATTAATAGGAATGTAGGATYGTG
	Tyk2_R	AACCTCCTCCCTACCAACTTC
31	Wnt2_F	TGAAGAGTTGATTTTAGGGGTGA
	Wnt2_R	AACTTTATCAATAAATCTCACCACTAACC

Sequencing

Libraries from different samples were quantified, pooled together, and used for sequencing on the IlluminaMiSeq platform according to the manufacturer's protocols.

Sequencing was performed with a 2x300bp paired-end mode.

Statistics

Quality control of sequencing reads was performed by FastQC. Filtered reads were mapped to genome by Blast after reads recalibration with USEARCH. All data are presented as mean ± SD and were analyzed with Independent samples t-test or U test to assess differences between groups. $P < 0.05$ was considered as statistically significant. Methylation and haplotype were analyzed using Perl script. Statistics were performed by t-test and ANOVA. Graphs were drawn with GraphPad Prism 5.0.

Results

Micro-CT, HE and ABH/OG staining

The reconstructed 3-dimensional image of the articular cartilage by Micro-CT showed a smooth surface of the articular cartilage with no osteophyte formation in the sham group (Fig. 1a1). The coronal section image (Fig. 1a2) showed thick, uniformly aligned trabeculae. However, the KOA group showed cartilage defects such as a rough surface, focal surface fissures and flaking, and exposure of the subchondral bone (Fig. 1b1). Round or oval-shaped osteophyteswere formed along the lining of joint. The coronal section image (Fig. 1b2) showed a thin cartilage layer, small, disorganized trabeculae, and subchondral bone cystic degeneration.

HE staining revealed a smooth surface of cartilage in the sham group, with even coloration of cartilage matrix into light pink and blue chondrocyte nuclei (Fig. 2). The cartilage had clear structural layers and a tidal line. The out layer of cartilage was composed of flat chondrocytes, the middle layer composed of round uniformly-aligned chondrocytes, and inner and calcification layers composed of proliferating chondrocytes. Meanwhile, the cartilage matrix was evenly stained into blue by ABH/OG staining (Fig. 3). In the KOA model group, HE staining a thin cartilage layer, superficial fibrillation, necrosis of chondrocytes, unclear nucleus and cytoplasm, a rough surface with fissures and flaking, portional loss of cartilage, exposure of the subchondral bone, uneven coloration, unclear structural layers and tidal line, proliferation of chondrocytes in the outlayer, disordered cell alignment, appearance of cell clusters, and blood vessels passing through the tide line. Meanwhile, weak and negative staining was seen by ABH/OG staining, with clear fibrillation (Fig. 3). These results suggest the successful modeling of KOA in rats with the Hulth method.

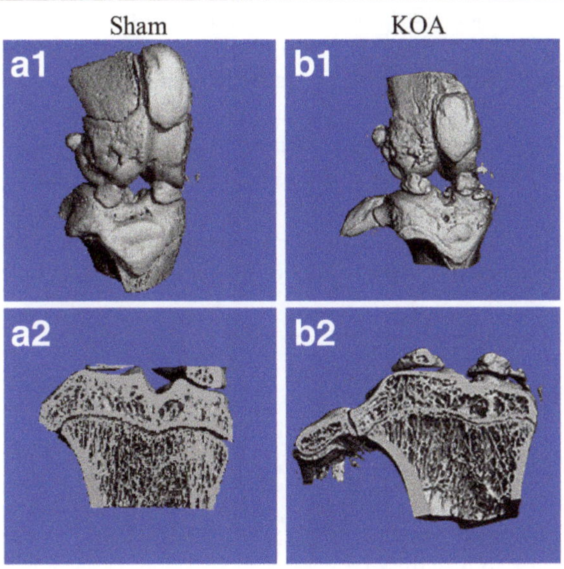

Fig. 1 Images of Micro-CT scanning of the rat knee joint. **a1** and **b1** are reconstructed 3-dimensional images; **a2** and **b2** are images of coronal sections

Immunohistochemistry and TUNNEL staining

Immunohistochemistry for apoptotic proteins Bax, Bcl-2, and Fas revealed brown positive cells. Six view fields were randomly selected under a microscope to count the positive cells and calculate the positive rate. Results showed significantly increased levels of Bax, Bcl-2, and Fas in the KOA group than in the sham group (Fig. 4, Table 1). TUNNEL staining revealed a significantly higher apoptosis rate in the KOA group than in the sham group (Fig. 4, Table 2).

Methylation analysis

A significantly decreased methylation rate was detected in the KOA group forC/ebpα-2 (within a CpG island -452 bp to the initiation codon on chromosome 1 91,363,511), Cdk2 (within a CpG island -55 bp to the initiation codon on chromosome 73,132,362), Bak1 (within a CpG island 6452 bp to the initiation codon on chromosome 20 5,622,277), and Fas (within CpG islands on the entire chromosome 1 gene), compared with the sham group (Fig. 6, Table 3).

Discussion

KOA is a multifactorial disease with multiple contributors including genetic aberrations and environmental factors apart from life style and healthy conditions. Pathologically, KOA mainly involves degeneration of the cartilage and alterations of the cartilage matrix. Abnormalities of gene regulation in chondrocytes may be implicated in the pathogenesis and progression of KOA. DNA methylation is a typical form of epigenetic modification of DNA, and it works with histone acetylation to affect the aging process. Abnormal epigenetic modification is closely associated with KOA pathology as a result of environmental changes or aging, and affects KOA occurrence and progression via epigenetic modification. As epigenetic modification is a reversible process, it is

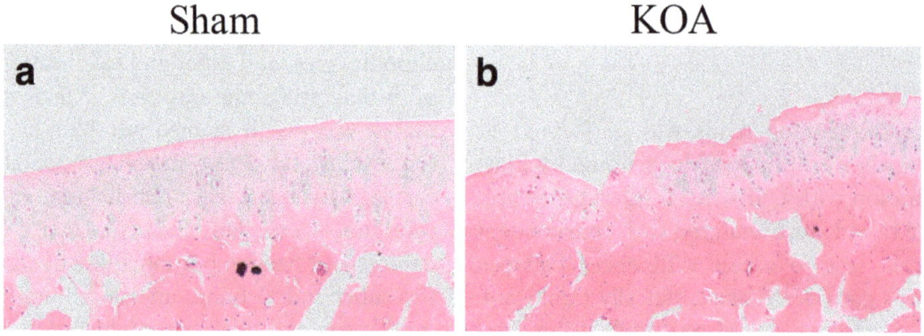

Fig. 2 HE staining of the knee joint. **a**, sham group; **b**, KOA model group

reasonable to discover its role in KOA pathology, in which it slows down the development or even prevents the occurrence of KOA. In this study, we selected 31 KOA-related genes by searching literatures, and sequence their methylated sites, in order to clarify the relationship between gene methylation and KOA.

Results of Micro-CT scanning (Fig. 1), HE staining (Fig. 2), ABH/OG staining (Fig. 3), immunohistochemistry (Fig. 4) and TUNNEL staining (Fig. 5) all confirmed the successful establishment of KOA model in rats. In addition, the methylation rate in the KOA group was significantly lower than that in the sham group for genes C/ebpα-2 (within a CpG island -452 bp to the initiation codon on chromosome 1 91,363,511), Cdk2 (within a CpG island -55 bp to the initiation codon on chromosome 7 3,132,362), Bak1 (within a CpG island 6452 bp to the initiation codon on chromosome 20 5,622,277), and Fas (within a CpG island on the entire chromosome 1 gene) (Fig. 6, Table 2). The decreased methylation in KOA chondrocytes may cause increased expression of these genes, which would further induce chondrocyte injury or apoptosis, leading to the pathogenesis and progression of KOA.

Aggravated chondrocyte injury or apoptosis occurs upon KOA onset [23]. Cartilage does not contain blood vessels. It has a low regeneration capacity and is therefore hard to repair after injury. When cartilage injury is so severe that the subchondral bone is damaged, rupture of small blood vessels would occur within the marrow cavity of cancellous bone. Then the blood forms a layer of fibrous clot on the surface of damaged cartilage area. In the absence of an external overload, the undifferentiated mesenchymal cells in bone marrow would move into this clot, whereby they differentiate into chondroblasts and proliferate into cells with chondrocyte morphology and typical features, in most cases fibrocartilage. Generally, an injury with a diameter < 3 mm can repair through generation of a hyaline cartilage, while a larger area of injury would repair by fibrous tissue [24]. Under normal conditions, C/ebpα can modulate the differentiation and proliferation of bone marrow mesenchymal stem cells into chondrocytes, and inhibit apoptosis of chondrocytes.

Here we found decreased methylation in promoter regions of C/ebpα and Cdk2 genes, which may induce overexpression of them. C/ebpα is present in multiple cell types, and participates in cell proliferation, differentiation, development, and tumorigenesis [25]. C/ebpα acts mainly to induce cell differentiation and inhibit cell proliferation [26]. The cyclin-dependent kinase Cdk2 can stimulate meiosis of germ cells and the G1-S transition during the mitotic cycle by interacting with cyclin E in early phases of DNA synthesis [27], thereby acting as a rate-limiting enzyme during cell proliferation [28]. Cdk2 activity peaks at S and G2 phases. In late phase of DNA replication, Cdk2 is activated by cyclin A2 to drive the S-G2 transition [29]. Wang H et al. found that C/ebpα directly interacts with Cdk2 to inhibit cell proliferation. In

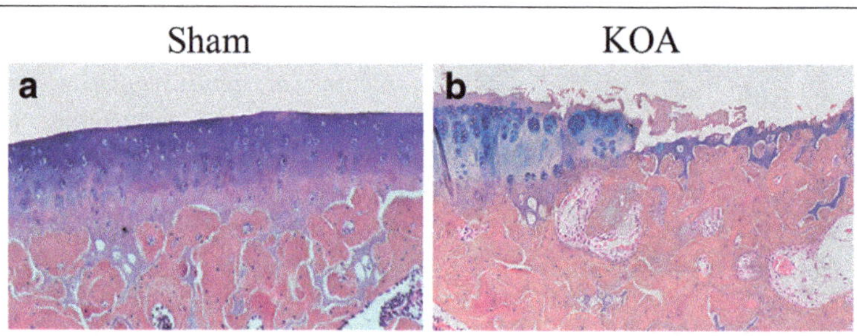

Fig. 3 ABH/OG staining of the knee joint. **a**, sham group; **b**, KOA model group

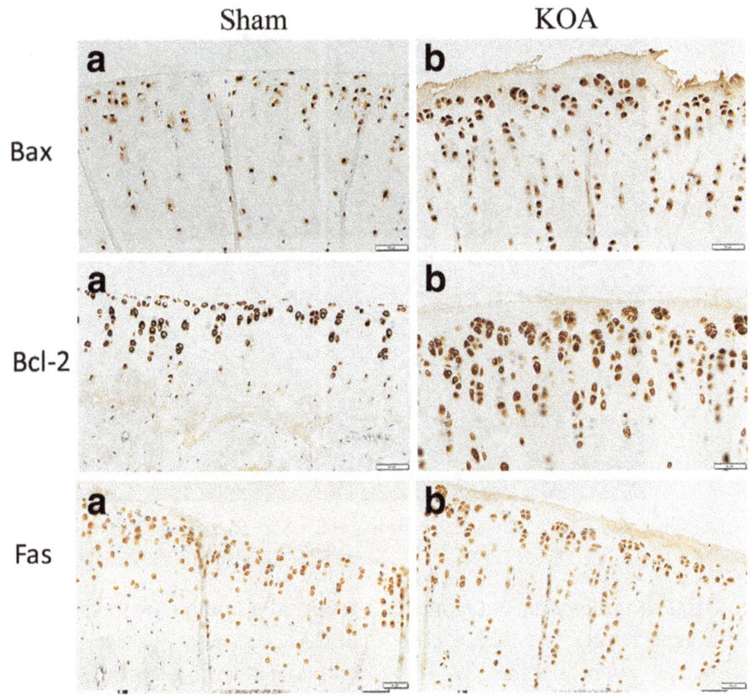

Fig. 4 Immunohistochemistry of Bax, Bcl-2 and Fas in the knee joint. **a**, sham group; **b**, KOA model group

C/ebpα knockout cells, they found significantly enhanced activity of Cdk2, resulting in increased proliferation [30]. In this study, the decreased methylation level in promoter region of C/ebpα-2 gene in chondrocytes may cause overproduction of C/ebpα-2, thereby inhibiting Cdk2 activity and chondrocyte proliferation. However, we also detected a lower level of methylation in the promoter region of Cdk2 gene. This may be compensation to the inhibition of Cdk2 activity, which would increase Cdk2 expression to attenuate the inhibitory effect of C/ebpα-2.

It has also been reported that changes in the time of expression and activity of Cdk2 are associated with cell apoptosis [31]. The relative expression level of cyclins varies according to specific phases of cell cycle. Cyclin E is highly expressed in G1/S phase, while cyclin B is highly expressed in M phase in normal cells. However, in apoptotic cells cyclin B can also be detected in G1 phase, and likely, other cyclins can be detected out of their specific phases. This alteration may be associated with the overexpression of Cdks [32], implying that cyclins and Cdks have other functions than that in cell cycling in apoptotic cells. In this study, the decreased methylation of Cdk2 in chondrocytes may cause overexpression of Cdk2, inducing abnormal activation of cyclins and resulting in failure of mitosis and finally apoptosis. In fact, there is report that apoptosis is a form of mitosis failure [33].

The apoptosis of chondrocytes in KOA is also mediated by the Fas/FasL death receptor pathway or Bak-induced mitochondrial mechanism [34]. Fas binds to its ligand FasL to activate the tyrosine kinase, inducing phosphorylation of intracellular serine/threonine, finally leading to DNA cleavage and cell apoptosis [35, 36]. Fas can also induce cell apoptosis by indirectly activating triphosphate inositol and diglycerides, which then cause a rapid calcium release from the endoplasmic reticulum into cytoplasm and an influx of extracellular calcium, resulting in DNA breakage and chromosome shrinkage, and finally

Table 2 Quantitative analysis of immunohistochemistry and TUNNEL staining

Staining	Positive rate (%)		*P* value
	Sham group	KOA group	
BAX	46.53 ± 3.86	88.62 ± 5.49	0.000
BCL-2	70.77 ± 7.61	85.99 ± 2.96	0.032
FAS	62.10 ± 1.68	89.77 ± 2.68	0.000
TUNNEL	50.65 ± 12.60	83.12 ± 13.79	0.040

Table 3 Methylation rate in the promoter region of selected genes

Target genes (distance to the initiationcodon)	sham group	KOA group	*P* value
	Methylation rate (mean ± SD)		
C/ebpα-2 (−452 bp)	0.01096 ± 0.0043	0.002572 ± 0.0024	0.005
Cdk2 (−55 bp)	0.013573 ± 0.0052	0.004166 ± 0.0030	0.008
Bak1 (6452 bp)	0.026212 ± 0.0139	0.007123 ± 0.0058	0.022
Fas	0.958532 ± 0.0063	0.944658 ± 0.0096	0.047

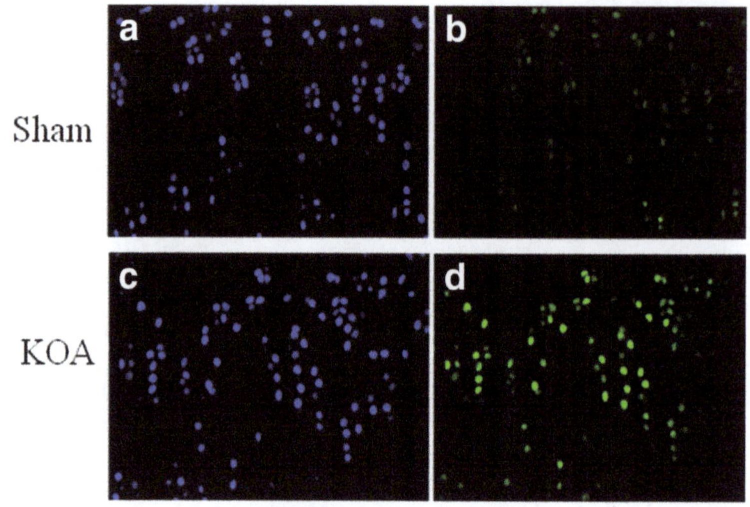

Fig. 5 TUNEL staining of the knee joint. **a** and **c**, nuclei of chondrocyte; **b** and **d**, nuclei of apoptotic cells

cell apoptosis [37]. Bak (Bcl-2 homologous antagonist/killer) is a member of Bcl-2 gene family, but with a contrast function of promoting cell apoptosis [36, 38, 39]. Machner et al. found that the expression of Fas mRNA in KOA patients was significantly higher than that in the control group by quantitative PCR [11]. Karaliotas et al. reported a notable overexpression of median mRNA levels of BAX was also observed in patients with stage III KOA compared with the control, while the BCL2/BAX ratio was markedlydecreased [40].Płucienniket al.found that the BCL2/BAX ratiomay regulate the gene promoter methylation [41]. Accumulating evidence has shown

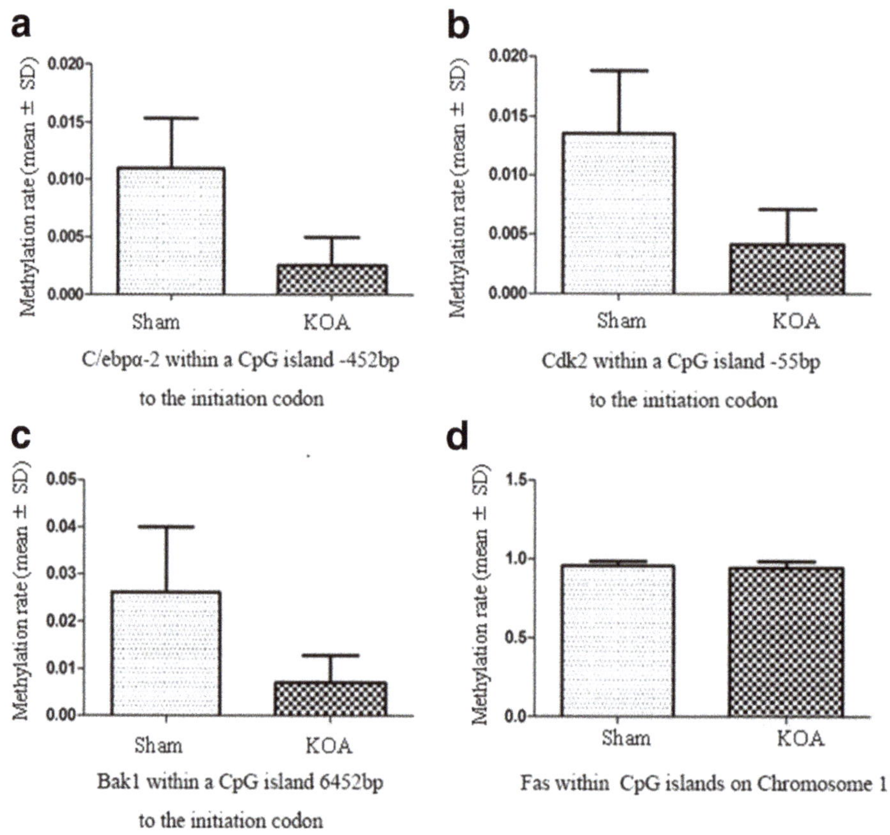

Fig. 6 Methylation rate in the promoter region of C/ebpα (**a**), Cdk2 (**b**), Bak1 (**c**), and Fas (**d**)

overproduction of pro-apoptotic factors like Fas and Bak in KOA chondrocytes, which causes increased cell apoptosis, while targeted inhibition of these factors reduces apoptosis [42–44]. Consistently, in this study we found increased expression of Fas, Bax and Bcl-2 in the KOA group than in the sham group using immunohistochemistry, and lower methylation levels in the promoter region of Fas and Bak1, which may induce their overexpression, thereby both leading to chondrocyte apoptosis. However, methylation in the promoter region of Fas genedid not play a key rolein the regulation at the level of its transcription, as the difference of the methylation of Fas gene between Sham and KOA groups was very slight. Li et al. reported that the transcription factors GA-binding protein (GABP) and activating protein-1 (AP-1) play a critical role in the induction of Fas mRNA [45]. Ryu et al.also found that Fas expression is transcriptionally induced by hypoxia-inducible factor (HIF)-2α [35]. In future, we will further study the transcriptional regulation of Fas gene by the transcription factors.

Conclusion

To sum up, genetic aberrations are involved in KOA. Apoptosis of chondrocytes is a major pathological event in KOA pathogenesis and progression. Cartilage degeneration is attributed to multiple rather than a single risk factor. Findings in this study suggest that decreased methylation in promoter region of C/ebpα, Cdk2, Fas, and Bak1 participates in the pathogenesis of KOA, but the underlying mechanisms and pathways involved remain to be determined.

Abbreviations

ABH/OG staining: Alcin blue/Orange G staining; Bak: Bcl-2 Homologous antagonist/killer; Bcl-2: B-cell lymphoma-2; C/ebpα: CCAAT/enhancer binding protein α; Cdk: Cyclin dependent kinase; EDTA: Ethylene DiamineTetraacetic Acid; Fas: Factor associated suicide; HE staining: Haematoxylin & eosin staining; KOA: Knee osteoarthritis; TUNNEL: Terminal-deoxynucleotidyltransferase mediated nick end labeling

Acknowledgements

We would like to thank for the person who gave assistance to this study.

Funding

This work was supported by the Three-Year Plan to Accelerate the Development of Chinese Medicine in Shanghai (ZY3-CCCX-3-3011, ZY3-LCPT-2-2003), the Twelfth Five-Year Key Project of the National Administration of Traditional Chinese Medicine; National Natural Science Foundation of China (81473701), and a project of Shanghai Key Laboratory of Geriatrics (13dz2260700).

Authors' contributions

XXW, PS, and HX performed the experiments and are responsible for data acquisition. HFQ and TW performed data analysis. DZT and XG are responsible for the conception and design of the study. DZT and XG drafted the article, and revised it critically for important intellectual content. All authors have participated actively in carrying out and improving the study and all have approved the submission of this article.

Consent for publication

Not applicable

Competing interests

The authors declare that they have no competing interest with other people or any organizations.

References

1. Crane DM, Oliver KS, Bayes MC. Orthobiologics and knee osteoarthritis: a recent literature review, treatment algorithm, and Pathophysiology discussion. Phys Med RehabilClin N Am. 2016;27(4):985–1002.
2. Reynard LN. Analysis of genetics and DNA methylation in osteoarthritis: what have we learnt about the disease? Semin Cell Dev Biol. 2017;62:57–66.
3. Xu YS, Jiang XJ, Chen JM. A single nucleotide polymorphism of AIRE gene located in the 21q22.3 increases the risk of rheumatoid arthritis. Oncotarget. 2017, published online. doi:10.18632/oncotarget.17746.
4. Shao L, Fujii H, Colmegna I, et al. Deficiency of the DNA repair enzyme ATM in rheumatoid arthritis. J Exp Med. 2009;206(6):1435–49.
5. Liang M, Russell G, Hulley PA. Bim, Bak, and Bax regulate osteoblast survival. J Bone Miner Res. 2008;23(5):610–20.
6. Lin MN, Liu XX, Wang SL, et al. Effect of OA kneepad on apoptosis genes Bcl-2 and p53 expression in articular cartilage cells of experimental knee osteoarthritis. Zhongguo Gu Shang. 2009;22(9):688–91.
7. Megyesi J, Tarcsafalvi A, Seng N, et al. Cdk2 phosphorylation of Bcl-xL after stress converts it to a pro-apoptotic protein mimicking Bax/Bak. Cell Death Discov. 2016;2:15066.
8. Roach HI, Aigner T. DNA methylation in osteoarthritic chondrocytes: a new molecular target. Osteoarthr Cartil. 2007;15(2):128–37.
9. Okada Y, Wu D, Trynka G, et al. Genetics of rheumatoid arthritis contributes to biology and drug discovery. Nature. 2014;506(7488):376–81.
10. Lv H, Ma X, Che T, et al. Methylation of the promoter a of estrogen receptor alpha gene in hBMSC and osteoblasts and its correlation with homocysteine. Mol Cell Biochem. 2011;355(1–2):35–45.
11. Machner A, Baier A, Wille A, et al. Higher susceptibility to Fas ligand induced apoptosis and altered modulation of cell death by tumor necrosis factor-alpha in periarticular tenocytes from patients with knee joint osteoarthritis. Arthritis Res Ther. 2003;5(5):R253–61.
12. Lee YH, Bae SC. Intercellular adhesion molecule-1 polymorphisms, K469E and G261R and susceptibility to vasculitis and rheumatoid arthritis: a meta-analysis. Cell Mol Biol (Noisy-le-grand). 2016;62(12):84–90.
13. Kurreeman FA, Stahl EA, Okada Y, et al. Use of a multiethnic approach to identify rheumatoid- arthritis-susceptibility loci, 1p36 and 17q12. Am J Hum Genet. 2012;90(3):524–32.
14. Sakao K, Takahashi KA, Arai Y, et al. Osteoblasts derived from osteophytes produce interleukin-6, interleukin-8, and matrix metalloproteinase-13 in osteoarthritis. J Bone Miner Metab. 2009;27(4):412–23.
15. Reynard LN, Loughlin J. Genetics and epigenetics of osteoarthritis. Maturitas. 2012;71(3):200–4.
16. Taniguchi T, Ogasawara K, Takaoka A, et al. IRF family of transcription factors as regulators of host defense. Annu Rev Immunol. 2001;19:623–55.
17. Ye L, Fan Z, Yu B, et al. Histone demethylases KDM4B and KDM6B promotes osteogenic differentiation of human MSCs. Cell Stem Cell. 2012;11(1):50–61.
18. Zhang Y, Ma C, Liu X, et al. Epigenetic landscape in PPARγ2 in the enhancement of adipogenesis of mouse osteoporotic bone marrow stromal cell. Biochimica et Biophysica Acta (BBA) - Mol Basis Dis. 2015;1852(11): 2504–16.
19. Baker EK, Taylor S, Gupte A, et al. Wnt inhibitory factor 1 (WIF1) is a marker of osteoblastic differentiation stage and is not silenced by DNA methylation in osteosarcoma. Bone. 2015;73:223–32.
20. Hulth A, Lindberg L. TelhagH. Experimental osteoarthritis in rabbits. Preliminary report. ActaOrthop Scand. 1970;41(5):522–30.

21. Feng H, Conneely KN, Wu H. A Bayesian hierarchical model to detect differentially methylated loci from single nucleotide resolution sequencing data. Nucleic Acids Res. 2014;42(8):e69.
22. Paul DS, Guilhamon P, Karpathakis A, et al. Assessment of RainDrop BS-seq as a method for large-scale, targeted bisulfite sequencing. Epigenetics. 2014;9(5):678–84.
23. Kim HA, Blanco FJ. Cell death and apoptosis in osteoarthritic cartilage. Curr Drug Targets. 2007;8(2):333–45.
24. Araki S, Imai S, Ishigaki H, et al. Improved quality of cartilage repair by bone marrow mesenchymal stem cells for treatment of an osteochondral defect in a cynomolgus macaque model. ActaOrthop. 2015;86(1):119–26.
25. Friedman AD. C/EBPalpha in normal and malignant myelopoiesis. Int J Hematol. 2015;101(4):330–41.
26. Zhao XY, Chen XY, Zhang ZJ, et al. Expression patterns of transcription factor PPARgamma and C/EBP family members during in vitro adipogenesis of human bone marrow mesenchymal stem cells. Cell Biol Int. 2015;39(4): 457–65.
27. Sun L, Huang Y, Wei Q, et al. Cyclin E-CDK2 protein phosphorylates plant homeodomain finger protein 8 (PHF8) and regulates its function in the cell cycle. J Biol Chem. 2015;290(7):4075–85.
28. Chauhan S, Diril MK, Lee JH, et al. Cdk2 catalytic activity is essential for meiotic cell division in vivo. Biochem J. 2016;473(18):2783–98.
29. Oakes V, Wang W, Harrington B, et al. Cyclin a/Cdk2 regulates Cdh1 and claspin during late S/G2 phase of the cell cycle. Cell Cycle. 2014;13(20):3302–11.
30. Wang H, Iakova P, Wilde M, et al. C/EBPalpha arrests cell proliferation through direct inhibition of Cdk2 and Cdk4. Mol Cell. 2001;8(4):817–28.
31. Roset R, Gil-Gomez G. Measurement of changes in Cdk2 and cyclin o-associated kinase activity in apoptosis. Methods Mol Biol. 2009;559:161–72.
32. Golsteyn RM. Cdk1 and Cdk2 complexes (cyclin dependent kinases) in apoptosis: a role beyond the cell cycle. Cancer Lett. 2005;217(2):129–38.
33. Vakifahmetoglu H, Olsson M, Zhivotovsky B. Death through a tragedy: mitotic catastrophe. Cell Death Differ. 2008;15(7):1153–62.
34. Hwang HS, Kim HA. Chondrocyte apoptosis in the pathogenesis of osteoarthritis. Int J Mol Sci. 2015;16(11):26035–54.
35. Ryu JH, Shin Y, Huh YH, et al. Hypoxia-inducible factor-2alpha regulates Fas-mediated chondrocyte apoptosis during osteoarthritic cartilage destruction. Cell Death Differ. 2012;19(3):440–50.
36. Musumeci G, Castrogiovanni P, Trovato FM, et al. Biomarkers of Chondrocyte apoptosis and Autophagy in osteoarthritis. Int J Mol Sci. 2015; 16(9):20560–75.
37. Lu Q, Wu Z, Li D. Single cell analysis of H (2) O (2) mediated Fas mRNA expression and ca (2+) influx in LO (2) cells. Zhonghua Yi XueZaZhi. 2000; 80(3):210–3.
38. Falah M, Najafi M, Houshmand M, et al. Expression levels of the BAK1 and BCL2 genes highlight the role of apoptosis in age-related hearing impairment. ClinInterv Aging. 2016;11:1003–8.
39. Lindqvist LM, Vaux DL. BCL2 and related prosurvival proteins require BAK1 and BAX to affect autophagy. Autophagy. 2014;10(8):1474–5.
40. Karaliotas GI, Mavridis K, Scorilas A, et al. Quantitative analysis of the mRNA expression levels of BCL2 and BAX genes in human osteoarthritis and normal articular cartilage: an investigation into their differential expression. Mol Med Rep. 2015;12(3):4514–21.
41. Płuciennik E, Nowakowska M, Wujcicka WI, et al. Genetic alterations of WWOX in Wilms' tumor are involved in its carcinogenesis. Oncol Rep. 2012;28(4):1417–22.
42. Tu Y, Xue H, Xia Z, et al. Effect of different concentrations of dexamethasone on apoptosis and expression of Fas/FasL in human osteoarthritis chondrocytes. ZhongguoXiu Fu Chong JianWaiKeZaZhi. 2012;26(5):536–41.
43. Sezgin M, Barlas IO, Yildir S, et al. Apoptosis-related Fas and FasL gene polymorphisms' associations with knee osteoarthritis. Rheumatol Int. 2013;33(8):2039–43.
44. Diaz-Gallo LM, Garcia S, Ortego-Centeno N, et al. Association study of BAK1 gene polymorphisms in Spanish rheumatoid arthritis and systemic lupus erythematosus cohorts. Ann RheumDis. 2012;71(2):314–6.
45. Li XR, Chong AS, Wu J, et al. Transcriptional regulation of Fas gene expression by GA-binding protein and AP-1 in T cell antigen receptor.CD3 complex-stimulated T cells. J Biol Chem. 1999;274(49):35203–10.

Association of frontal plane knee alignment with foot posture in patients with medial knee osteoarthritis

Hiroshi Ohi[1,2†], Hirotaka Iijima[3,4,5*†], Tomoki Aoyama[3], Eishi Kaneda[6], Kazuko Ohi[1,2] and Kaoru Abe[1]

Abstract

Background: To examine the association of radiographic frontal plane knee alignment with three-dimensional foot posture in patients with medial knee osteoarthritis (OA).

Methods: Participants in orthopedic clinics with Kellgren/Lawrence (K/L) grade ≥1 (88 patients and 88 knees; age, 61–91 years; 65.9% female) were enrolled. An anteroposterior radiographic view was used to assess the anatomical axis angle (AAA) after subtracting a sex-specific correction factor. The three-dimensional foot posture was also evaluated.

Results: Multiple regression analyses showed that increased corrected AAA (i.e., valgus direction) was independently associated with a decrease in the hallux valgus angle (regression coefficient: −0.40 per degree, 95% confidence interval [CI]: −0.72, −0.09; $P = 0.013$) and increase in the pronation angle of the calcaneus relative to floor (regression coefficient: 0.33 per degree, 95% CI: 0.10, 0.56; $P = 0.005$) adjusted for age, sex, and body mass index. The relationship between the corrected AAA and hallux valgus angle strengthened (regression coefficient: −0.60 per degree, 95% CI: −1.08, −0.13; $P = 0.014$) in varus-aligned knees examined separately (63 knees). The other foot postures (navicular height, navicular height/foot length, and rearfoot angle) were not significantly associated with corrected AAA.

Conclusions: Radiographic frontal plane knee alignment was associated with hallux valgus angle and calcaneus angle relative to the floor in patients with medial knee OA, particularly in varus-aligned knees. These results indicate a connection between altered frontal knee alignment and foot posture, which may be helpful in understanding the pathogenesis of altered foot posture observed in patients with knee OA.

Keywords: Osteoarthritis, Foot posture, Anatomical alignment, Hallux valgus

Background

Knee osteoarthritis (OA) is one of the leading diseases responsible for knee pain and disability [1, 2]. Progression of the disease is widely believed to result from local mechanical factors, [3] and much of the previous research has focused on local knee malalignment [4, 5]. However, people with knee OA exhibit an altered foot posture including flatfoot, pronated foot, and hallux valgus more frequently than healthy adults [6–9]. Flatfoot is associated with the presence of knee pain and medial cartilage damage in patients with knee OA [10]. Hallux valgus is associated with both knee and foot pain as well as the presence of nodal OA [11] and an increase in disability levels in women with knee OA [12]. A recent study showed that approximately 13–39% of individuals with knee OA, or at-risk of knee OA, have concurrent foot pain that adversely affects their functional status [13], knee symptoms [14], and clinical outcomes 1 year following total knee arthroplasty (TKA) [15].

The foot is thought to play an important role in knee OA from a biomechanical perspective owing to rotational

* Correspondence: iijima.hirotaka.4m@yt.sd.keio.ac.jp
†Equal contributors
[3]Department of Physical Therapy, Human Health Sciences, Graduate School of Medicine, Kyoto University, Kyoto, Japan
[4]Department of System Design Engineering, Keio University, Yokohama, Japan
Full list of author information is available at the end of the article

coupling between the rearfoot and tibia [16, 17]. A simulated genu varum walking pattern increases the subtalar pronation moment, whereas a simulated genu valgum walking pattern increases the subtalar supination moment [18]. Furthermore, accumulated evidence shows that realignment of the knee following TKA results in changes in hindfoot alignment [19–21] and foot kinematics during gait [22]. Although this evidence suggests the existence of a biomechanical link between altered frontal plane knee alignment and altered foot posture in patients with knee OA, we are unaware of any studies that have investigated the direct relationship of frontal plane knee alignment and foot posture, including forefoot, midfoot, and rearfoot postures, within this population. Since some patients with knee OA persistent hindfoot pain after TKA, [23] this knowledge would be helpful to understand the altered foot morphology related to knee OA pathology and to provide the basis for establishing the pathogenesis of concurrent foot pain in patients with knee OA. This may be important, given that patients with knee OA already have knee pain and disability, [1, 24] and the coexistence of altered foot posture may aggravate these symptoms.

Currently, the gold standard measure of knee alignment is the mechanical axis (or hip-knee-ankle) angle. However, it requires full-limb radiographs and the expertise of a radiology technologist to overcome the inherent technical difficulty. Alternatively, the measure of the anatomical axis angle (AAA) has been validated as a comparable measure to the full-limb radiographs, [25, 26] has been used for evaluating knee alignment, is less technically difficult and less costly. Thus, this study aimed to examine the association of radiographic frontal plane knee alignment measured as AAA with three-dimensional foot posture in patients with medial knee OA. General hypothesis was that increased frontal plane knee varus alignment independently associated with increases in the hallux valgus angle and rearfoot valgus angle and decreases in medial arch (navicular) height.

Methods

Patients

This cross-sectional study included outpatients with knee OA diagnosed by their treating physician in community orthopedic clinics. This study is the same cohort of subjects of recently published article [27]. For recruitment, an advertisement was distributed to patients who sought conservative treatment for knee OA in January 2015.

The eligibility criteria included (i) age ≥50 years; (ii) knees with radiographic OA (i.e., Kellgren/Lawrence [K/L] [28] grade ≥1) in one or both knees, as evaluated by weight-bearing anteroposterior radiographs; and (iii) an ability to walk independently on a flat surface without any ambulatory assistive device. The exclusion criteria were (i) a history of knee surgery, (ii) inflammatory arthritis, (iii) periarticular fracture, (iv) neurological problems, or (v) lateral compartment knee OA. Lateral knee OA was defined as a knee having a K/L grade ≥1 along with joint space narrowing (JSN) >0 in the lateral compartment with JSN = 0 in the medial compartment [29, 30]. Since medial and lateral knee OA have distinct characteristics, and most knee OA in Japan is medial type, [31] lateral knee OA was excluded in this study. Because pre-radiographically defined knee OA, particularly K/L grade 1, predicts radiographic OA progression to at least grade 2, [32, 33] we included patients with K/L grades ≥1. Patients with either bilateral or unilateral knee OA were considered.

Measurements

Radiographic evaluation of the knee joint

The radiographic OA severity of both knees in each patient was assessed in the anteroposterior short view in the weight-bearing position by experienced examiners using the original version of the K/L grading system [28, 34]. Specifically, the K/L grade was scored as follows: 0 = normal; 1 = doubtful JSN and possible osteophyte; 2 = definite osteophyte and possible JSN; 3 = multiple osteophytes, definite JSN, and some sclerosis and possible deformity of bone ends; and 4 = large osteophyte, marked JSN, severe sclerosis, and definite deformity of bone ends. The interrater agreements for the K/L grade determination were excellent (κ: 0.84, 95% confidence interval [CI]: 0.79, 0.90).

Frontal plane knee alignment was evaluated by measurement of the AAA on an anteroposterior radiograph by a trained examiner (HI) using the Nazca software (Astrostage Inc., Tokyo, Japan). The AAA was defined as the internal angle formed by the intersection of two lines originating 10 cm from the knee joint surfaces bisecting the femur and tibia, and converging at the center of the tibial spine tips [35]. The exact distance from the knee joint surface at which the femur or tibia was to be bisected was determined on the basis of the size of the patients; a length 1.3 times that of the epicondylar line from the medial epicondyle to the lateral epicondyle was used. Measurements of the AAA were modified to better reflect mechanical alignment by subtracting a sex-specific correction factor of 3.5° for women and 6.4° for men according to Kraus; [25] throughout the text, the corrected AAA is described. Sex-specific corrections on AAA has also been shown to be important [36, 37]. Increase and decrease in corrected AAA signifies valgus and varus postures, respectively. The need for sex-specific correction has been proposed because women have more distal femoral valgus than men [38]. The knees were categorized based on corrected AAA into three groups: neutral (corrected AAA ≥179° but <182°), varus (corrected AAA <179°), and valgus (corrected AAA ≥182°) alignments. The intrarater reliability for measuring the AAA was excellent (intraclass correlation coefficient [ICC]: 0.98, 95% CI, 0.98, 0.99).

Evaluation of the three-dimensional foot posture and rearfoot angle

Three-dimensional foot posture was evaluated using a three-dimensional footprint automatic measurement apparatus (CUTE, JMS-2100CU; Dream GP Inc., Osaka, Japan) (Figure 1a). The details regarding the measurement setup are provided in the previous study [27]. This foot-scanning system is based on laser line triangulation where the measuring head moves around a single foot in an oval trajectory [39]. The laser scanner rotates around the patient's foot and measures >30,000 points, including the ankle, instep, heel, and toes as well as the sole, recreating the patient's foot shape precisely. This scanning system has a high accuracy for measurements of foot posture; the measurement error of foot length is −0.27 to 0.36 mm (accuracy within ± 0.2%) and that of foot width is 0.51–1.22 mm (accuracy within ± 0.5%) [39].

Before each capture session, the patients stood on bare feet with feet shoulder-width apart as straight as possible with little movement, and black round seal markers, which correspond to three anatomical landmarks to detect foot alignment, were attached to skin. This placed 50% of their body weight on the foot being assessed. The anatomical landmarks were the (i) navicular tuberosity, (ii) bottom of the calcaneal tuberosity, and (iii) enthesis of the Achilles tendon. The markers were attached by an experienced prosthetist and orthotist (HO) who had

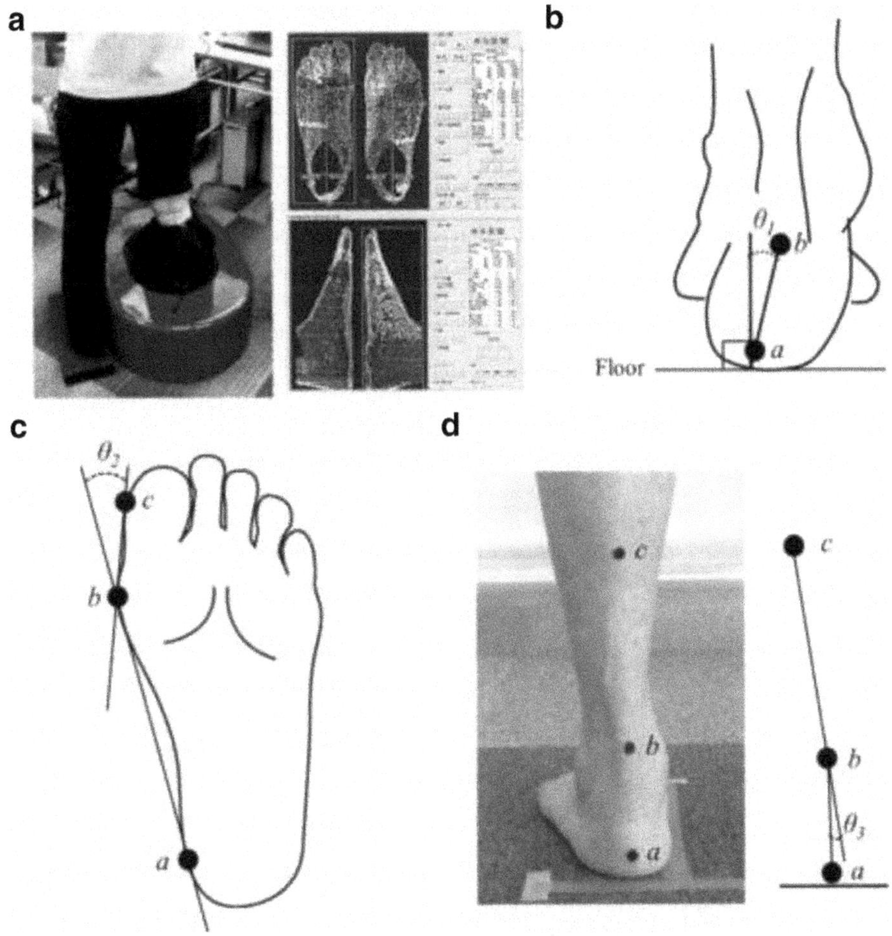

Fig. 1 Evaluation of foot posture and rearfoot angle. **a** Foot-scanning system to evaluate three-dimensional foot posture. **b** Measurement of calcaneus angle relative to the floor (*θ1*), which was defined as the angle formed by a line joining the bottom of the calcaneal tuberosity (*a*) with the enthesis of the Achilles tendon (*b*) and a line perpendicular to floor. **c**, Measurement of the hallux valgus angle (*θ2*). The hallux valgus angle (*θ2*) was defined as two lines intersecting between a line connecting the medial side of the first metatarsophalangeal joint (*b*) with the medial side of the heel (*a*) and a line connecting the medial side of the first metatarsophalangeal joint (*b*) with the medial side of the hallux (*c*). **d** Measurement of rearfoot angle (*θ3*), which was defined as the angle between the bisection of the lower one-third of the leg (*bc*) and the bisection of the calcaneus (*ab*). Note that the measurement procedures of foot length and navicular height are not indicated in this figure

>15 years of clinical experience in the orthopaedic field, with no knowledge of each patient's clinical status, such as OA severity. The measurement procedure consisted of consecutive right and left foot scanning, with each taking approximately 13 s.

After the measurement step, the following foot postures were automatically calculated by the system: calcaneus angle relative to the floor, foot length, hallux valgus angle, navicular height, and navicular height/foot length. The calcaneus angle relative to the floor was defined as the angle formed by a line joining the bottom of the calcaneal tuberosity with the enthesis of the Achilles tendon and a line perpendicular to floor (Figure 1B). The foot-scanning system defined the floor line and automatically calculated the line perpendicular to the floor. Increases and decreases in calcaneus angle relative to the floor indicate pronation and supination, respectively. Throughout the manuscript, "pronation/supination" indicates posture on a single frontal plane. As hallux valgus is often found in patients with knee OA, [9] foot length was defined as the distance from the most posterior portion of the calcaneus to the end of the second toe. The hallux valgus angle was defined as two lines intersecting between a line connecting the medial side of the first metatarsophalangeal joint with the medial side of the heel and a line connecting the medial side of the first metatarsophalangeal joint with the medial side of the hallux (Figure 1C). Hallux valgus was defined as a hallux valgus angle ≥20° [40]. Navicular height was defined as the distance from the floor to the navicular tuberosity.

After evaluation of the three-dimensional foot posture, the rearfoot (calcaneus) angle relative to the lower leg in a relaxed standing position was also evaluated to provide information about the subtalar joint. Before each evaluation, the patients stand as straight as possible as in the evaluation of the three-dimensional foot posture, and an additional black round seal marker was attached onto the skin of the midline of the lower one-third of the leg. The lower leg and rearfoot images from the back view were recorded using a digital camera (IXY DIGITAL 22015; Canon Inc., Tokyo, Japan). Two trained examiners measured the rearfoot angle as the angle between the bisection of the lower one-third of the leg and the bisection of the calcaneus, [41] referring to the three anatomical landmarks mentioned above (i.e., midline of lower one-third of the leg, enthesis of the Achilles tendon, and bottom of the calcaneal tuberosity) using ImageJ software. The interrater reliability for measuring the rearfoot angle was excellent (ICC: 0.92, 95% CI: 0.89, 0.94).

Assessment of covariates

Data on age, sex, and height were self-reported by the patients. Weight was measured on a scale, with the participants wearing their clothes but without their shoes. Body mass index (BMI) was calculated by dividing the weight by the square of height.

Statistical analysis

To minimize any bias produced by similarities between the right and left knees of the same patients, [42] only one knee per patient was analyzed, the "index knee." The index knee was defined as the more painful knee in the present or past. If patients felt that their knees were equally painful, the index knee was randomly selected using computer-generated block randomization.

To clarify the associations between frontal knee alignment and three-dimensional foot posture when standing, regression coefficients (betas) and their 95% CIs were calculated using two models (a crude model and adjusted model) of multiple regression analyses. In the crude model, each foot posture (hallux valgus angle, navicular height, navicular height/foot length, calcaneus angle relative to floor, and rearfoot angle) was included as a dependent variable and the corrected AAA (continuous) was included as a predictor. The multiple regression analyses were done first with a crude model, which was then adjusted for age (continuous), sex (0: male, 1: female), and BMI (continuous) for adjusted model. These covariates were chosen because they might be associated with the alterations of the frontal plane knee alignment and foot posture and not on the causal pathway [11, 43, 44].

Sensitivity analyses were performed to assess whether the relationship between the corrected AAA and foot posture is influenced by the subsample of knees with K/L grade ≥2. Furthermore, to address the possibility that the relationship of the corrected AAA with foot posture differs when patients are subdivided into those with (corrected AAA <179°) and without (corrected AAA ≥179°) varus alignment, additional multiple regression analyses were performed in each subgroup separately. In these analyses, we replicated the same multiple logistic regression analyses as mentioned earlier. Data analyses were performed with JMP version 11 (SAS Institute, Cary, NC, USA). *P*-values <0.05 were considered statistically significant.

Results

A flow chart describing the distribution of study patients is shown in Figure 2. In this study, 102 patients were initially enrolled. However, 4 patients were excluded (owing to use of an ambulatory assistive device on a flat surface and lateral knee OA), and 10 patients were also excluded owing to invalid data (missing data) of outcome variables; the remaining 88 patients with 88 index knees of K/L grade ≥1 (86.3% of the initial cohort) were included in the final analysis. Table 1 shows the person-level and knee-level characteristics of the study patients.

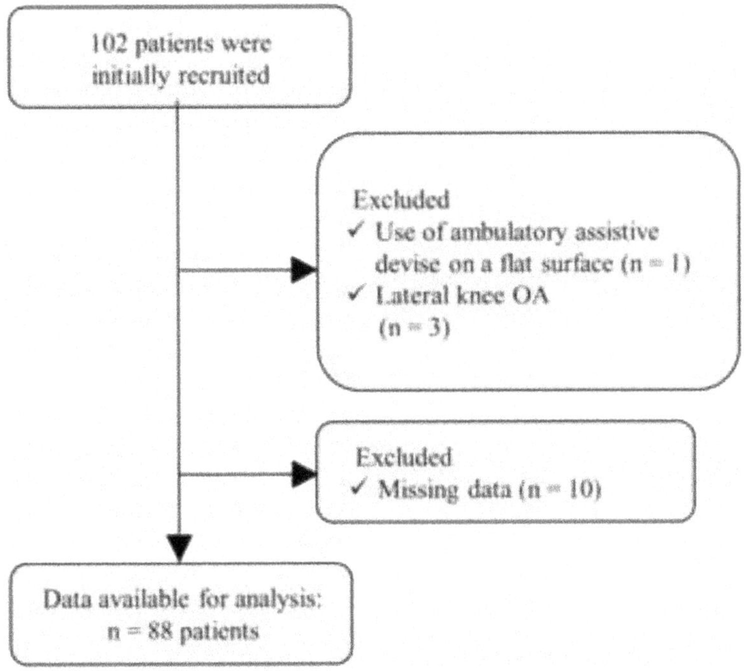

Fig. 2 Flow chart describing the distribution of study patients

Corrected AAA was independently associated with the hallux valgus and calcaneus angles

The results of the multiple regression analyses characterizing the association between the corrected AAA and three-dimensional foot posture are shown in Table 2. An increased corrected AAA (i.e., valgus direction) was significantly associated with a decrease in the hallux valgus angle (beta: −0.40 per degree, 95% CI: −0.71, −0.09; $R^2 = 0.07$; $P = 0.012$) even when adjusted for age, sex, and BMI (beta: −0.40 per degree, 95% CI: −0.72, −0.09; $R^2 = 0.14$; $P = 0.013$). These relationships were still significant even when the calcaneus angle and navicular height were further included as predictors (data not shown).

An increased corrected AAA was significantly associated with increases (i.e., pronation direction) in the calcaneus angle relative to the floor (beta: 0.31 per degree, 95% CI: 0.09, 0.53; $R^2 = 0.08$; $P = 0.006$) even when adjusted for age, sex, and BMI (beta: 0.33 per degree, 95% CI: 0.10, 0.56; $R^2 = 0.10$; $P = 0.005$). However, the other foot postures (i.e., navicular height and navicular height/foot length) were not significantly associated with corrected AAA with the numbers available (navicular height, beta: 0.08 per degree, 95% CI: −0.21, 0.38; $R^2 = 0.16$; $P = 0.566$; navicular height/foot length, beta: 0.03 per degree, 95% CI: −0.10, 0.15; $R^2 = 0.07$; $P = 0.688$). Also, an increased corrected AAA was not significantly associated with rearfoot angle with the numbers available (beta: −0.09 per degree, 95% CI: −0.26, 0.08; $R^2 = 0.07$; $P = 0.290$).

Sensitivity analysis showed that these relationships were comparable; there were significant associations between the increased corrected AAA and decrease in the hallux valgus angle (beta: −0.46 per degree, 95% CI: −0.83, −0.08; $R^2 = 0.23$; $P = 0.018$) as well as calcaneus angle relative to the floor (beta: 0.33 per degree, 95% CI: 0.06, 0.60; $R^2 = 0.11$; $P = 0.015$) adjusted for age, sex, and BMI in knees with K/L grade ≥2 ($n = 58$).

The association of corrected AAA with the hallux valgus and calcaneus angles became stronger in varus-aligned knees

When only the varus knees ($n = 63$) were analyzed, the association between the increased corrected AAA and the decrease in hallux valgus angle became strong adjusted for age, sex, and BMI (beta: −0.60 per degree, 95% CI: −1.08, −0.13; $R^2 = 0.17$; $P = 0.014$). The association between the increased corrected AAA and the increase in calcaneus angle relative to floor also became stronger when adjusted for age, sex, and BMI (beta: 0.45 per degree, 95% CI: 0.13, 0.76; $R^2 = 0.14$; $P = 0.006$). However, the associations between the corrected AAA and the other foot postures as well as the rearfoot angle in varus-aligned knees were similar (data not shown) compared to values shown in Table 2. Moreover, when only the non-varus knees ($n = 25$) were analyzed, the association of the corrected AAA with the hallux valgus was not significant adjusted for age, sex, and BMI with the numbers available (beta: −0.35 per degree, 95% CI: −2.12, 1.42; $R^2 = 0.16$; $P = 0.682$).

Table 1 Demographic characteristics, knee alignment, and three-dimensional foot posture of the study patients ($n = 88$ patients, 88 knees)

Person-level characteristics	
Age, years	74.8 ± 7.58
Female, no. (%)	58 (65.9)
Height, m	1.56 ± 7.89
Weight, kg	59.2 ± 10.5
Body mass index, kg/m^2	24.3 ± 3.54
Knee-level characteristics	
Corrected AAA, degree	176.6 ± 4.77
Tibiofemoral joint alignment, no. (%)	
Neutral (corrected AAA ≥179 degrees but <182 degrees)	20 (22.7)
Valgus (corrected AAA ≥182 degrees)	5 (5.7)
Varus (corrected AAA <179 degrees)	63 (71.6)
Tibiofemoral joint K/L grade, no. (%)	
Grade 1	30 (34.1)
Grade 2	35 (39.8)
Grade 3	14 (15.9)
Grade 4	9 (10.2)
Hallux valgus angle, degree	13.6 ± 7.22
Presence of hallux valgus, no. (%)[a]	11 (12.5)
Navicular height, mm	30.1 ± 6.75
Navicular height/foot length, %[b]	12.7 ± 2.75
Calcaneus angle relative to floor, degree[c]	1.35 ± 5.09
Rear foot angle, degree[d]	6.01 ± 3.76

Values are mean ± standard deviation unless indicated otherwise. AAA = anatomical axis angle; K/L = Kellgren/Lawrence
[a]Presence of hallux valgus is defined as the hallux valgus angle ≥20°
[b]Navicular height/foot length is calculated by the navicular height divided by the foot length
[c]A positive value indicates pronation direction of the calcaneus
[d]A positive value indicates valgus direction of the rearfoot

Discussion

Alterations of foot morphology in patients with knee OA are associated with knee pain, disability, and cartilage damage [10–12]. Although several studies suggest the existence of a biomechanical connection between frontal knee alignment and rearfoot angle, [16–22] the relationship of frontal plane alignment and foot posture of patients with knee OA has not been fully elucidated. The current study first revealed that an increased corrected AAA (i.e., valgus direction) was independently associated with decreases in the hallux valgus angle and decreases in the calcaneus angle relative to the floor. Furthermore, increased corrected AAA was more closely associated with decreases in the hallux valgus angle as well as increases in the calcaneus angle relative to floor in varus-aligned knee, examined separately. However, there were no significant associations in non-varus-aligned knee. Although variance in the multiple regression model was relatively small ($R^2 < 0.2$), even on the association between corrected AAA and hallux valgus, our data may suggest that altered frontal knee alignment is associated with altered foot posture, particularly the hallux valgus angle in varus-aligned knee.

Hallux valgus is a common deformity with a wide prevalence rate ranging from 23 to 64% [9, 11, 40]. Lower prevalence rate of hallux valgus in this study (12.5%) could be attributed to the definitions of hallux valgus used; previous studies used physical examination, [9] self-reported questionnaire, [11] or foot radiograph in the weight-bearing position [40]. Hallux valgus is associated with a higher risk of foot and knee pain, [11] increased disability in women with knee OA, [12] and was linked to the progression of knee OA in a case study [45]. Although nonsurgical care is the first option for patients who have hallux valgus deformity, [46] many patients require surgery, [47] which increases healthcare costs [48]. The current study first revealed that a frontal plane knee alignment was independently associated

Table 2 Regression coefficient from multiple regression analysis, characterizing the association between increased corrected AAA (per degree) and three-dimensional foot posture ($n = 88$ knees)

Dependent variables	Beta (95% CI) of corrected AAA, per degree*	
	Crude model	Adjusted model
Hallux valgus angle	**−0.40 (−0.71, −0.09)***	**−0.40 (−0.72, −0.09)***
Navicular height	−0.02 (−0.32, 0.29)	0.08 (−0.21, 0.38)
Navicular height/foot length	−0.002 (−0.13, 0.12)	0.03 (−0.10, 0.15)
Calcaneus angle relative to floor	**0.31 (0.09, 0.53)****	**0.33 (0.10, 0.56)****
Rearfoot angle	−0.10 (−0.27, 0.06)	−0.09 (−0.26, 0.08)

95% CI = 95% confidence interval; AAA = anatomical axis angle
The value of regression of coefficient (beta) for each dependent variable is described per degree of AAA (continuous) to indicate the predictive ability using 2 cumulative models of multiple regression analyses
Adjusted model includes values derived from multiple regression analysis with age, (continuous), sex (0: male, 1: female), and body mass index (continuous) entered simultaneously (one-step model) as predictors
*$P < 0.05$, **$P < 0.01$. Bold indicates a statistically significant result

with the hallux valgus angle, which is comparable to a subsample of knees with a K/L grade ≥2, and this relationship became stronger in varus-aligned knees. Although the current study cannot elucidate the mechanism to explain the relationship between knee alignment and hallux valgus angles, several studies showed that patients with hallux valgus have an altered foot pressure pattern during gait in patients with medial knee OA [49–52]. The AAA was correlated with the coronal location of the center of pressure, [51] and realignment of the knee following TKA results in a foot pressure pattern, particularly in the hallux [53]. These results indicate a correlation between altered frontal plane knee alignment and altered pressure on the hallux.

The altered rearfoot posture of pronation in patients with knee OA has been proposed to be a compensatory response to the varus alignment to allow the foot to be plantigrade [54]. However, contrary to our initial hypothesis, we found that increased varus knee alignment (decreased corrected AAA) was associated with an increase in the supination angle of the calcaneus relative to the floor. This discrepancy is possibly attributed to a reduced compensatory capacity of the ankle/subtalar joint complex or a restricted range of motion in subtalar pronation. Hindfoot varus deformity exists in 30% of cases of end-stage varus knee OA, [21, 55] and hindfoot varus is believed to occur as a result of the loss of this compensatory capacity of the hindfoot. A prospective study to follow-up on the foot posture in patients with knee OA who had varus alignment would help address this question.

Interestingly, the relationship of the corrected AAA with the rearfoot angle, an indicator of varus or valgus alignment of the subtalar joint, was not significant when adjusted for possible confounders. On the other hand, the significant relationship of the corrected AAA with the calcaneus angle relative to the floor indicates that the calcaneus angle might be more sensitive to the altered frontal plane alignment. These discrepancies of assessment techniques for calcaneus and rearfoot angles might explain why there is no significant relationship of the rearfoot angle with altered frontal knee alignment in this study. Norton et al. showed that the relationship of the mechanical axis and the hindfoot valgus angle was stronger in severe varus alignment, but this relationship was rather diminished in patients with a milder varus alignment [20]. We also found no significant relationship between the corrected AAA and calcaneus angle relative to the floor or the rearfoot angle in the non-varus-aligned knee, supporting their finding.

We found that navicular height and navicular height/foot length, two of the midfoot alignments, were not significantly associated with the corrected AAA. Navicular height in patients with knee OA is similar to that in healthy adults, [8] even in patients diagnosed to have a pronated foot according to foot posture index and arch index [6, 56]. The association of the rearfoot with navicular drop was only moderate even in healthy adults [57]. Furthermore, we found only a weak relationship between the calcaneus angle and navicular height/foot length (data not shown), which might explain why the corrected AAA was associated only with the calcaneus angle but not navicular height in this study.

Rearfoot pronation results in an increase in loading to the first metatarsal, [58] which might contribute to the degenerative changes in the first metatarsophalangeal joint on the same side as medial knee OA [45, 59]. However, we also found that including navicular height (i.e., an indicator of medial arch) and calcaneus angle (i.e., an indicator of rearfoot alignment) in the multiple regression model as a predictor did not affect the regression coefficient of the corrected AAA on the hallux valgus angle, indicating a weak influence of the medial arch and rearfoot alignment on the association of frontal plane knee alignment and the hallux valgus angle. Nix et al. recently reviewed 37 papers to detect foot structure associated with hallux valgus and found inconsistent results regarding flat foot as a risk factor [60]. Thus, there is a possibility that systemic factors, rather than biomechanical factors, might contribute to the association of frontal plane knee alignment and the hallux valgus angle. Radiography-detected first metatarsophalangeal joint OA is associated with radiographic OA at the distal and proximal interphalangeal joint, first carpometacarpal joint, and knee joint, suggesting hallux valgus as a component of generalized OA [61].

This study has some limitations. First, this is a cross-sectional study without any sample size calculation. As such, the causal relationship of frontal plane knee alignment and foot postures cannot be inferred, and the results should be interpreted with caution because of a wide 95% CI of beta. Furthermore, without a control group, it is unclear whether these changes are the result of OA degenerative process, or merely a reflection of a normal relationship between foot posture and knee alignment. We found that significant relationships between foot posture and knee alignment were independent from K/L grade of index knee (data not shown), which counters the theory that all of these changes are the results of some OA process. Our data sets the foundation for a prospective cohort study with the aim of clarifying the pathogenesis of altered foot posture observed in patients with knee OA. Second, since study participants were limited to medial knee OA (94.3% with varus or neutral alignment), these results may not directly translate to a general population with knee OA. Third, evaluation of three-dimensional foot posture is based on laser line triangulation, which captures foot morphology

[39]. This skin-based scanning system may be affected by body composition, such as BMI. In this way, radiography-based evaluation would facilitate the identification of an exact relationship between frontal plane knee alignment and foot posture. Fourth, we used short anteroposterior radiographs to assess the AAA as opposed to the accepted gold standard of using long-limb radiographs to measure the mechanical axis angle. Furthermore, our methods do not account for the transverse plane, which may have an impact on the association between knee alignment and foot postures. Given that varus alignment may need greater offset than valgus alignment on the prediction of mechanical axis from AAA, and offset depends on degree of knee deformity [36], the true mechanical axis angle considering knee rotational alignment would be helpful to understand the altered foot morphology related to knee OA pathology. Nevertheless, AAA with sex-specific correction is well correlated with the mechanical axis angle, [25, 36, 37] and it can be used even when a full-limb radiograph is not available. Furthermore, we found that other offsets such as sex-specific correction factors of 3.0° or 4.6° for women and 4.7° or 6.5° for men [36, 37] and regression analysis (mechanical axis = 0.915 × AAA + 13.895), [26] did not change the relationship between knee and foot alignments (data not shown). Fifth, this study lacks reproducibility data of black seal marker attachments on foot, which may impact the relationship between knee alignment and foot posture. Unblinding marker attachments due to observation of the patients during markers attachment is also an important limitation. However, we performed a pilot study and found good reproducibility of marker attachments on navicular tuberosity in healthy adult (data not shown). Furthermore, an experienced prosthetist and orthotist clinician performed these marker attachments without knowledge of each patient's clinical status, which is a strength point in this study. Finally, the foot scanning system used in this study only evaluated static measurements while standing. This may explain why variance explained in the model was relatively small, particularly on the association between corrected AAA and hallux valgus. Small variance limits the ability to determine the clinical impact of relationships between knee alignment and foot posture. While standing, approximately half of the external loading applied to the talus is transmitted to the heel [58]. Measurements that capture dynamic alignment (e.g., higher loading phase onto the toe, such as in terminal stance during gait) might provide practical information about the association of altered frontal knee alignment and forefoot alignment. Indeed, patients with medial knee OA display altered hallux and midfoot kinematics, particularly in the terminal stance phase of gait compared to healthy adults [62].

Conclusions

Corrected AAA evaluated by radiography was independently associated with the hallux valgus angle and calcaneus angle relative to the floor in patients with medial knee OA, particularly in varus-aligned knees. These results indicate the existence of a connection between altered frontal knee alignment and foot posture, which would be helpful to understand the pathogenesis of altered foot posture observed in patients with knee OA.

Abbreviations

OA: Knee osteoarthritis; TKA: Total knee arthroplasty; AAA: Anatomical axis angle; K/L: Kellgren/Lawrence; JSN: Joint space narrowing; ICC: Intraclass correlation coefficient; BMI: Body mass index.

Acknowledgements

The authors acknowledge the staff of Nozomi Orthopaedic Clinic in Hiroshima for their contribution to data collection.

Funding

This work was supported by Grants-in-Aid for Scientific Research from the Japan Society for the Promotion of Science; from the Ministry of Education, Culture, Sports, Science, and Technology; and from the Ministry of Health, Labor, and Welfare.

Authors' contributions

All authors have made substantial contributions to (1) substantial contributions to research design, or the acquisition, analysis or interpretation of data; (2) drafting the paper or revising it critically; (3) approval of the submitted and final versions; and (4) agreed to be accountable for all aspects of the work. The specific contributions of the authors are as follows: HO, HI, TA, EK, KO, and KA conceived and designed the study; HO, HI, TA, and KA analyzed and interpreted the data; HO, HI, KO, and KA drafted the article; HO, HI, and TA critically revised the article for important intellectual content; HO, HI, TA, EK, KO, and KA finally approved the article; HI and TA advised statistical analysis method; TA and EK obtained funding; HO, HI, EK, and KA collected and assembled the data.

Competing interests

The authors declare that they have no competing interests.

Consent for publication

Not applicable.

Author details

[1]Graduate School of Health and Welfare, Niigata University of Health and Welfare, Niigata, Japan. [2]Ohi Manufacturing Co., Ltd., Kyoto, Japan. [3]Department of Physical Therapy, Human Health Sciences, Graduate School of Medicine, Kyoto University, Kyoto, Japan. [4]Department of System Design

Engineering, Keio University, Yokohama, Japan. [5]Japan Society for the Promotion of Science, Tokyo, Japan. [6]Nozomi Orthopaedic Clinic, Hiroshima, Japan.

References

1. Guccione AA, Felson DT, Anderson JJ, Anthony JM, Zhang Y, Wilson PW, Kelly-Hayes M, Wolf PA, Kreger BE, Kannel WB. The effects of specific medical conditions on the functional limitations of elders in the Framingham Study. Am J Public Health. 1994;84(3):351–8.
2. Peat G, McCarney R, Croft P. Knee pain and osteoarthritis in older adults: a review of community burden and current use of primary health care. Ann Rheum Dis. 2001;60(2):91–7.
3. Hunter DJ, Sharma L, Skaife T. Alignment and osteoarthritis of the knee. J Bone Joint Surg Am. 2009;91 Suppl 1:85–9.
4. Sharma L. The role of varus and valgus alignment in knee osteoarthritis. Arthritis Rheum. 2007;56(4):1044–7.
5. Felson DT, Niu J, Gross KD, Englund M, Sharma L, Cooke TD, Guermazi A, Roemer FW, Segal N, Goggins JM, et al. Valgus malalignment is a risk factor for lateral knee osteoarthritis incidence and progression: findings from the Multicenter Osteoarthritis Study and the Osteoarthritis Initiative. Arthritis Rheum. 2013;65(2):355–62.
6. Levinger P, Menz HB, Fotoohabadi MR, Feller JA, Bartlett JR, Bergman NR. Foot posture in people with medial compartment knee osteoarthritis. J Foot Ankle Res. 2010;3:29.
7. Reilly K, Barker K, Shamley D, Newman M, Oskrochi GR, Sandall S. The role of foot and ankle assessment of patients with lower limb osteoarthritis. Physiotherapy. 2009;95(3):164–9.
8. Anne Reilly K, Louise Barker K, Shamley D, Sandall S. Influence of foot characteristics on the site of lower limb osteoarthritis. Foot Ankle Int. 2006;27(3):206–11.
9. Golightly YM, Hannan MT, Dufour AB, Renner JB, Jordan JM. Factors associated with hallux valgus in a community-based cross-sectional study of adults with and without osteoarthritis. Arthritis Care Res (Hoboken). 2015;67(6):791–8.
10. Gross KD, Felson DT, Niu J, Hunter DJ, Guermazi A, Roemer FW, Dufour AB, Gensure RH, Hannan MT. Association of flat feet with knee pain and cartilage damage in older adults. Arthritis Care Res (Hoboken). 2011;63(7):937–44.
11. Roddy E, Zhang W, Doherty M. Prevalence and associations of hallux valgus in a primary care population. Arthritis Rheum. 2008;59(6):857–62.
12. Guler H, Karazincir S, Turhanoglu AD, Sahin G, Balci A, Ozer C. Effect of coexisting foot deformity on disability in women with knee osteoarthritis. J Am Podiatr Med Assoc. 2009;99(1):23–7.
13. Paterson KL, Hinman RS, Hunter DJ, Wrigley TV, Bennell KL. Impact of concurrent foot pain on health and functional status in people with knee osteoarthritis: data from the osteoarthritis initiative. Arthritis Care Res (Hoboken). 2015;67(7):989–95.
14. Paterson KL, Kasza J, Hunter DJ, Hinman RS, Menz HB, Peat G, Bennell KL. The relationship between foot and ankle symptoms and risk of developing knee osteoarthritis: data from the osteoarthritis initiative. Osteoarthritis Cartilage. 2017;25(5):639–46.
15. Gates LS, Bowen CJ, Sanchez-Santos MT, Delmestri A, Arden NK. Do foot & ankle assessments assist the explanation of 1 year knee arthroplasty outcomes? Osteoarthritis Cartilage. 2017;25(6):892–8.
16. Souza TR, Pinto RZ, Trede RG, Kirkwood RN, Fonseca ST. Temporal couplings between rearfoot-shank complex and hip joint during walking. Clin Biomech (Bristol, Avon). 2010;25(7):745–8.
17. Lafortune MA, Cavanagh PR, Sommer 3rd HJ, Kalenak A. Foot inversion-eversion and knee kinematics during walking. J Orthop Res. 1994;12(3):412–20.
18. Van Gheluwe B, Kirby KA, Hagman F. Effects of simulated genu valgum and genu varum on ground reaction forces and subtalar joint function during gait. J Am Podiatr Med Assoc. 2005;95(6):531–41.
19. Mullaji A, Shetty GM. Persistent hindfoot valgus causes lateral deviation of weightbearing axis after total knee arthroplasty. Clin Orthop Relat Res. 2011;469(4):1154–60.
20. Norton AA, Callaghan JJ, Amendola A, Phisitkul P, Wongsak S, Liu SS, Fruehling-Wall C. Correlation of knee and hindfoot deformities in advanced knee OA: compensatory hindfoot alignment and where it occurs. Clin Orthop Relat Res. 2015;473(1):166–74.
21. Hara Y, Ikoma K, Arai Y, Ohashi S, Maki M, Kubo T. Alteration of hindfoot alignment after total knee arthroplasty using a novel hindfoot alignment view. J Arthroplasty. 2015;30(1):126–9.
22. Levinger P, Menz HB, Morrow AD, Bartlett JR, Feller JA, Fotoohabadi MR, Bergman NR. Dynamic foot function changes following total knee replacement surgery. Knee. 2012;19(6):880–5.
23. Okamoto Y, Otsuki S, Jotoku T, Nakajima M, Neo M. Clinical usefulness of hindfoot assessment for total knee arthroplasty: persistent post-operative hindfoot pain and alignment in pre-existing severe knee deformity. Knee Surg Sports Traumatol Arthrosc. 2016. Epub ahead of print.
24. Muraki S, Oka H, Akune T, Mabuchi A, En-yo Y, Yoshida M, Saika A, Suzuki T, Yoshida H, Ishibashi H, et al. Prevalence of radiographic knee osteoarthritis and its association with knee pain in the elderly of Japanese population-based cohorts: the ROAD study. Osteoarthritis Cartilage. 2009;17(9):1137–43.
25. Kraus VB, Vail TP, Worrell T, McDaniel G. A comparative assessment of alignment angle of the knee by radiographic and physical examination methods. Arthritis Rheum. 2005;52(6):1730–5.
26. Hinman RS, May RL, Crossley KM. Is there an alternative to the full-leg radiograph for determining knee joint alignment in osteoarthritis? Arthritis Rheum. 2006;55(2):306–13.
27. Iijima H, Ohi H, Isho T, Aoyama T, Fukutani N, Kaneda E, Ohi K, Abe K, Kuroki H, Matsuda S. Association of bilateral flat feet with knee pain and disability in patients with knee osteoarthritis: A cross-sectional study. J Orthop Res. 2017. Epub ahead of print.
28. Kellgren JH, Lawrence JS. Radiological assessment of osteo-arthrosis. Ann Rheum Dis. 1957;16(4):494–502.
29. Wise BL, Kritikos L, Lynch JA, Liu F, Parimi N, Tileston KL, Nevitt MC, Lane NE. Proximal femur shape differs between subjects with lateral and medial knee osteoarthritis and controls: the Osteoarthritis Initiative. Osteoarthritis Cartilage. 2014;22(12):2067–73.
30. Altman RD, Gold GE. Atlas of individual radiographic features in osteoarthritis, revised. Osteoarthritis Cartilage. 2007;15(Suppl A):A1–A56.
31. Muraki S, Akune T, En-Yo Y, Yoshida M, Suzuki T, Yoshida H, Ishibashi H, Tokimura F, Yamamoto S, Tanaka S, et al. Joint space narrowing, body mass index, and knee pain: the ROAD study (OAC1839R1). Osteoarthritis Cartilage. 2015;23(6):874–81.
32. Hart DJ, Spector TD. Kellgren & Lawrence grade 1 osteophytes in the knee–doubtful or definite? Osteoarthritis Cartilage. 2003;11(2):149–50.
33. Cibere J, Sayre EC, Guermazi A, Nicolaou S, Kopec JA, Esdaile JM, Thorne A, Singer J, Wong H. Natural history of cartilage damage and osteoarthritis progression on magnetic resonance imaging in a population-based cohort with knee pain. Osteoarthritis Cartilage. 2011;19(6):683–8.
34. Schiphof D, de Klerk BM, Kerkhof HJ, Hofman A, Koes BW, Boers M, Bierma-Zeinstra SM. Impact of different descriptions of the Kellgren and Lawrence classification criteria on the diagnosis of knee osteoarthritis. Ann Rheum Dis. 2011;70(8):1422–7.
35. McDaniel G, Mitchell KL, Charles C, Kraus VB. A comparison of five approaches to measurement of anatomic knee alignment from radiographs. Osteoarthritis Cartilage. 2010;18(2):273–7.
36. Sheehy L, Felson D, Zhang Y, Niu J, Lam YM, Segal N, Lynch J, Cooke TD. Does measurement of the anatomic axis consistently predict hip-knee-ankle angle (HKA) for knee alignment studies in osteoarthritis? Analysis of long limb radiographs from the multicenter osteoarthritis (MOST) study. Osteoarthritis Cartilage. 2011;19(1):58–64.
37. Issa SN, Dunlop D, Chang A, Song J, Prasad PV, Guermazi A, Peterfy C, Cahue S, Marshall M, Kapoor D, et al. Full-limb and knee radiography assessments of varus-valgus alignment and their relationship to osteoarthritis disease features by magnetic resonance imaging. Arthritis Rheum. 2007;57(3):398–406.
38. Cooke D, Scudamore A, Li J, Wyss U, Bryant T, Costigan P. Axial lower-limb alignment: comparison of knee geometry in normal volunteers and osteoarthritis patients. Osteoarthritis Cartilage. 1997;5(1):39–47.
39. Fujita H, Fukumoto S, Yoshida H, Wakasugi Y, Kano H. A 3D Foot Scanning System with a Sensor Head Guided around the Foot (Japanese Title: 単一の計測ヘッドで足の全体形状計測を行う三次元足型自動計測機). Trans Inst Syst Control Inf Eng. 2004;17:330–7.
40. Nishimura A, Kato K, Fukuda A, Nakazora S, Yamada T, Uchida A, Sudo A. Prevalence of hallux valgus and risk factors among Japanese community dwellers. J Orthop Sci. 2014;19(2):257–62.
41. Root ML, Orien WP, Weed JH. Normal and abnormal function of the foot: Clinical Biomechanics. 1977.
42. Zhang Y, Glynn RJ, Felson DT. Musculoskeletal disease research: should we analyze the joint or the person? J Rheumatol. 1996;23(7):1130–4.

43. Matsumoto T, Hashimura M, Takayama K, Ishida K, Kawakami Y, Matsuzaki T, Nakano N, Matsushita T, Kuroda R, Kurosaka M. A radiographic analysis of alignment of the lower extremities–initiation and progression of varus-type knee osteoarthritis. Osteoarthritis Cartilage. 2015;23(2):217–23.
44. Uritani D, Fukumoto T, Matsumoto D, Shima M. Associations between toe grip strength and hallux valgus, toe curl ability, and foot arch height in Japanese adults aged 20 to 79 years: a cross-sectional study. J Foot Ankle Res. 2015;8:18.
45. Ozguclu E, Kilic E, Kaymak B. A knee osteoarthritis connected with hallux valgus-related pes planus. J Biomech. 2008;41(16):3523–4.
46. Coughlin MJ. Hallux valgus. J Bone Joint Surg Am. 1996;78(6):932–66.
47. Coughlin MJ, Thompson FM. The high price of high-fashion footwear. Instr Course Lect. 1995;44:371–7.
48. Torkki M, Malmivaara A, Seitsalo S, Hoikka V, Laippala P, Paavolainen P. Surgery vs orthosis vs watchful waiting for hallux valgus: a randomized controlled trial. JAMA. 2001;285(19):2474–80.
49. Lidtke RH, Muehleman C, Kwasny M, Block JA. Foot center of pressure and medial knee osteoarthritis. J Am Podiatr Med Assoc. 2010;100(3):178–84.
50. Saito I, Okada K, Nishi T, Wakasa M, Saito A, Sugawara K, Takahashi Y, Kinoshita K. Foot pressure pattern and its correlation with knee range of motion limitations for individuals with medial knee osteoarthritis. Arch Phys Med Rehabil. 2013;94(12):2502–8.
51. Otsuki T, Nawata K, Okuno M. Quantitative evaluation of gait pattern in patients with osteoarthrosis of the knee before and after total knee arthroplasty. Gait analysis using a pressure measuring system. J Orthop Sci. 1999;4(2):99–105.
52. Shih KS, Chien HL, Lu TW, Chang CF, Kuo CC. Gait changes in individuals with bilateral hallux valgus reduce first metatarsophalangeal loading but increase knee abductor moments. Gait Posture. 2014;40(1):38–42.
53. Voronov ML, Pinzur MS, Havey RM, Carandang G, Gil JA, Hopkinson WJ. The relationship between knee arthroplasty and foot loading. Foot Ankle Spec. 2012;5(1):17–22.
54. Riegger-Krugh C, Keysor JJ. Skeletal malalignments of the lower quarter: correlated and compensatory motions and postures. J Orthop Sports Phys Ther. 1996;23(2):164–70.
55. Takenaka T, Ikoma K, Ohashi S, Arai Y, Hara Y, Ueshima K, Sawada K, Shirai T, Fujiwara H, Kubo T. Hindfoot alignment at one year after total knee arthroplasty. Knee Surg Sports Traumatol Arthrosc. 2016;24(8):2442–6.
56. Abourazzak F, Kadi N, Azzouzi H, Lazrak F, Najdi A, Nejjari C, Harzy T. A Positive Association Between Foot Posture Index and Medial Compartment Knee Osteoarthritis in Moroccan People. Open Rheumatol J. 2014;8:96.
57. Buchanan KR, Davis I. The relationship between forefoot, midfoot, and rearfoot static alignment in pain-free individuals. J Orthop Sports Phys Ther. 2005;35(9):559–66.
58. Arangio GA, Phillippy DC, Xiao D, Gu WK, Salathe EP. Subtalar pronation–relationship to the medial longitudinal arch loading in the normal foot. Foot Ankle Int. 2000;21(3):216–20.
59. Mahiquez MY, Wilder FV, Stephens HM. Positive hindfoot valgus and osteoarthritis of the first metatarsophalangeal joint. Foot Ankle Int. 2006;27(12):1055–9.
60. Nix SE, Vicenzino BT, Collins NJ, Smith MD. Characteristics of foot structure and footwear associated with hallux valgus: a systematic review. Osteoarthritis Cartilage. 2012;20(10):1059–74.
61. Wilder FV, Barrett JP, Farina EJ. The association of radiographic foot osteoarthritis and radiographic osteoarthritis at other sites. Osteoarthritis Cartilage. 2005;13(3):211–5.
62. Arnold J, Mackintosh S, Jones S, Thewlis D. Altered dynamic foot kinematics in people with medial knee osteoarthritis during walking: a cross-sectional study. Knee. 2014;21(6):1101–6.

23

Disability due to knee pain and somatising tendency in Japanese adults

Tomoko Fujii[1], Hiroyuki Oka[1*], Junji Katsuhira[2], Juichi Tonosu[3], Satoshi Kasahara[4], Sakae Tanaka[5] and Ko Matsudaira[1]

Abstract

Background: Knee pain is common and related to knee osteoarthritis. However, there is a discrepancy between knee pain and radiographic osteoarthritis. In the general population, knee pain is associated with psychological and cognitive factors, which would be one explanation for the discrepancy. Limited evidence demonstrates that somatization is associated with knee pain. This study examined the association between disability due to knee pain and a high somatising tendency.

Methods: Japanese adults (aged 20–64 years) who had experienced knee pain in the past four weeks were included in this study ($n = 14{,}695$, 50% women). Data were extracted from a large internet survey. Somatising tendency was assessed using the Somatic Symptom Scale-8 (SSS-8). Disability due to knee pain was categorized into three levels: 1) knee pain without difficulty with activities of daily living (ADL), 2) knee pain with ADL difficulty but without requiring sick leave, and 3) knee pain requiring sick leave. The association between ≥ high somatising tendency (SSS-8 score ≥ 12) as well as very high somatising tendency (SSS-8 score ≥ 16) and disability due to knee pain was examined using logistic regression models adjusted for age, sex, body mass index, depressive symptoms, education level, regular exercise, chronicity of knee pain (≥3 months), osteoarthritis, rheumatoid arthritis, and fibromyalgia.

Results: Greater disability due to knee pain was associated with a higher odds ratio for ≥ high somatising tendency (adjusted odds ratio (aOR) = 2.36 [2.10–2.66] in group 2 vs. group 1, aOR = 3.23 [2.66–3.92] in group 3 vs. group 1). Stronger associations were found for a very high somatising tendency (aOR = 2.80 [2.42–3.23] in group 2 vs. group 1, aOR = 4.51 [3.64–5.58] in group 3 vs. group 1).

Conclusions: Somatization may play a role in disability due to knee pain in the general adult population with knee pain, similar to the role of somatization in low back pain.

Keywords: Knee pain, Osteoarthritis of the knee, Somatising tendency

Background

Knee pain is a common symptom. The 12-month prevalence of knee pain was reported to be 29% in people who were 40–79 years old in Nottingham, UK [1]. In Japan, the prevalence of knee pain was reported to be 33% (men 28%, women 35%) in an integrated cohort in which most participants were 60 years of age or older [2]. In a cohort study of Japanese workers who were 19–64 years old, the one-month prevalence of knee pain was 12% [3].

One cause of knee pain is osteoarthritis (OA). However, there is a discrepancy between radiographic knee OA and knee pain; not all people with knee pain have radiographic knee OA, and not all people with knee OA have knee pain [4]. Recently, magnetic resonance imaging (MRI) of the knee has been studied in relation to knee pain [5, 6]. However, even the structural changes assessed via MRI may not always explain knee pain [7]. Felson et al. emphasized the importance of separating the disease process of OA and the syndrome of musculoskeletal pain and disability, which is a common concept in low back pain [8].

Psychological factors predict the incidence, chronicity, and disability of low back pain [9–11]. Similarly, some evidence indicates that psychological factors are also

* Correspondence: okah-tky@umin.ac.jp
[1]Department of Medical Research and Management for Musculoskeletal Pain, 22nd Century Medical & Research Center, Faculty of Medicine, The University of Tokyo, 7-3-1 Hongo, Bunkyo-ku, Tokyo 113-8655, Japan
Full list of author information is available at the end of the article

associated with knee pain, which could be one of the explanations for the discrepancy between radiographic changes and knee pain [12, 13]. Somatization, one psychological factor, is "a tendency to experience and communicate somatic distress in response to psychosocial stress and to seek medical help for it" [14]. Somatization often coexists with depression and anxiety [15]. Somatising tendency is a predisposition to be more aware of and to worry about, common somatic symptoms [16]. Longitudinal studies have shown that somatising tendency is not merely a consequence of musculoskeletal pain but a risk factor for multisite musculoskeletal pain [3, 17]. A few studies have reported that somatising tendency was associated with knee pain [3, 18, 19]. However, evidence is limited regarding whether somatising tendency is associated with disability due to knee pain in the general population. This study aimed to examine whether the severity of disability due to knee pain is associated with a high somatising tendency in the general population of adults with knee pain.

Methods

Participants

Japanese adults aged 20–64 years with knee pain in the past four weeks ($n = 14{,}695$) were included in the present study. Data were extracted from a large internet survey of physical and mental health, which was conducted in February 2015. Participants were recruited by an internet research company, United Inc. (Tokyo, Japan), with which more than 1.37 million individuals across Japan have voluntarily registered. The only inclusion criterion for the survey was an age of 20–64 years. Of the approximately 1.25 million eligible individuals, 270,000 individuals were randomly selected and invited by e-mail to complete an online questionnaire. All respondents ($n = 52{,}353$) provided web-based informed consent and were compensated. Because the focus of this internet survey was not knee pain, the question regarding knee pain, which we created based on the typical question regarding low back pain, was generic. The question with an illustration showing the area of pain asked whether a participant had knee pain persisting for ≥1 day in the past four weeks. The possible responses were as follows: 1) I did not have knee pain (KP0), 2) I had knee pain without difficulty with activities of daily living (ADL) (KP1), 3) I had knee pain with ADL difficulty but without requiring absence from social activities, such as work or school (KP2), and 4) I had knee pain requiring absence from social activities, such as work or school (KP3). Twenty-eight percent of the respondents ($n = 14{,}695$) answered that they had knee pain (KP1, 2, or 3). Only the individuals with knee pain were included in this analysis. Additionally, respondents were asked whether their knee pain lasted for ≥3 months. The Institutional Review Board of the University of Tokyo approved this study.

Assessments

Somatising tendency

Somatising tendency was assessed using the Japanese version of the Somatic Symptom Scale-8 (SSS-8) [20]. The SSS-8 is a self-administered questionnaire that assesses somatic symptom burden. The SSS-8 was developed as an abbreviated 8-item version of the Patient Health Questionnaire-15 (PHQ-15) to assess the presence and severity of common somatic symptoms [21]. The following somatic symptoms were assessed: 1) stomach or bowel problems; 2) back pain; 3) pain in the arms, legs, or joints; 4) headaches; 5) chest pain or shortness of breath; 6) dizziness; 7) feeling tired or having low energy; and 8) having trouble sleeping. The SSS-8 was used as a reference measure in the Diagnostic and Statistical Manual of Mental Disorders (Fifth Edition) (DSM-5) field trials to facilitate the diagnosis of somatic symptom disorder [22]. The German version of the SSS-8 has good reliability and validity for the general German population [20]. We translated the English version of the SSS-8 into Japanese [23], and the Japanese version of the SSS-8 has been linguistically and psychometrically validated [24]. The total SSS-8 score was categorized, as in Gierk et al., into the following five groups: no to minimal (0–3); low (4–7); medium (8–11); high (12–15); and very high (16–32) [20].

Covariates

Demographic information was also collected in the survey. Body mass index (BMI) was calculated based on self-reported body weight and height as weight (kg)/height $(m)^2$. BMI was categorized into 3 levels (< 25, 25–29, and ≥30). The participants were asked whether they engaged in exercise regularly over the past year, such as walking and jogging, that lasted for ≥30 min. The possible responses were none, 1–2 times per month, once per week, or more than twice per week. Engaging in regular exercise was defined as exercising more than twice per week. We also collected self-reported information on the chronic conditions for which the respondents were seeking treatment, including OA, rheumatoid arthritis (RA), and fibromyalgia.

Depressive symptoms were assessed using the Patient Health Questionnaire-2 (PHQ-2), an assessment composed of two questions from the Patient Health Questionnaire-9 [25]. The Japanese version of the Patient Health Questionnaire was previously validated [26]. The PHQ-2 assesses whether an individual has experienced depression and anhedonia within the past two weeks. Although each item is rated on a scale of 0–3 in the original PHQ-2, the present study used the National

Center of Neurology and Psychiatry version of the Japanese PHQ-2, which gives each item a binary response of yes or no (1/0) [26]. Therefore, the possible scores for the PHQ-2 were 0, 1, or 2. Individuals who answer yes to at least one question are suspected of experiencing depression, and closer assessment of these individuals is recommended.

Statistical analysis

Initially, the demographic data were examined using descriptive statistics. The characteristics of the participants were compared according to three knee pain groups using the chi-square test. Whether the severity of disability due to knee pain was associated with ≥ high somatising tendency (SSS-8 score ≥ 12) and very high somatising tendency (SSS-8 score ≥ 16) was examined using logistic regression models. The outcome variables were 1) ≥ high and 2) very high somatising tendency, and they were analyzed in separate regression models. The independent variable was disability due to knee pain (3 levels). The participants who had knee pain without any ADL difficulty (KP1) were treated as the reference group. The chronicity of knee pain was also examined as an independent variable. The final multiple models were adjusted for age (5 levels), sex, BMI (3 levels), PHQ-2 (3 levels), education level (any college or no college), regular exercise (yes/no), and whether the participant was seeking treatment for OA, RA, or fibromyalgia. These potential confounders, which would be associated with both somatising tendency and knee pain and/or were adjusted for in previous studies, were chosen a priori based on the literature [12, 16, 27, 28]. Multicollinearity was not suspected as all variance inflation factors (VIFs) were < 2. The odds ratios (ORs) and their 95% confidence intervals (CIs) were estimated. Analyses were conducted using SAS version 9.4 (SAS Institute, Inc., Cary, NC, USA). All analyses were two-sided, and an α-level of 0.05 was considered statistically significant.

Results

Participant characteristics are shown in Table 1. The mean age (± standard deviation) was 45.6 ± 11.9 years, and half of the participants (49.5%) were women. Among the participants with knee pain, most (82.8%, $n = 12{,}161$) had knee pain without any ADL difficulty (KP1), 13.3% ($n = 1954$) had knee pain with ADL difficulty but without requiring sick leave (KP2), and only 4.0% ($n = 580$) reported using sick leave due to knee pain (KP3). Individuals in the greater disability group were more likely to be men, unmarried, and lack a college education. The proportion of participants with a PHQ-2 score of 2 was higher in the greater disability groups, and the proportion of participants with OA, RA, and fibromyalgia was also higher in the greater disability groups. The proportion of participants with a high or very high somatising tendency was higher in the greater disability groups.

The results of the final logistic regression model are shown in Table 2. Disability due to knee pain was significantly associated both with ≥ high and very high somatising tendency after adjusting for age, sex, BMI, PHQ-2, education, regular exercise, OA, RA, fibromyalgia, and the chronicity of knee pain. The participants who had knee pain with ADL difficulty were more than twice as likely to have at least a high somatising tendency compared to those who had knee pain without difficulty (adjusted OR = 2.36 [2.10–2.66], $p < 0.001$). Individuals who had knee pain requiring sick leave were more than three times as likely to have at least a high somatising tendency compared to those who had knee pain without ADL difficulty (adjusted OR = 3.23 [2.66–3.92], $p < 0.001$). The results for very high somatising tendency were similar, but stronger associations were found. The odds ratios for very high somatising tendency were 2.80 (95% CI [2.42–3.23], $p < 0.001$) in the participants who had knee pain with ADL difficulty and 4.51 (95% CI [3.64–5.58], $p < 0.001$) in the individuals who had knee pain requiring sick leave compared with those who had knee pain without ADL difficulty. Chronicity of knee pain was significantly associated with ≥ high somatising tendency (OR = 1.28 [1.16, 1.41], $p < 0.001$) but not with very high somatising tendency (OR = 1.12 [0.98, 1.28], $p = 0.103$).

Discussion

This study is the first to report a significant association between disability due to knee pain and high somatising tendency in Japanese adults. Individuals who had knee pain with difficulty in ADL were more than twice as likely to have a very high somatising tendency compared with those who had knee pain without difficulty in ADL, and those who had knee pain requiring sick leave were more than four times as likely to have a high somatising tendency.

Knee pain is a common symptom, one cause of which is knee OA. However, a discrepancy between knee pain and radiographic knee OA has been observed [4]. A systematic review reported that this discordance can be partly explained by the fact that radiographic knee OA is often defined only based on anterior-posterior and/or lateral views, without a skyline view, which would miss knee OA in the patella-femoral joint [29]. The review also reported that the discordance varied according to the knee pain definition. However, the authors concluded that there was still discordance between knee pain and radiographic knee OA. Therefore, one approach involves separating knee pain and its related disability from the disease process of OA [8], which is a

Table 1 Characteristics of the participants with knee pain

	All (*n* = 14,695)	Knee pain without difficulty in ADL (*n* = 12,161)	Knee pain with difficultly but without sick leave (*n* = 1954)	Knee pain with sick leave (*n* = 580)	*p-value**
Age (%)					< 0.001
20–29	1942 (13.2)	1569 (12.9)	271 (13.9)	102 (17.6)	
30–39	2903 (19.8)	2345 (19.3)	411 (21.0)	147 (25.3)	
40–49	3462 (23.6)	2875 (23.6)	441 (22.6)	146 (25.2)	
50–59	4322 (29.4)	3599 (29.6)	588 (30.1)	135 (23.3)	
60–64	2066 (14.1)	1773 (14.6)	243 (12.4)	50 (8.6)	
Sex (%)					0.0003
Men	7421 (50.5)	6082 (50.0)	1000 (51.2)	339 (58.5)	
Women	7274 (49.5)	6079 (50.0)	954 (48.8)	241 (41.6)	
BMI (%)					0.0003
< 25	11,078 (75.4)	9228 (75.9)	1431 (73.2)	419 (72.2)	
25–29	2811 (19.1)	2311 (19.0)	381 (19.5)	119 (20.5)	
≥ 30	806 (5.5)	622 (5.1)	142 (7.3)	42 (7.2)	
Marital status (%)					< 0.001
Not married	6249 (42.5)	5069 (41.7)	884 (45.2)	296 (51)	
Married	8446 (57.5)	7092 (58.3)	1070 (54.8)	284 (49)	
Education (%)					0.003
No college	7820 (53.2)	6402 (52.6)	1077 (55.1)	341 (58.8)	
Some college	6875 (46.8)	5759 (47.4)	877 (44.9)	239 (41.2)	
Exercise (%)					0.016
No regular exercise	11,585 (78.8)	9577 (78.8)	1524 (78)	484 (83.5)	
Regular exercise	3110 (21.2)	2584 (21.3)	430 (22)	96 (16.6)	
PHQ-2 (%)[a]					< 0.001
0	9415 (64.1)	8028 (66.0)	1060 (54.3)	327 (56.4)	
1	2546 (17.3)	2054 (16.9)	399 (20.4)	93 (16.0)	
2	2734 (18.6)	2079 (17.1)	495 (25.3)	160 (27.6)	
Chronic knee pain (%)					< 0.001
No	4906 (33.4)	4096 (33.7)	509 (26.1)	301 (51.9)	
Yes	9789 (66.6)	8065 (66.3)	1445 (74.0)	279 (48.1)	
Osteoarthritis (%)	607 (4.1)	328 (2.7)	209 (10.7)	70 (12.1)	< 0.001
Rheumatoid arthritis (%)	229 (1.6)	138 (1.1)	67 (3.4)	24 (4.1)	< 0.001
Fibromyalgia (%)	81 (0.6)	38 (0.3)	27 (1.4)	16 (2.8)	< 0.001
SSS-8 (%)					< 0.001
No to minimal	5262 (35.8)	4679 (38.5)	418 (21.4)	165 (28.5)	
Low	4175 (28.4)	3542 (29.1)	526 (26.9)	107 (18.5)	
Medium	2510 (17.1)	2069 (17.0)	363 (18.6)	78 (13.5)	
High	1434 (9.8)	1079 (8.9)	284 (14.5)	71 (12.2)	
Very high	1314 (8.9)	792 (6.5)	363 (18.6)	159 (27.4)	

ADL activities of daily living, *BMI* body mass index, *PHQ-2* Patient Health Questionnaire-2, *SSS-8* Somatic Symptom Scale-8
**p-value* from the chi-square test
[a]PHQ-2 items are commonly scored 0 to 3, but the items in the Japanese PHQ-2 were scored yes/no (0/1)

concept similar to that used for low back pain. Knee pain and knee OA share some risk factors, such as older age, being overweight, and having previous knee injuries [28, 30]. In addition, psychological factors, such as depression and somatising tendency, seem to play some role in knee pain, which could be one explanation for

Table 2 Associations between high (SSS-8 ≥ 12) or very high somatising tendency (SSS-8 ≥ 16) and disability due to knee pain from multiple logistic regression models (n = 14,695)

	SSS8 ≥ 12			SSS8 ≥ 16		
	OR [95% CI][a]	*p-value*	Type 3 *p-value*	OR [95% CI][a]	*p-value*	Type 3 *p-value*
Disability due to pain			< 0.001			< 0.001
Knee pain without difficulty in ADL	1			1		
Knee pain with difficulty but without sick leave	2.36 [2.10, 2.66]	< 0.001		2.80 [2.42, 3.23]	< 0.001	
Knee pain with sick leave	3.23 [2.66, 3.92]	< 0.001		4.51 [3.64, 5.58]	< 0.001	
Chronic knee pain yes vs. no	1.28 [1.16, 1.41]	< 0.001		1.12 [0.98, 1.28]	0.103	

SSS-8 Somatic Symptom Scale-8, *OR* odds ratio, *CI* confidence interval, *ADL* activities of daily living
[a]Adjusted for age, sex, body mass index, depressive symptoms (Patient Health Questionnaire-2 (PHQ-2)), education, regular exercise, osteoarthritis, rheumatoid arthritis, and fibromyalgia

the discrepancy between radiographic changes and knee pain [12, 13]. Assessing these psychological factors may help predict the onset and prognosis of knee pain in general and occupational health practices.

The results of the current study add to those of the few previous studies that found an association between somatising tendency and knee pain. As part of a large international survey of musculoskeletal symptoms (the Cultural and Psychosocial Influences on Disability [CUPID] study), Matsudaira et al. used a self-administered questionnaire in Japanese to examine pain in six anatomical regions [3]. Somatising tendency was assessed using a subset of items from the Brief Symptom Inventory [31]. The odds of experiencing any knee pain or disabling knee pain in the past month was approximately three times higher in the participants who had ≥2 distressing somatic symptoms compared to those who had no such somatic symptoms. In the CUPID study in Sri Lanka, a similar but weaker association was found, with a prevalence ratio of 1.8 [19]. These two studies were cross-sectional reports, and the causal direction was unknown. Palmer et al. followed working-aged subjects for 18 months in a postal survey in the UK [18]. A higher somatising tendency was associated with new onset of knee pain and its persistence. The present study further suggests the possibility that a high somatising tendency may lead to greater disability and sick leave utilization in people with knee pain.

The factors associated with disability in knee OA patients have been reported in the literature. Older age, female sex, lower social class, obesity, lower quadriceps strength, comorbid health problems, helplessness, and knee pain severity (rather than radiographic severity) were associated with disability or worsening of physical function in people with knee OA [32–36]. Reduced work productivity is typically assessed in terms of absenteeism (days off from work) and presentieesm (productivity loss while at work). A study on reduced work productivity due to knee problems found that a low 12-Item Short Form Health Survey (SF-12) Physical Component Summary score, semi-manual labor or manual labor, and a high maximum knee pain score were associated with presenteeism in people with chronic knee pain and joint space narrowing [37]. A low SF-12 Mental Component Summary score was associated with absenteeism in this study, although reduced work productivity was primarily attributed to presenteeism. For low back pain, the risk factors for chronicity/disability have been extensively studied and are reflected in the guidelines for the management of low back pain [38]. Psychological distress, depressive mood, somatization, work-related factors, pain severity, functional impact, and prior episodes of low back pain have all been reported as prognostic factors [38]. In a recent prospective study, baseline disability, age, and somatization were independently associated with follow-up disability in patients with chronic low back pain [39]. Our results suggest that the factors associated with disability due to knee pain in the general population may not be the same as those in knee OA patients. Somatising tendency may play some role in disability due to knee pain, which is similar to low back pain. When there is a large discrepancy between radiographic changes and knee pain-related disability, it may be useful for clinicians to assess the patient's somatising tendency and consider a potential psychological approach.

It is plausible that individuals with a high somatising tendency are more aware of and worry about their knee symptoms and consequently avoid activities that may exacerbate their symptoms [40]. Avoidance behavior may result in disuse and disability. In a previous study, somatising tendency was associated with knee pain especially when the pain was chronic or disabling, although the study was cross-sectional [41]. Therefore, somatising tendency is speculated to be more important for disability related to knee pain rather than the occurrence of knee pain. However, due to the cross-sectional design of the current study, this conclusion cannot be determined. Future longitudinal studies are needed.

Chronicity of knee pain was associated with ≥ high somatising tendency but not with a very high somatising tendency. A prospective study found an association between baseline somatising tendency and knee pain persistence [18]. Chronic pain should lead to greater concern regarding the symptom. Determining a conclusion from our results is difficult. People often experience knee pain intermittently. We inquired only about knee pain occurring within the past four weeks. Therefore, it is possible that a participant who did not have chronic knee pain in the past four weeks experienced chronic knee pain previously. Prospective studies are needed to examine the association between somatising tendency and the course of disability due to knee pain.

The strength of the present study is its large sample size with information on relevant covariables. The participants were not recruited in clinical settings; therefore, the possibility of bias due to seeking medical treatment should be low. However, some limitations should be noted. Due to the cross-sectional study design, the causal direction of the association between disability due to knee pain and somatising tendency is unknown. In the survey participants who did not have knee pain and were not included in this study ($n = 37,658$), the proportions of subjects in the SSS-8 categories of no to minimal, low, medium, high, and very high were 63.8%, 21.4%, 8.6%, 3.4%, and 2.8% respectively, and the proportions of these subjects with high and very high somatising tendencies were much lower than those of the subjects with knee pain. Because the SSS-8 questions assess joint pain, SSS-8 scores should be higher in people with knee pain than those in people without knee pain. In addition, we suspected that chronicity of knee pain was an important covariate that should be examined with disability due to knee pain simultaneously in the regression models. Therefore, we included only the participants with knee pain. Individuals with more disabling knee pain would have had higher SSS-8 scores than those who had knee pain without ADL difficulty. However, the definition of a very high somatising tendency was a high SSS-8 score (≥16). Therefore, we believe that the very high somatising tendency in these participants would not be solely attributed to knee pain. Because the focus of our internet survey was not knee pain, standard questionnaires regarding knee pain and function, such as the Western Ontario and McMaster Universities Osteoarthritis Index (WOMAC), were not used [42]. The questions and responses regarding knee pain and disability in the survey were generic to reduce the burden on the survey participants. Usually, PHQ-2 items are scored 0–3, but the Japanese version of the PHQ-2 used in our study has only binary responses. Although this questionnaire is recommended as a screening tool to assess the necessity of further evaluation for depression by the National Center of Neurology and Psychiatry, misclassification is possible, which would be non-differential. Finally, the participants in the present study were recruited online; therefore, our results may not be generalizable to the general Japanese population.

Conclusion

High somatising tendency was associated with greater disability due to knee pain in adults. Assessing and addressing somatising tendency may help predict patient outcomes and facilitate the treatment of patients with knee pain in general clinical practice.

Abbreviations

ADL: Activities of daily living; BMI: Body mass index; CI: Confidence interval; CUPID study: Cultural and Psychosocial Influences on Disability study; DSM-5: Diagnostic and Statistical Manual of Mental Disorders (Fifth Edition); MRI: Magnetic resonance imaging; OA: Osteoarthritis; OR: Odds ratio; PHQ-15: Patient Health Questionnaire-15; PHQ-2: Patient Health Questionnaire-2; RA: Rheumatoid arthritis; SF-12: 12-Item Short Form Health Survey; SSS-8: Somatic Symptom Scale-8; VIFs: Variance inflation factors; WOMAC: Western Ontario and McMaster Universities Osteoarthritis Index

Acknowledgements

We would like to thank American Journal Experts for providing editorial assistance.

Funding

This study was conducted as a collaborative research study between the University of Tokyo and Eli Lilly Japan (https://www.lilly.co.jp/). Eli Lilly Japan K.K. funded this study. The funder had no role in the study design, data collection and analysis, decision to publish, or preparation of the manuscript.

Authors' contributions

KM conceived and planned the internet survey of physical and mental health. HO contributed to the data acquisition. TF analyzed and interpreted the data and drafted the manuscript. KM, HO, ST, JK, JT, and SK critically reviewed the manuscript. All authors read and approved the final manuscript.

Consent for publication

Not applicable.

Competing interests

All authors have declared the following potential conflicts of interest. KM received the following support: a research grant from the Ministry of Health, Labour and Welfare for the submitted work; grant support, including an endowed chair from Sumitomo Dainippon Pharma Co., Ltd. and Okamura Corporation; grant support, including an endowed chair and lecture fees from AYUMI Pharmaceutical Corporation, Nippon Zoki Pharmaceutical Co., Ltd., Ono Pharmaceutical Co., LTD., Eli Lilly Japan K.K., Astellas Pharma Inc., TOTO LTD., and Eisai Co., Ltd.; lecture fees from Pfizer Japan Inc., Hisamitsu Pharmaceutical Co., Inc., Janssen Pharmaceutical K.K., Kaken Pharmaceutical Co., LTD., and Teijin Pharma Limited; and lecture fees and advisory fees from Shionogi & Co., Ltd. outside the submitted work. HO received grants from Teijin Pharma Limited, Pfizer Inc., and Fujifilm Medical Co., Ltd.; grants and personal fees from AYUMI Pharmaceutical Corporation, Nippon Zoki Pharmaceutical Co., Ltd., and Ono Pharmaceutical Co., LTD.; and grants from Eli Lilly Japan K.K. outside the submitted work. ST received personal fees for expert testimony from Amgen Inc., Asahi Kasei Pharma Corporation, Amgen Astellas BioPharma K.K., Ono Pharmaceutical Co., LTD., Kyocera Medical Corporation, Daiichi Sankyo Company, Limited, Teijin Pharma Limited, Eli Lilly Japan K.K., and Pfizer Japan Inc.; endowments from Astellas Pharma Inc., AYUMI Pharmaceutical Corporation, Pfizer Japan Inc., Bristol-Myers Squibb, Daiichi Sankyo Company, Limited, and Chugai Pharmaceutical Co., Ltd.; and grants from the Japan Agency for Medical Research and Development (AMED), the Japan Society for the Promotion of Science (JSPS)/Grant-in-aid for Scientific Research (A), and the Japan Society for the Promotion of Science (JSPS)/Grant-in-aid for Exploratory Research outside the submitted work. TF, JK, JT, and SK have no competing interests to report.

Author details

[1]Department of Medical Research and Management for Musculoskeletal Pain, 22nd Century Medical & Research Center, Faculty of Medicine, The University of Tokyo, 7-3-1 Hongo, Bunkyo-ku, Tokyo 113-8655, Japan. [2]Department of Prosthetics & Orthotics and Assistive Technology, Faculty of Medical Technology, Niigata University of Health and Welfare, 1398 Shimami-cho, Kita-ku, Niigata-shi, Niigata 950-3198, Japan. [3]Department of Orthopaedic Surgery, Kanto Rosai Hospital, 1-1 Kizukisumiyoshi-cho, Nakahara-ku, Kawasaki City, Kanagawa 211-8510, Japan. [4]Department of Pain and Palliative Medicine, Faculty of Medicine, The University of Tokyo, 7-3-1 Hongo, Bunkyo-ku, Tokyo 113-8655, Japan. [5]Department of Orthopaedic Surgery, Faculty of Medicine, The University of Tokyo, 7-3-1 Hongo, Bunkyo-ku, Tokyo 113-8655, Japan.

References

1. O'Reilly SC, Muir KR, Doherty M. Knee pain and disability in the Nottingham community: association with poor health status and psychological distress. Br J Rheumatol. 1998;37(8):870–3.
2. Yoshimura N, Akune T, Fujiwara S, Shimizu Y, Yoshida H, Omori G, Sudo A, Nishiwaki Y, Yoshida M, Shimokata H, et al. Prevalence of knee pain, lumbar pain and its coexistence in Japanese men and women: the longitudinal cohorts of motor system organ (LOCOMO) study. J Bone Miner Metab. 2014;32(5):524–32.
3. Matsudaira K, Palmer KT, Reading I, Hirai M, Yoshimura N, Coggon D. Prevalence and correlates of regional pain and associated disability in Japanese workers. Occup Environ Med. 2011;68(3):191–6.
4. Hannan MT, Felson DT, Pincus T. Analysis of the discordance between radiographic changes and knee pain in osteoarthritis of the knee. J Rheumatol. 2000;27(6):1513–7.
5. Hunter DJ, Guermazi A, Roemer F, Zhang Y, Neogi T. Structural correlates of pain in joints with osteoarthritis. Osteoarthr Cartil. 2013;21(9):1170–8.
6. Joseph GB, Hou SW, Nardo L, Heilmeier U, Nevitt MC, McCulloch CE, Link TM. MRI findings associated with development of incident knee pain over 48 months: data from the osteoarthritis initiative. Skelet Radiol. 2016;45(5): 653–60.
7. Javaid MK, Kiran A, Guermazi A, Kwoh CK, Zaim S, Carbone L, Harris T, McCulloch CE, Arden NK, Lane NE, et al. Individual magnetic resonance imaging and radiographic features of knee osteoarthritis in subjects with unilateral knee pain: the health, aging, and body composition study. Arthritis Rheum. 2012; 64(10):3246–55.
8. Felson DT, Lawrence RC, Dieppe PA, Hirsch R, Helmick CG, Jordan JM, Kington RS, Lane NE, Nevitt MC, Zhang Y, et al. Osteoarthritis: new insights. Part 1: the disease and its risk factors. Ann Intern Med. 2000;133(8):635–46.
9. Pinheiro MB, Ferreira ML, Refshauge K, Ordonana JR, Machado GC, Prado LR, Maher CG, Ferreira PH. Symptoms of depression and risk of new episodes of low back pain: a systematic review and meta-analysis. Arthritis care & research. 2015;67(11):1591–603.
10. Taylor JB, Goode AP, George SZ, Cook CE. Incidence and risk factors for first-time incident low back pain: a systematic review and meta-analysis. Spine J. 2014;14(10):2299–319.
11. Pincus T, Burton AK, Vogel S, Field AP. A systematic review of psychological factors as predictors of chronicity/disability in prospective cohorts of low back pain. Spine. 2002;27(5):E109–20.
12. Phyomaung PP, Dubowitz J, Cicuttini FM, Fernando S, Wluka AE, Raaijmaakers P, Wang Y, Urquhart DM. Are depression, anxiety and poor mental health risk factors for knee pain? A systematic review. BMC Musculoskelet Disord. 2014;15:10.
13. Urquhart DM, Phyomaung PP, Dubowitz J, Fernando S, Wluka AE, Raajmaakers P, Wang Y, Cicuttini FM. Are cognitive and behavioral factors associated with knee pain? A systematic review. Semin Arthritis Rheum. 2015;44(4):445–55.
14. Lipowski ZJ. Somatization: the concept and its clinical application. Am J Psychiatry. 1988;145(11):1358–68.
15. Lowe B, Spitzer RL, Williams JB, Mussell M, Schellberg D, Kroenke K. Depression, anxiety and somatization in primary care: syndrome overlap and functional impairment. Gen Hosp Psychiatry. 2008;30(3):191–9.
16. Vargas-Prada S, Coggon D. Psychological and psychosocial determinants of musculoskeletal pain and associated disability. Best Pract Res Clin Rheumatol. 2015;29(3):374–90.
17. Solidaki E, Chatzi L, Bitsios P, Markatzi I, Plana E, Castro F, Palmer K, Coggon D, Kogevinas M. Work-related and psychological determinants of multisite musculoskeletal pain. Scand J Work Environ Health. 2010;36(1):54–61.
18. Palmer KT, Reading I, Calnan M, Linaker C, Coggon D. Does knee pain in the community behave such as a regional pain syndrome? Prospective cohort study of incidence and persistence. Ann Rheum Dis. 2007;66(9):1190–4.
19. Warnakulasuriya SS, Peiris-John RJ, Coggon D, Ntani G, Sathiakumar N, Wickremasinghe AR. Musculoskeletal pain in four occupational populations in Sri Lanka. Occupational medicine (Oxford, England). 2012;62(4):269–72.
20. Gierk B, Kohlmann S, Kroenke K, Spangenberg L, Zenger M, Brahler E, Lowe B. The somatic symptom scale-8 (SSS-8): a brief measure of somatic symptom burden. JAMA Intern Med. 2014;174(3):399–407.
21. Kroenke K, Spitzer RL, Williams JB. The PHQ-15: validity of a new measure for evaluating the severity of somatic symptoms. Psychosom Med. 2002; 64(2):258–66.
22. Narrow WE, Clarke DE, Kuramoto SJ, Kraemer HC, Kupfer DJ, Greiner L, Regier DA. DSM-5 field trials in the United States and Canada, part III: development and reliability testing of a cross-cutting symptom assessment for DSM-5. Am J Psychiatry. 2013;170(1):71–82.
23. Matsudaira K, Kawaguchi M, Murakami M, Fukudo S, Hashizume M, Oka H, Löwe B. Development of a linguistically validated Japanese version of the somatic symptom Scale-8 (SSS-8). Jpn J Psychosom Med. 2016;56(9):931–7.
24. Matsudaira K, Oka H, Kawaguchi M, Murakami M, Fukudo S, Hashizume M, Lowe B. Development of a Japanese version of the somatic symptom Scale-8: psychometric validity and internal consistency. Gen Hosp Psychiatry. 2017;45:7–11.
25. Kroenke K, Spitzer RL, Williams JB. The patient health Questionnaire-2: validity of a two-item depression screener. Med Care. 2003;41(11):1284–92.
26. Muramatsu K, Miyaoka H, Kamijima K, Muramatsu Y, Yoshida M, Otsubo T, Gejyo F. The patient health questionnaire, Japanese version: validity according to the mini-international neuropsychiatric interview-plus. Psychol Rep. 2007; 101(3 Pt 1):952–60.
27. Vargas-Prada S, Coggon D, Ntani G, Walker-Bone K, Palmer KT, Felli VE, Harari R, Barrero LH, Felknor SA, Gimeno D, et al. Descriptive epidemiology of Somatising tendency: findings from the CUPID study. PLoS One. 2016;11(4): e0153748.
28. Miranda H, Viikari-Juntura E, Martikainen R, Riihimaki H. A prospective study on knee pain and its risk factors. Osteoarthr Cartil. 2002;10(8):623–30.
29. Bedson J, Croft PR. The discordance between clinical and radiographic knee osteoarthritis: a systematic search and summary of the literature. BMC Musculoskelet Disord. 2008;9:116.
30. Blagojevic M, Jinks C, Jeffery A, Jordan KP. Risk factors for onset of osteoarthritis of the knee in older adults: a systematic review and meta-analysis. Osteoarthritis and cartilage / OARS, Osteoarthritis Research Society. 2010;18(1):24–33.
31. Derogatis LR, Melisaratos N. The brief symptom inventory: an introductory report. Psychol Med. 1983;13(3):595–605.
32. Creamer P, Lethbridge-Cejku M, Hochberg MC. Factors associated with functional impairment in symptomatic knee osteoarthritis. Rheumatology (Oxford, England). 2000;39(5):490–6.
33. McAlindon TE, Cooper C, Kirwan JR, Dieppe PA. Determinants of disability in osteoarthritis of the knee. Ann Rheum Dis. 1993;52(4):258–62.
34. Jordan JM, Luta G, Renner JB, Linder GF, Dragomir A, Hochberg MC, Fryer JG. Self-reported functional status in osteoarthritis of the knee in a rural southern community: the role of sociodemographic factors, obesity, and knee pain. Arthritis Care Res. 1996;9(4):273–8.
35. Peters TJ, Sanders C, Dieppe P, Donovan J. Factors associated with change in pain and disability over time: a community-based prospective observational study of hip and knee osteoarthritis. Br J Gen Pract. 2005;55(512):205–11.
36. de Rooij M, van der Leeden M, Heymans MW, Holla JF, Hakkinen A, Lems WF, Roorda LD, Veenhof C, Sanchez-Ramirez DC, de Vet HC, et al. Prognosis of pain and physical functioning in patients with knee osteoarthritis: a systematic review and meta-analysis. Arthritis care & research. 2016;68(4):481–92.

37. Agaliotis M, Fransen M, Bridgett L, Nairn L, Votrubec M, Jan S, Heard R, Mackey M. Risk factors associated with reduced work productivity among people with chronic knee pain. Osteoarthr Cartil. 2013;21(9):1160–9.
38. Airaksinen O, Brox JI, Cedraschi C, Hildebrandt J, Klaber-Moffett J, Kovacs F, Mannion AF, Reis S, Staal JB, Ursin H, et al. Chapter 4. European guidelines for the management of chronic nonspecific low back pain. Eur Spine J. 2006;15(Suppl 2):S192–300.
39. Jegan NR, Brugger M, Viniol A, Strauch K, Barth J, Baum E, Leonhardt C, Becker A. Psychological risk and protective factors for disability in chronic low back pain - a longitudinal analysis in primary care. BMC Musculoskelet Disord. 2017;18(1):114.
40. Vargas-Prada S, Martinez JM, Coggon D, Delclos G, Benavides FG, Serra C. Health beliefs, low mood, and somatising tendency: contribution to incidence and persistence of musculoskeletal pain with and without reported disability. Scand J Work Environ Health. 2013;39(6):589–98.
41. Palmer KT, Calnan M, Wainwright D, Poole J, O'Neill C, Winterbottom A, Watkins C, Coggon D. Disabling musculoskeletal pain and its relation to somatization: a community-based postal survey. Occupational medicine (Oxford, England). 2005;55(8):612–7.
42. Bellamy N, Buchanan WW, Goldsmith CH, Campbell J, Stitt LW. Validation study of WOMAC: a health status instrument for measuring clinically important patient relevant outcomes to antirheumatic drug therapy in patients with osteoarthritis of the hip or knee. J Rheumatol. 1988;15(12):1833–40.

24

A 12-week randomized, double-blind, placebo-controlled multicenter study of choline-stabilized orthosilicic acid in patients with symptomatic knee osteoarthritis

Piet Geusens[1,2,3*], Karel Pavelka[4], Jozef Rovensky[5], Johan Vanhoof[3], Nathalie Demeester[6], Mario Calomme[6] and Dirk Vanden Berghe[7]

Abstract

Background: The aim of this study was to assess the efficacy of choline-stabilized orthosilicic acid (ch-OSA) in patients with symptomatic knee osteoarthritis (OA).

Methods: In a multicenter, double-blind, placebo-controlled study, 211 patients with knee OA (Kellgren and Lawrence grade II or III) and moderate to moderately severe pain were randomly allocated to ch-OSA or placebo for 12 weeks. The primary outcome was the change in the WOMAC pain subscale from baseline to week 12. Secondary outcomes were changes from baseline to week 12 in WOMAC total, WOMAC stiffness, WOMAC physical function, Subject Global Assessment and levels of cartilage degradation biomarkers C-terminal telopeptide of collagen type II (CTX-II) and cartilage oligomeric matrix protein (COMP). Pre-specified subgroup analyses included the effect of gender.

Results: A total of 166 (120 women, 46 men) patients were included in the analysis (87 and 79 in the ch-OSA and placebo group, respectively). In the total study population, no differences were observed between the two treatment groups for the different outcomes but significant treatment x gender interactions were found. In men taking ch-OSA, a significant improvement in WOMAC total, WOMAC stiffness and WOMAC physical function as well as a lower increase in biomarker levels of cartilage degradation was observed, but not in women. The change in WOMAC pain showed a similar positive trend in men taking ch-OSA.

Conclusion: After 12 weeks of treatment, no effect was found of ch-OSA in the total study population on clinical parameters and biomarkers, but a gender interaction was observed. In men, ch-OSA was found effective in reducing symptoms of knee OA, which was associated with a slight but significant reduction of biomarkers that are related to cartilage degradation.

Keywords: Osteoarthritis, Knee, Choline-stabilized orthosilicic acid, WOMAC, Cartilage degradation marker, Silicon, Choline

* Correspondence: drpgeusens@gmail.com
[1]Biomedical Research Institute (BIOMED), Hasselt University, Diepenbeek, Belgium
[2]Rheumatology, Maastricht UMC, Maastricht, The Netherlands
Full list of author information is available at the end of the article

Background

Osteoarthritis (OA) is one of the leading causes of functional disability and compromised quality of life in the elderly worldwide [1]. It is a chronic and slowly progressive disease, with the knee being the most affected weight-bearing joint [2, 3]. OA is a complex disease of joints, characterised by degradation of articular cartilage, changes of the subchondral bone and inflammation, leading to pain and stiffness in the joint [4, 5]. At present, there are no safe OA therapeutic strategies approved that result in a concurrent structural modification and symptom improvement [6, 7]. The treatment of OA is therefore, besides exercise and physiotherapy, still mainly based on analgesics, non-steroidal anti-inflammatory drugs (NSAIDs) and surgical procedures [8].

Several risk factors for the development of knee OA have been identified, including age, obesity, injury and genetic profiles. Sex differences in knee OA incidence and prevalence have been reported as well, with females generally at higher risk [7, 9]. Moreover, the meta-analysis performed by Srikanth et al. demonstrated that women tend to have more severe knee OA, particularly after menopausal age [9].

Given the limitations of plain radiography and the high charges for magnetic resonance imaging (MRI), biochemical markers have gained considerable interest over the past 15 years [10, 11]. However, in contrast to the well-established biochemical markers for bone diseases, the value of biomarkers in OA still needs further elucidation [12]. To this respect, Bauer et al. proposed the BIPED – burden of disease, investigative, prognostic, efficacy of intervention and diagnostic – categories, providing a classification system for biochemical markers [13]. Among numerous candidates, C-terminal telopeptide of collagen type II (CTX-II) and cartilage oligomeric matrix protein (COMP), which are two markers of cartilage degradation, have been reported to be the best performing biochemical markers across all BIPED categories [11].

Choline-stabilized orthosilicic acid (ch-OSA) is a specific complex of orthosilicic acid and choline that has been previously demonstrated to stimulate collagen synthesis which positively affects bone turnover [14] as well as surface and mechanical properties of the skin [15]. The choline component of ch-OSA was suggested to contribute to this effect [14], as it lowers plasma homocysteine levels [16]. More specifically, hyperhomocysteinemia has been shown to interfere with collagen cross-linking, leading to connective tissue pathology [17]. To this respect, it may be hypothesized that ch-OSA acts on both cartilage and subchondral bone, consequently rendering it a candidate for the treatment of OA. The aim of this study was to evaluate the symptomatic effects of the oral intake of ch-OSA on knee OA over a 12-week period. Additionally, CTX-II and COMP were analysed to assess the influence of ch-OSA on cartilage degradation.

Methods

A 12-week, international, multicenter, double-blind, randomized, parallel-group, placebo-controlled single-joint study in outpatients with symptomatic knee OA was performed. Participants were recruited either directly from the investigation centres (situated in Belgium (Reuma*Clinic*, Genk and Diagnosecentrum, Lommel; both private hospitals in co-operation with Biomedical Research Institute, Hasselt University, Hasselt, Belgium and Rheumatology, Maastricht UMC, Maastricht, The Netherlands), Slovakia (National Institute of Rheumatic Diseases, Piestany; public hospital) and Czech Republic (Institute of Rheumatology, Prague; public hospital) or following pre-screening by general practitioners (Belgium).

Patients

Potential participants were initially assessed during a screening visit. The inclusion criteria defined eligible patients as men and women between 50 and 75 years of age with a diagnosis of primary knee OA according to the American College of Rheumatology criteria [18] for at least 12 weeks prior to randomization i.e. knee pain plus at least three of the following characteristics: > 50 years, < 30 min of morning stiffness, crepitus on active motion, bony tenderness, bony enlargement, no palpable warmth of the synovium. Additional inclusion criteria comprised a radiographic confirmed Kellgren and Lawrence grade II or III (mild to moderate osteophytes and joint space narrowing) in the previous 6 months [19]; a knee OA pain intensity score, assessed by the question "How would you describe your maximum OA knee pain when not taking analgesic medications in the 24 h prior to this visit", of "moderate (2)" or "moderately severe (3)" on a 5-point Likert Scale; a Western Ontario and McMaster University OA Index (WOMAC) physical function subscale score > 0 on a 100 mm horizontal visual analogue scale (VAS) [20]. In case both knees were affected, the knee with the highest pain score was selected as the target knee. In order to avoid interference with the subject's pain perception, the use of paracetamol within a 48 h period prior to the screening visit was not allowed.

The major exclusion criteria were the following: secondary OA of the target knee; morning stiffness of ≥ 30 min; a swollen or warm joint suspected to be secondary to gout, pseudo gout or sepsis; significant injury in the target joint within 6 months before the start of the trial; arthroplasty and joint surgery of the target knee within 2 years prior to the start of the study. Additionally, specified previous medications led to exclusion from the trial.

Following a wash-out period during which the use of pain medication and OA-related treatments were not allowed, eligible subjects were scheduled for a baseline visit. The duration of the wash-out period was at least five drug half-lives of the corresponding drug, or as described in the exclusion criteria.

Design, randomisation and blinding

At the baseline visit, patients were randomly assigned to take a capsule of either ch-OSA (520 mg ch-OSA beadlets containing 5 mg of silicon and 100 mg of choline; Bio Minerals N.V., Belgium) or placebo (520 mg microcrystalline cellulose beadlets; Pharmatrans Sanaq AG, Switzerland) twice daily by oral route for 12 weeks. The treatment allocation occurred sequentially in a 1:1 ratio using a randomization list, which was generated by an independent statistician in R (software version 2.10.1 for Windows; The R Foundation for Statistical Computing, Vienna, Austria). More specifically, block randomization was stratified by site, applying randomly selected block sizes of 2 or 4. The individual code was kept in a sealed envelope by the investigator to be opened only in case of medical emergency.

Patients were assessed by the investigator at baseline and at 2, 6 and 12 weeks after randomization. At the first three visits, the study dietary supplement was delivered in bottles labelled with the subject's randomization number (according to the allocation sequence) and the instructions to take one capsule in the morning and another in the evening with a glass of water or juice. Blinding among subjects, investigators and monitors was maintained by providing identical packaging, appearance, taste and odour for ch-OSA and placebo capsules, respectively. Treatment compliance was verified at subsequent visits by counting the number of unused doses. In this respect, the limit for an acceptable compliance was set at 75%.

Pain medication and OA-related treatments were not allowed throughout the trial. However, subjects were allowed to take up to 2 g of paracetamol per day as rescue medication in case of intolerable pain, except during a 48 h period before each evaluation.

Assessments and outcome measures

At each visit, allocated patients were requested to complete a 100 mm horizontal VAS WOMAC questionnaire based on symptoms in the target knee in the preceding 48 h. This 24-item questionnaire resulted in a total WOMAC score and three WOMAC subscores, based on the following subscales: pain (5 questions), stiffness (2 questions) and physical function (17 questions). For each WOMAC score, a 0–100 mm range was generated by averaging across the respective items, with lower scores indicating better outcomes. The Subject Global Assessment was evaluated on a 100 mm horizontal VAS as well (0–100 mm range), by asking the following question: "Considering all the ways your knee OA affects you, how are you doing today?". Finally, fasting serum and second void urine were collected at the baseline and final visit to assess biochemical markers of cartilage degradation (urine, serum), baseline serum estradiol and serum silicon concentration. For the collection of serum, silicon free polypropylene syringes (Sarstedt, Germany) and needles (Microlance, Becton Dickinson, Spain) were used as published elsewhere [15]. Aliquots of both samples were stored at −20 °C until analysis. More specifically, urinary CTX-II concentrations were determined using the Urine CartiLaps EIA from IDS (Boldon, UK). These concentrations were corrected for urinary creatinine concentrations, which were determined with a creatinine assay (R&D Systems, Abingdon, UK). Serum COMP levels were measured using AnaMar Medical's (Lund, Sweden) COMP ELISA. Serum Estradiol levels were measured with Estradiol III electrochemiluminescense immunoassay from Roche (Mannheim, Germany). All analyses were performed according to the manufacturers' protocols. Serum silicon concentration was measured using electrothermal atomic absorption spectrometry with inverse longitudinal Zeeman background correction (AAnalyst 800, Perkin Elmer, Bodenseewerk, Germany) and the analytical features (temperature program, matrix modifier, sample preparation method) were published elsewhere [15].

The primary outcome measure was the change in the WOMAC pain subscale from baseline to week 12. Secondary outcome measures included the changes from baseline to 12 weeks in the total WOMAC score, the WOMAC stiffness subscale, the WOMAC physical function subscale, the Subject Global Assessment and CTX-II and COMP levels.

Statistical analysis

The sample size calculation estimated that a group size of 100 subjects was necessary to ensure at least 80% power to detect differences of 16% between the ch-OSA and placebo group with respect to pain and physical function (quantified according to the WOMAC pain and function subscale, assuming a relative standard deviation of 40% (based on data of 13 studies; Additional file 2: Table S2)), considering a dropout rate of 10% and a 0.05 two-sided significance level.

Statistical analyses were performed using the per-protocol population, defined as all randomized patients meeting the inclusion criteria, who completed the trial and who did not have major protocol violations. Results are presented as mean ± standard deviation (SD).

For WOMAC total, WOMAC subscales and Subject Global Assessment scores, a repeated measures (RM) univariate analysis of covariance (ANCOVA) model was applied in which the baseline value was treated as a covariate while treatment and gender were treated as fixed factors. Between and within treatment differences were assessed and the models also included interaction terms between treatment and gender. Differences in serum silicon and biomarker values (baseline versus final visit) were analysed between and within treatments using RM analysis of variance (ANOVA), albeit after removal of outliers. These outliers were identified using the median absolute deviation and a critical value of 4.5 [21]. In case of a significant interaction between time and treatment, post hoc t-tests with Bonferroni correction were performed.

Additionally, as specified in the study protocol, subgroup analyses by gender were performed for all outcome measures. Due to the smaller group sizes, non-parametric tests were used. More specifically, differences between treatment groups were analysed with Mann-Whitney U, whereas differences within treatment groups were analysed using Friedman's test with post hoc Bonferroni-corrected Wilcoxon signed-ranks. Correlation of serum silicon with clinical parameters was analysed in subgroups with the Spearman rank correlation test.

Significance levels were set at $P < 0.05$ (two-sided), except for interaction tests ($P < 0.10$) [22]. All statistical analyses were performed using SPSS software (version 21.0 for Windows, IBM Corp., Armonk, NY, USA).

Results

Patients

Between June 2010 and April 2012, a total of 211 eligible subjects were randomized and allocated to receive ch-OSA ($n = 106$) or a placebo ($n = 105$). As demonstrated in Fig. 1, 166 patients were ultimately included in the per-protocol analysis. Demographic variables, baseline disease characteristics and baseline outcome measures were similar in both groups (Table 1). Mean age of the randomized patients was 61.9 ± 7.1 years with a majority of postmenopausal women. The mean baseline serum level of estradiol was significantly ($P < 0.0005$) lower in women compared to men (Table 1). Baseline CTX-II levels showed a higher trend ($P = 0.1$) in women compared to men (Table 1).

Compliance and safety

Compliance throughout the study was excellent as 98% of the patients reached the minimum compliance of 75%. Overall, the mean compliance was 106 ± 12% in the per-protocol population and > 100% both in men and women. No adverse events related to the treatment were reported in either treatment group.

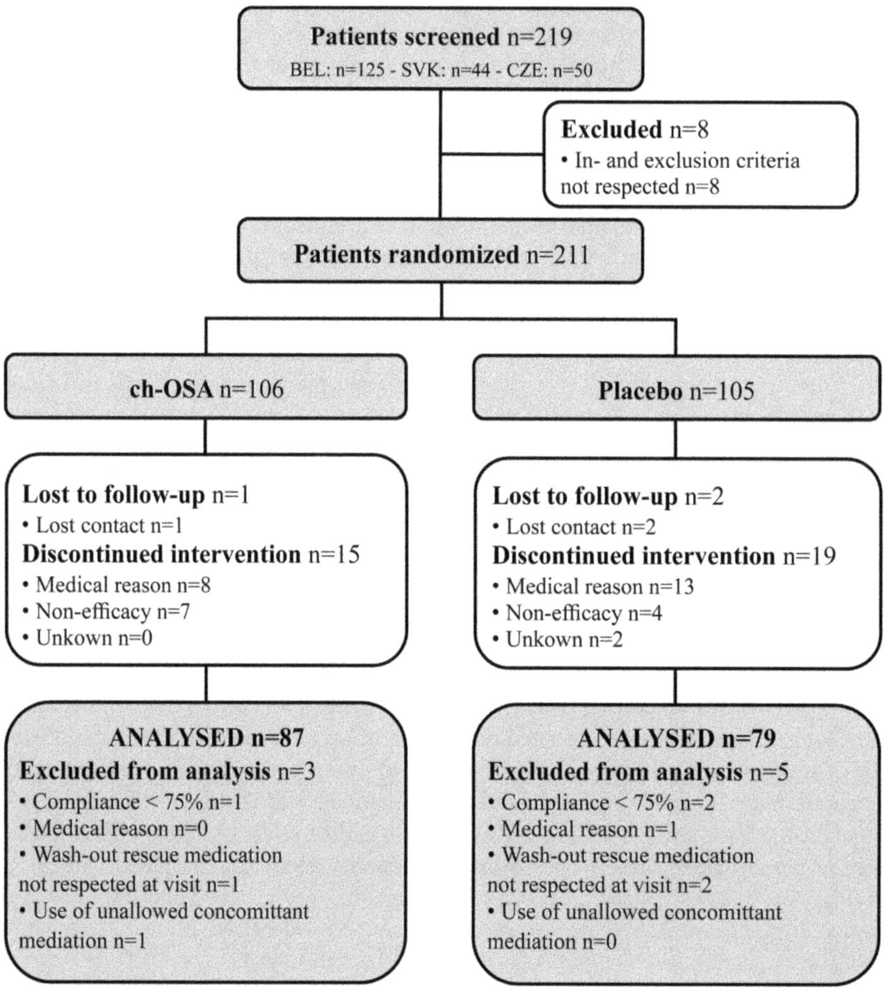

Fig. 1 Flow diagram of study enrolment, allocation, follow-up and analysis

Table 1 Baseline characteristics of the study population by treatment group and gender

Characteristic	Placebo ($n = 79$)	ch-OSA ($n = 87$)	Male ($n = 46$)	Female ($n = 120$)
Age (years)	62.2 ± 7.7	61.7 ± 6.5	61.0 ± 7.2	62.3 ± 7.0
Women	55 (69.6)	65 (74.7)	0	120 (100)
Body mass index (kg/m^2)	29.5 ± 5.2	29.5 ± 5.4	29.1 ± 4.7	29.6 ± 5.6
Menopausal Status	1 pre (1.5)	1 pre (1.8)	-	2 pre (1.7)
	0 peri (1.5)	1 peri		1 peri (0.8)
	54 post (98.2)	63 post (96.9)		117 post (97.5)
Kellgren and Lawrence grade II	48 (60.8)	59 (67.8)	26 (56.5)	81 (67.5)
Kellgren and Lawrence grade III	31 (39.2)	28 (32.2)	20 (43.5)	39 (32.5)
Likert pain score 2	38 (48.1)	32 (36.8)	19 (41.3)	51 (42.5)
Likert pain score 3	41 (51.9)	55 (63.2)	27 (58.7)	69 (57.5)
WOMAC Total (/100 mm)	43.1 ± 20.3	40.9 ± 19.4	42.2 ± 21.5	41.9 ± 19.2
WOMAC Pain (/100 mm)	41.2 ± 20.3	38.2 ± 19.8	41.9 ± 20.9	38.7 ± 19.7
WOMAC Stiffness (/100 mm)	45.3 ± 24.6	44.0 ± 23.5	44.9 ± 23.4	44.5 ± 24.3
WOMAC Function (/100 mm)	43.4 ± 21.2	41.4 ± 19.8	42.0 ± 22.5	42.5 ± 19.7
Subject Global Assessment (/100 mm)	49.4 ± 21.8	50.1 ± 18.2	51.3 ± 22.4	49.2 ± 19.0
CTX-II/Creatinine (ng/mmol)	413.1 ± 189.6	430.4 ± 212.7	378.5 ± 162.8	441.0 ± 213.9
COMP (U/L)	10.8 ± 2.8	10.7 ± 2.8	11.0 ± 2.8	10.6 ± 2.8
Estradiol (ng/L)	-	-	35.5 ± 31.0	22.0 ± 36.2 [a]

Data expressed as mean ± SD or n (%);-: not applicable; [a] significant difference between groups (men versus women); Number of patients without outliers for CTX-II: Placebo ($n = 66$), ch-OSA ($n = 68$); Number of patients without outliers for COMP: Placebo ($n = 74$), ch-OSA ($n = 80$)

Efficacy

The primary and secondary outcome measures are shown in Table 2, along with the absolute values of the assessed clinical outcome measures at the different visits. After 12 weeks of treatment, the change from baseline in silicon serum levels was significantly higher in the ch-OSA group compared to the placebo group (Table 2). The statistical analyses demonstrated no significant differences between the two treatment groups with respect to the primary and secondary outcome measures. Nevertheless, significant treatment x gender interactions were found for all clinical outcomes (ANCOVA).

Subsequently, pre-specified subgroup analyses by gender were performed. Table 3 provides an overview of the assessed parameters in men and women in the placebo and ch-OSA group, respectively. There was a superior effect of ch-OSA in men after 12 weeks of treatment as the mean changes from baseline in WOMAC total, WOMAC stiffness and WOMAC physical function were significantly higher with ch-OSA compared to placebo (Fig. 2). The corresponding mean differences (95% CI) between placebo and ch-OSA in men were the following: WOMAC total 11.0 mm (0.1 to 21.9), WOMAC stiffness 16.5 mm (3.0 to 30.0) and WOMAC physical function 10.6 mm (−0.5 to 21.6). A similar, yet non-significant trend was observed for WOMAC pain and Subject Global Assessment: 10.2 mm (−1.7 to 22.1) and 8.4 mm (−5.5 to 22.3), respectively. As shown in Fig. 3, increases in biomarkers of cartilage degradation (CTX-II and COMP) were significantly lower after 12 weeks in the male ch-OSA group, resulting in the following mean differences (95% CI) between placebo and ch-OSA: CTX-II 102.0 ng/mmol (12.6 to 191.4) (Fig. 3a) and COMP 2.1 U/L (0.3 to 3.9) (Fig. 3b). The statistical analysis of the female subgroups, on the other hand, demonstrated no significant treatment differences (data not shown). Similar as in the total study population, the change from baseline in silicon serum levels was significantly higher in the ch-OSA group compared to the placebo group for both women and men. The following observed mean differences (95% CI) between placebo and ch-OSA were observed: men, 26.1 μg/L (3.15 to 49.4) and women, 46.0 μg/L (27.0 to 65.0). No significant correlations were found between clinical parameters and serum silicon in neither women nor men (data not shown).

Discussion

This is the first clinical study to evaluate the symptom relief effect of ch-OSA in patients with knee OA. Although the intake of the dietary supplement for 12 weeks failed to show a statistically significant benefit over placebo regarding the clinical outcome scores and biomarker values in the per-protocol population, pre-specified subgroup analyses demonstrated a significant effect of ch-OSA in men. Accordingly, WOMAC total, stiffness and physical function scores were significantly reduced in men taking ch-OSA compared to men in the placebo group. While

Table 2 Overview of the primary and secondary outcome measures and the absolute clinical outcome scores at baseline, week 2, week 6 and week 12 in the placebo and choline-stabilized orthosilicic acid (ch-OSA) group

	Placebo ($n = 79$)					ch-OSA ($n = 87$)					Treatment difference at 12 weeks (95% CI)	*P* value	*P* value treatment x gender interaction
	Baseline (mean ± SD)	Week 2 (mean ± SD)	Week 6 (mean ± SD)	Week 12 (mean ± SD)	Change week 12 – baseline (mean ± SD)	Baseline (mean ± SD)	Week 2 (mean ± SD)	Week 6 (mean ± SD)	Week 12 (mean ± SD)	Change week 12 – baseline (mean ± SD)			
WOMAC total score (/100 mm)	43.1 ± 20.3	39.1 ± 21.3	32.7 ± 21.2	32.3 ± 23.9	−10.8 ± 20.5	40.9 ± 19.4	37.3 ± 20.9	29.5 ± 21.5	29.3 ± 22.9	−11.6 ± 15.8	0.8 (−4.8 to 6.4)	0.78	0.06
WOMAC pain score (/100 mm)	41.2 ± 20.3	36.6 ± 21.1	30.3 ± 21.1	29.7 ± 23.9	−11.5 ± 22.1	38.2 ± 19.8	34.7 ± 21.4	27.7 ± 21.8	26.1 ± 22.2	−12.1 ± 17.5	0.6 (−5.5 to 6.7)	0.85	0.07
WOMAC stiffness score (/100 mm)	45.3 ± 24.6	39.7 ± 24.3	32.7 ± 23.4	34.0 ± 25.0	−11.3 ± 24.2	44.0 ± 23.5	38.8 ± 23.1	30.5 ± 22.8	30.0 ± 24.9	−14.0 ± 19.5	2.7 (−4.0 to 9.4)	0.43	0.04
WOMAC function score (/100 mm)	43.4 ± 21.2	39.8 ± 21.8	33.4 ± 21.8	32.9 ± 24.3	−10.6 ± 20.8	41.4 ± 19.8	37.9 ± 21.2	29.9 ± 21.8	30.2 ± 23.6	−11.2 ± 16.5	0.6 (−5.1 to 6.3)	0.84	0.09
Subject Global Assessment (/100 mm)	49.4 ± 21.8	39.0 ± 19.9	33.4 ± 20.7	32.5 ± 22.7	−16.9 ± 24.3	50.1 ± 18.2	41.2 ± 22.4	33.5 ± 24.4	32.1 ± 24.5	−18.0 ± 22.7	1.2 (−6.0 to 8.4)	0.75	0.05
CTX-II/Creatinine (ng/mmol)	413.1 ± 189.6	-	-	528.0[a] ± 261.8	114.9 ± 174.7	430.4 ± 212.7	-	-	533.6[a] ± 263.2	103.2 ± 178.6	11.7 (−48.7 to 72.1)	0.70	-
COMP (U/L)	10.8 ± 2.8	-	-	11.3 ± 3.4	0.6 ± 2.9	10.7 ± 2.8	-	-	11.1 ± 2.8	0.4 ± 2.6	0.1 (−0.7 to 1.0)	0.75	-
Silicon (μg/L)	50.9 ± 33.6	-	-	65.4[a] ± 42.2	14.6 ± 40.9	59.9 ± 36.1	-	-	115.8 [a, b] ± 56.0	55.8 ± 52.1	41.2 (25.8 to 56.8)	0.0005	-

[a]significant difference from baseline within the group; [b]significant difference between groups (placebo versus ch-OSA); -: not applicable; Number of patients without outliers for CTX-II: placebo ($n = 66$), ch-OSA ($n = 68$); Number of patients without outliers for COMP: placebo ($n = 74$), ch-OSA ($n = 80$); Number of patients without outliers for Silicon: placebo ($n = 69$), ch-OSA ($n = 75$)

levels of cartilage degradation related biomarkers increased over 12 weeks in men in the placebo group and in women in both groups, these levels were significantly lower in the male ch-OSA group at the final visit. More specifically, the increase in CTX-II was less pronounced and COMP levels remained unchanged. The former suggests that ch-OSA can slow the ongoing progression of cartilage degradation in men.

The management of knee OA remains a major challenge. The key objective is to cease or delay disease progression by controlling cartilage degradation, inflammation and changes of subchondral bone. Nevertheless, most published recommendations primarily aim to control OA symptoms since safe and effective disease-modifying OA drugs (DMOADs) are currently lacking [23–26]. NSAIDs, for instance, are still among the most commonly used medicines to relieve OA pain, regardless of their well-known side-effects in prolonged therapy [24, 27]. The rationale for studying the effectiveness of ch-OSA in knee OA was consequently based on its previously demonstrated effect on collagen synthesis and its safety in long-term use [14, 15]. The components of ch-OSA, choline and orthosilicic acid (OSA), have both been mentioned with respect to collagen metabolism. Firstly, choline lowers plasma homocysteine levels through its precursor-function in the biochemical conversion of homocysteine to methionine [16]. This reduction positively affects collagen cross-linking, since homocysteine has been shown to interfere with post-translational modifications of collagen through direct and indirect inhibition of lysyl oxidase as well as through down regulation of other genes involved in collagen cross-linking [28]. Indeed, Zhang et al. recently reported elevated serum homocysteine levels in patients with severe OA compared to those with mild OA or healthy controls [29]. Secondly, although the exact role of silicon in bone and connective tissue health remains unclear, its involvement in collagen synthesis and/or stabilisation was recently put forward by Jugdaohsingh et al. [30]. In the present study, the lack of correlation between the change in serum silicon and clinical parameters in men taking ch-OSA, suggests that the effect of ch-OSA cannot be explained as an effect of silicon only. ch-OSA was previously shown to have a positive effect on markers of bone formation, with a significant increase of procollagen type I N-terminal propeptide (PINP) in osteopenic women following a supplementation period of 12 months [14]. In an animal model for postmenopausal osteoporosis, it was demonstrated that ch-OSA partially prevented femoral bone loss [31].

The former supports the hypothesis of a possible effect of ch-OSA on collagen in both cartilage and subchondral bone and consequently on knee OA, particularly in view of increasing evidence of a close interrelationship between subchondral bone and articular cartilage [32, 33]. A positive effect of ch-OSA was indeed confirmed in the present study, already after 12 weeks of treatment, yet only in men. Several hypotheses can be suggested with respect to this gender difference. In general, women report more pain and disability from knee OA [34, 35]. The perception of pain, however, has been demonstrated to depend on the estrogen state. In fact, a low estrogen state was found to be related to hyperalgesia [36]. Consequently, the possibility that the enhanced pain

Table 3 Gender-specific subgroups: Overview of the absolute clinical outcome scores and biomarker values at baseline, week 2, week 6 and week 12 in the placebo and choline-stabilized orthosilicic acid (ch-OSA) group

	Placebo (n = 79)							
	Male (n = 24)				Female (n = 55)			
	Baseline (mean ± SD)	Week 2 (mean ± SD)	Week 6 (mean ± SD)	Week 12 (mean ± SD)	Baseline (mean ± SD)	Week 2 (mean ± SD)	Week 6 (mean ± SD)	Week 12 (mean ± SD)
WOMAC total score (/100 mm)	42.0 ± 22.4	37.5^{a} ± 26.2	34.1^{a} ± 24.3	34.7 ± 30.7	43.6 ± 19.6	39.8 ± 19.0	32.1$^{a, b}$ ± 19.9	31.2 ^{a} ± 20.5
WOMAC pain score (/100 mm)	42.5 ± 22.7	35.1^{a} ± 24.5	32.6^{a} ± 24.0	33.0 ± 31.2	40.6 ± 19.4	37.2 ± 19.7	29.3$^{a, b}$ ± 19.8	28.2 ^{a} ± 20.1
WOMAC stiffness score (/100 mm)	43.8 ± 25.3	40.0 ± 27.3	33.5 ± 26.4	38.2 ± 29.6	45.9 ± 24.5	39.5^{a} ± 23.2	32.4$^{a, b}$ ± 22.2	32.2 ^{a} ± 22.8
WOMAC function score (/100 mm)	41.7 ± 23.3	37.9 ± 27.3	34.6 ± 25.2	34.9 ± 31.0	45.9 ± 24.5	39.5 ± 23.2	32.4$^{a, b}$ ± 22.2	32.2 ^{a} ± 22.8
Subject Global Assessment (/100 mm)	51.1 ± 26.0	41.7 ± 22.4	33.3 ^{a} ± 23.4	33.8^{a} ± 24.3	48.6 ± 19.9	37.9^{a} ± 18.8	33.5$^{a, b}$ ± 19.7	32.0 ^{a} ± 22.2
CTX-II/Creatinine (ng/mmol)	389.8 ± 178.0	-	-	565.2^{a} ± 267.8	425.6 ± 196.5	-	-	508.1^{a} ± 259.5
COMP (U/L)	11.1 ± 3.0	-	-	13.0^{a} ± 3.6	10.6 ± 2.7	-	-	10.6 ± 3.2
Silicon (μg/L)	54.4 ± 28.1	-	-	59.2 ± 36.0	49.5 ± 35.6			67.8 ^{a} ± 44.4

[a]significant difference from baseline within the group; [b] significant difference from week 2 within the group; [c] significant difference between groups (placebo versus ch-OSA); -: not applicable; Number of patients without outliers for CTX-II: placebo males (n = 23), placebo females (n = 43), ch-OSA males (n = 18), ch-OSA females (n = 50); Number of patients without outliers for COMP: placebo males (n = 22), placebo females (n = 52), ch-OSA males (n = 21), ch-OSA females (n = 59); Number of patients without outliers for Silicon: placebo males (n = 19), placebo females (n = 50), ch-OSA males (n = 19), ch-OSA females (n = 56)

Table 3 Gender-specific subgroups: Overview of the absolute clinical outcome scores and biomarker values at baseline, week 2, week 6 and week 12 in the placebo and choline-stabilized orthosilicic acid (ch-OSA) group *(Continued)*

	ch-OSA (*n* = 87)							
	Male (*n* = 22)				Female (*n* = 65)			
	Baseline (mean ± SD)	Week 2 (mean ± SD)	Week 6 (mean ± SD)	Week 12 (mean ± SD)	Baseline (mean ± SD)	Week 2 (mean ± SD)	Week 6 (mean ± SD)	Week 12 (mean ± SD)
WOMAC total score (/100 mm)	42.5 ± 20.9	36.1[a] ± 22.1	26.8[a] ± 22.8	24.2[a] ± 21.3	40.4 ± 19.0	37.7 ± 20.7	30.4[a, b] ± 21.2	31.1[a] ± 23.4
WOMAC pain score (/100 mm)	41.3 ± 19.3	32.2[a] ± 20.0	24.3[a] ± 21.5	21.6[a] ± 19.6	37.1 ± 20.0	35.5 ± 21.9	28.8[a, b] ± 22.0	27.6[a] ± 22.9
WOMAC stiffness score (/100 mm)	46.2 ± 21.8	37.2[a] ± 25.3	28.8[a] ± 23.8	24.1[a] ± 23.4	43.3 ± 24.1	39.4 ± 22.5	31.1[a, b] ± 22.6	32.0[a] ± 25.3
WOMAC function score (/100 mm)	42.4 ± 22.2	27.1 ± 22.9	27.3[a] ± 23.5	25.0[a] ± 22.3	43.3 ± 24.1	39.4 ± 22.5	31.1[a, b] ± 22.6	32.0[a] ± 25.3
Subject Global Assessment (/100 mm)	51.5 ± 18.3	36.6[a] ± 20.9	24.6[a, b] ± 20.8	25.8 [a] ± 23.7	49.6 ± 18.3	42.7[a] ± 22.8	36.5[a, b] ± 24.9	34.2[a] ± 24.6
CTX-II/Creatinine (ng/mmol)	364.0 ± 144.7	-	-	437.4[a] ± 171.8	454.3 ± 229.0	-	-	568.3[a] ± 282.6
COMP (U/L)	10.9 ± 2.7	-	-	10.6 ± 2.7	10.6 ± 2.9	-	-	11.3[a] ± 2.8
Silicon (µg/L)	68.4 ± 38.0	-	-	99.3[a, c] ± 42.7	57.0 ± 35.3	-	-	121.3[a, c] ± 59.1

perception masked the effect of ch-OSA in women in the present study cannot be ruled out given the predominance of postmenopausal women (98%) with low endogenous estrogen levels, of which only 7% was on hormone replacement therapy (HRT), a contraceptive, a selective estrogen receptor modulator (SERM) or phytoestrogens. In fact, the mean serum estradiol level of women in the present study was significantly lower compared to that of the male study population.

Besides the fact that postmenopausal women have a different pain perception than man, it has also been confirmed that the severity of knee OA is higher in women as well, and principally in postmenopausal women [9, 37]. Accordingly, urinary CTX-II levels were found to be significantly higher in postmenopausal women than in men [38]. The latter is in correspondence with the trend towards higher baseline CTX-II concentrations observed in – predominantly postmenopausal – women in the present study. Again, decreased estrogen levels might be of importance. Several in vitro, in vivo, genetic and clinical studies indeed designate a potential protective role for estrogens against the development of OA, given the various actions of estrogen on articular tissues [39]. Additionally, considerable experimental models indicate that estrogen deficiency-related increases in bone turnover contribute to the progression of OA [40, 41]. Therefore, in view of the more severe OA forms in women, it can be suggested that the 12-week supplementation period could have been insufficient to result in a clinical benefit.

Given the apparent extensive involvement of estrogen deficiency in the development and progression of knee OA, the use of HRTs or SERMs in women seems plausible. Nevertheless, it has been concluded that the health risks of HRTs may outweigh the potential benefits and that HRTs

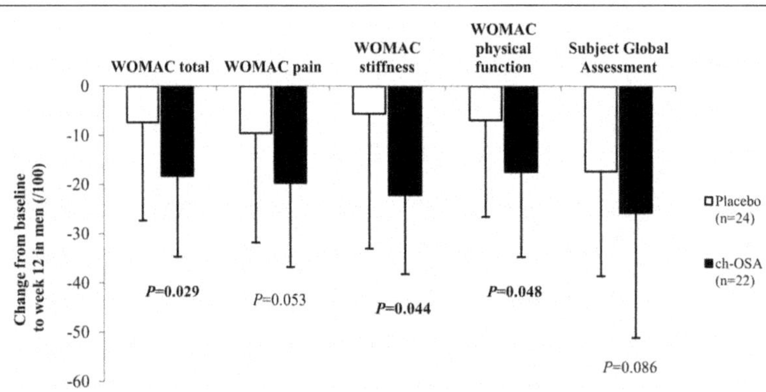

Fig. 2 Mean change (± SD) from baseline to week 12 in WOMAC total, WOMAC pain, WOMAC stiffness, WOMAC physical function and Subject Global Assessment in men. *P* values refer to differences between placebo and choline-stabilized orthosilicic acid (ch-OSA)

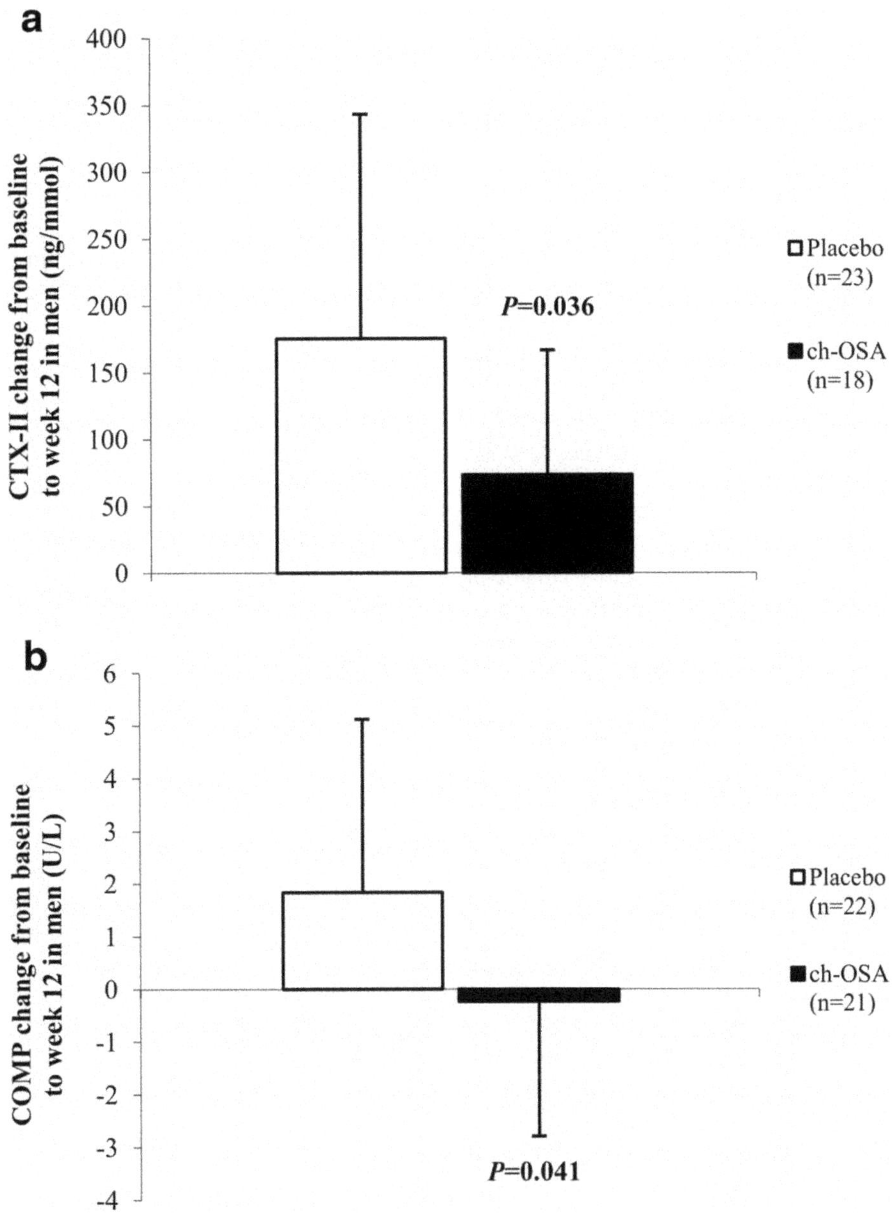

Fig. 3 Mean change (± SD) from baseline to week 12 in CTX-II (**a**) and COMP (**b**) levels in men. *P* values refer to differences between placebo and choline-stabilized orthosilicic acid (ch-OSA)

and SERMs should not be recommended as first-line treatments for OA [42, 43]. Several other pharmacological therapies have been studied with respect to knee OA, including symptomatic slow-acting drugs for OA (SYSADOAs) like glucosamine sulphate, chondroitin sulphate, hyaluronic acid and diacerein. Due to the frequently inconsistent conclusions of these studies, the appropriateness of the former therapies has been recently designated as uncertain [26]. Furthermore, therapeutic approaches that target subchondral bone resorption and/or formation have gained attention [32, 43]. Bisphosphonates, strontium ranelate and calcitonin have been studied in this context, yet none of these treatments has been approved as a DMOAD since evidence of concomitant structural and symptomatic effects is still pending [6, 26]. Additionally, safety issues are of importance, such as the risk of cardiovascular events associated with strontium ranelate [44]. The safety of ch-OSA in prolonged therapy, on the other hand, has been previously demonstrated [45].

Although the relevance of biochemical markers in OA has not yet been proven to be of definite clinical importance, Lotz et al. described their value as secondary outcomes [12]. More specifically, effects on biomarkers can support the primary outcome and provide evidence of pharmacodynamics and mechanisms of action of OA drugs. This is indeed valid in the present study, given that the trend observed for the primary outcome (WOMAC pain) in ch-OSA-treated men was associated with significantly lower biomarker levels, the latter referring to decreased cartilage degradation.

The present study has a number of limitations. Firstly, the evaluation of the magnitude of pain changes is ambiguous. This is related to the relatively high placebo effect – which is however common in OA trials – on the one hand, and to the complicated interpretation of changes evaluated as means rather than individual improvements, on the other hand [46]. Furthermore, the dropout rate was higher than assumed in the sample size calculation (18% in contrast to the postulated 10%), which negatively affected the statistical power in the subgroup analyses, particularly in the male subgroups.

In conclusion, this randomized, placebo-controlled trial provided a first indication of a potential benefit of ch-OSA in the treatment of knee OA in men, particularly in view of the need for a safe long-term treatment. Future research is however needed to further elucidate the observed effects and gender difference since no benefit was found in women. Considering the hypothesis that the 12-week supplementation period may have been insufficient in women, an extension of the treatment duration to at least 6 months would be valuable [47]. Additionally, the inclusion of younger, premenopausal women could, at least in part, contribute to the clarification of the role of estrogen in OA. The potential disease-modifying effects of ch-OSA at the level of the knee, on the other hand, could be evaluated after a prolonged treatment period using reliable and sensitive imaging technologies, such as MRI or high-resolution peripheral quantitative computed tomography (HRpQCT) [43, 48]. Determination of biochemical markers of bone metabolism could also extend the knowledge on the mechanisms of action of ch-OSA. Finally, application of the former research suggestions would also contribute to the identification of different subgroups. These subgroups could then be subjected to separate statistical analyses, which could provide evidence for the further assessment of ch-OSA's potentials in view of individualized targeted treatments for knee OA.

Conclusions

Choline-stabilized orthosilicic acid did not improve symptoms of knee osteoarthritis in the total study population but a gender effect was observed. A symptomatic improvement was found in men but not in women, after 12 weeks of supplementation, which was associated with a slight but significant reduction of biomarkers which are related to cartilage degradation. In view of the need for a safe long-term therapy for the treatment of knee osteoarthritis, this study provided first evidence on the potential benefit of choline-stabilized orthosilicic acid. Future research is however needed to further elucidate the observed effects and gender difference. Considering the hypothesis that the 12-week supplementation period may have been insufficient in women, an extension of the treatment duration to at least 6 months would be valuable.

Abbreviations

ANCOVA: Univariate analysis of covariance; BIPED: Burden of disease, investigative, prognostic, efficacy of intervention and diagnostics; ch-OSA: choline-stabilized orthosilicic acid; COMP: Cartilage oligomeric matrix protein; CTX-II: C-terminal telopeptide of collagen type II; DMOADs: Disease-modifying osteoarthritis drugs; ELISA: Enzyme-linked immuno sorbent assay; HRpQCT: High-resolution peripheral quantitative computed tomography; HRT: Hormone replacement therapy; MRI: Magnetic resonance imaging; NSAIDs: Non-steroidal anti-inflammatory drugs; OA: Osteoarthritis; OSA: Orthosilicic acid; PINP: Procollagen type I N-terminal propeptide; RM: Repeated measures; SERM: Selective estrogen receptor modulator; SYSADOAs: Symptomatic slow-acting drugs for osteoarthritis; VAS: Visual analogue scale; WOMAC: Western Ontario and McMaster University osteoarthritis Index

Acknowledgements

The authors thank Veronika Sebkova, Eva Kracmarova, Marianna Provazníková, Eva Jančušková, Adéla Suchá and Marcela Kadlecová from MKS Research s.r.o. for monitoring activities and trial coordination in Slovakia and the Czech Republic; and Atlantic Bone Screen for the analysis of cartilage degradation markers. The following investigators participated in the trial: (Belgium) Marleen Coppens, Hubert Berghs, Willy Pardon, Sonja Poesen, Pascal Duysters, Jan Huysmans, Theo Vansummeren; (Slovakia) Roman Fano, Marián Kovalančík, Pavol Masaryk, Zuzana Popracová, Jozef Zvarka, Roman Stančik; (Czech Republic) Hana Jarošová, Martina Votavová, Simona Skácelová. The help of the study nurses was also appreciated by the authors: (Belgium) Luc Emonds, Carine Swinnen, Els Binnemans; (Slovakia) Gabriela Klementová; (Czech Republic) Kateřina Kohoutová.

Funding

Bio Minerals N.V. provided the study medication (ch-OSA and placebo) and funding.

Authors' contributions

Concept and study design, data interpretation, drafting and revising of the manuscript, final approval of the manuscript, agreement to be accountable for accuracy and integrity of the work: PG, KP, JR, JVH, ND, MC, DVB.

Competing interests

Dr. Geusens provides lectures, consulting advice and collaboration in clinical studies with Amgen, Eli Lilly, Merck Sharp and Dohme, Novartis, Sanofi-Aventis, Abbvie, Will, Pfizer, UCB, Bristol-Myers-Squibb, and Menarini.

Dr. Pavelka received honoraria for speaking and consultations from BMS, AbbVie, MSD, Roche, Amgen, UCB, Egis, Pfizer, IBSA, GBC.
Dr. Demeester and Dr. Calomme are employees of the study sponsor Bio Minerals N.V.

Consent for publication
Not applicable.

Author details
[1]Biomedical Research Institute (BIOMED), Hasselt University, Diepenbeek, Belgium. [2]Rheumatology, Maastricht UMC, Maastricht, The Netherlands. [3]ReumaClinic, Bretheistraat 149, Genk 3600, Belgium. [4]Institute of Rheumatology, Prague, Czech Republic. [5]Nábrežie I. Krasku 4782/4, Piešťany, Slovakia. [6]Research & Development, Bio Minerals NV, Destelbergen, Belgium. [7]Department of Pharmaceutical Sciences, University of Antwerp, Antwerp-Wilrijk, Belgium.

References
1. Woolf AD, Pfleger B. Burden of major musculoskeletal conditions. Bull World Health Organ. 2003;81:646–56.
2. Zhang W, Moskowitz RW, Nuki G, Abramson S, Altman RD, Arden N, et al. OARSI recommendations for the management of hip and knee osteoarthritis, part I: critical appraisal of existing treatment guidelines and systematic review of current research evidence. OsteoarthrCartil. 2007;15:981–1000.
3. Kraus VB, Burnett B, Coindreau J, Cottrell S, Eyre D, Gendreau M, et al. Application of biomarkers in the development of drugs intended for the treatment of osteoarthritis. Osteoarthr Cartil. 2011;19:515–42.
4. Felson DT, Lawrence RC, Dieppe PA, Hirsch R, Helmick CG, Jordan JM, et al. Osteoarthritis: new insights. Part 1: the disease and its risk factors. Ann Intern Med. 2000;133:635–46.
5. Bijlsma JW, Berenbaum F, Lafeber FP. Osteoarthritis: an update with relevance for clinical practice. Lancet. 2011;377:2115–26.
6. Lafeber FP, van Laar JM. Strontium ranelate: ready for clinical use as disease-modifying osteoarthritis drug? Ann Rheum Dis. 2013;72:157–61.
7. Losina E, Weinstein AM, Reichmann WM, Burbine SA, Solomon DH, Daigle ME, et al. Lifetime risk and age at diagnosis of symptomatic knee osteoarthritis in the US. Arthritis Care Res. 2013;65:703–11.
8. Thysen S, Luyten FP, Lories RJ. Targets, models and challenges in osteoarthritis research. Dis Model Mech. 2015;8:17–30.
9. Srikanth VK, Fryer JL, Zhai G, Winzenberg TM, Hosmer D, Jones G. A meta-analysis of sex differences prevalence, incidence and severity of osteoarthritis. Osteoarthr Cartil. 2005;13:769–81.
10. Guermazi A, Hunter DJ, Roemer FW. Plain radiography and magnetic resonance imaging diagnostics in osteoarthritis: validated staging and scoring. J Bone Joint Surg Am. 2009;91 Suppl 1:54–62.
11. van Spil WE, DeGroot J, Lems WF, Oostveen JC, Lafeber FP. Serum and urinary biochemical markers for knee and hip-osteoarthritis: a systematic review applying the consensus BIPED criteria. Osteoarthr Cartil. 2010;18:605–12.
12. Lotz M, Martel-Pelletier J, Christiansen C, Brandi ML, Bruyere O, Chapurlat R, et al. Value of biomarkers in osteoarthritis: current status and perspectives. Ann Rheum Dis. 2013;72:1756–63.
13. Bauer DC, Hunter DJ, Abramson SB, Attur M, Corr M, Felson D, et al. Classification of osteoarthritis biomarkers: a proposed approach. Osteoarthr Cartil. 2006;14:723–7.
14. Spector TD, Calomme MR, Anderson SH, Clement G, Bevan L, Demeester N, et al. Choline-stabilized orthosilicic acid supplementation as an adjunct to calcium/vitamin D3 stimulates markers of bone formation in osteopenic females: a randomized, placebo-controlled trial. BMC Musculoskelet Disord. 2008;9:85.
15. Barel A, Calomme M, Timchenko A, De Paepe K, Demeester N, Rogiers V, et al. Effect of oral intake of choline-stabilized orthosilicic acid on skin, nails and hair in women with photodamaged skin. Arch Dermatol Res. 2005;297:147–53.
16. Ueland PM. Choline and betaine in health and disease. J Inherit Metab Dis. 2011;34:3–15.
17. Toohey JI. Homocysteine toxicity in connective tissue: theories, old and new. Connect Tissue Res. 2008;49:57 61.
18. Altman R, Asch E, Bloch D, Bole G, Borenstein D, Brandt K, et al. Development of criteria for the classification and reporting of osteoarthritis. Classification of osteoarthritis of the knee. Diagnostic and Therapeutic Criteria Committee of the American Rheumatism Association. Arthritis Rheum. 1986;29:1039–49.
19. Kellgren JH, Lawrence JS. Radiological assessment of osteo-arthrosis. Ann Rheum Dis. 1957;16:494–502.
20. Bellamy N, Buchanan WW, Goldsmith CH, Campbell J, Stitt LW. Validation study of WOMAC: a health status instrument for measuring clinically important patient relevant outcomes to antirheumatic drug therapy in patients with osteoarthritis of the hip or knee. J Rheumatol. 1988;15:1833–40.
21. Leys C, Ley C, Klein O, Bernard P, Licata L. Detecting outliers: do not use standard deviation around the mean, use absolute deviation around the median. J Exp Soc Psychol. 2013;49:764–6.
22. Ziegler D, Pritchett YL, Wang F, Desaiah D, Robinson MJ, Hall JA, et al. Impact of disease characteristics on the efficacy of duloxetine in diabetic peripheral neuropathic pain. Diabetes Care. 2007;30:664–9.
23. Jordan KM, Arden NK, Doherty M, Bannwarth B, Bijlsma JW, Dieppe P, et al. EULAR Recommendations 2003: an evidence based approach to the management of knee osteoarthritis: report of a Task Force of the Standing Committee for International Clinical Studies Including Therapeutic Trials (ESCISIT). Ann Rheum Dis. 2003;62:1145–55.
24. Zhang W, Moskowitz RW, Nuki G, Abramson S, Altman RD, Arden N, et al. OARSI recommendations for the management of hip and knee osteoarthritis, part II: OARSI evidence-based, expert consensus guidelines. Osteoarthr Cartil. 2008;16:137–62.
25. Hochberg MC, Altman RD, April KT, Benkhalti M, Guyatt G, McGowan J, et al. American College of Rheumatology 2012 recommendations for the use of nonpharmacologic and pharmacologic therapies in osteoarthritis of the hand, hip, and knee. Arthritis Care Res. 2012;64:465–74.
26. McAlindon TE, Bannuru RR, Sullivan MC, Arden NK, Berenbaum F, Bierma-Zeinstra SM, et al. OARSI guidelines for the non-surgical management of knee osteoarthritis. Osteoarthr Cartil. 2014;22:363–88.
27. Geusens P, Lems W. Efficacy and tolerability of lumiracoxib, a highly selective cyclo-oxygenase-2 (COX2) inhibitor, in the management of pain and osteoarthritis. Ther Clin Risk Manag. 2008;4:337–44.
28. Thaler R, Agsten M, Spitzer S, Paschalis EP, Karlic H, Klaushofer K, et al. Homocysteine suppresses the expression of the collagen cross-linker lysyl oxidase involving IL-6, Fli1, and epigenetic DNA methylation. J Biol Chem. 2011;286:5578–88.
29. Zhang Q, Li H, Zhang Z, Yang F, Chen J. Serum metabolites as potential biomarkers for diagnosis of knee osteoarthritis. Dis Markers. 2015;2015:684794.
30. Jugdaohsingh R, Watson AI, Pedro LD, Powell JJ. The decrease in silicon concentration of the connective tissues with age in rats is a marker of connective tissue turnover. Bone. 2015;75:40–8.
31. Calomme M, Geusens P, Demeester N, Behets GJ, D'Haese P, Sindambiwe JB, et al. Partial prevention of long-term femoral bone loss in aged ovariectomized rats supplemented with choline-stabilized orthosilicic acid. Calcif Tissue Int. 2006;78:227–32.
32. Spector TD, Conaghan PG, Buckland-Wright JC, Garnero P, Cline GA, Beary JF, et al. Effect of risedronate on joint structure and symptoms of knee osteoarthritis: results of the BRISK randomized, controlled trial [ISRCTN01928173]. Arthritis Res Ther. 2005;7:R625–33.
33. Lories RJ, Luyten FP. The bone-cartilage unit in osteoarthritis. Nat Rev Rheumatol. 2011;7:43–9.
34. McAlindon TE, Snow S, Cooper C, Dieppe PA. Radiographic patterns of osteoarthritis of the knee joint in the community: the importance of the patellofemoral joint. Ann Rheum Dis. 1992;51:844–9.
35. O'Connor MI, Hooten EG. Breakout session: gender disparities in knee osteoarthritis and TKA. Clin Orthop Relat Res. 2011;469:1883–5.
36. Smith YR, Stohler CS, Nichols TE, Bueller JA, Koeppe RA, Zubieta JK. Pronociceptive and antinociceptive effects of estradiol through endogenous opioid neurotransmission in women. J Neurosci. 2006;26:5777–85.
37. Hanna FS, Teichtahl AJ, Wluka AE, Wang Y, Urquhart DM, English DR, et al. Women have increased rates of cartilage loss and progression of cartilage defects at the knee than men: a gender study of adults without clinical knee osteoarthritis. Menopause. 2009;16:666–70.
38. van Spil WE, Drossaers-Bakker KW, Lafeber FP. Associations of CTX-II with biochemical markers of bone turnover raise questions on its tissue origin: data from CHECK, a cohort study of early osteoarthritis. Ann Rheum Dis. 2013;72:29–36.

39. Roman-Blas JA, Castaneda S, Largo R, Herrero-Beaumont G. Osteoarthritis associated with estrogen deficiency. Arthritis Res Ther. 2009;11:241.
40. Calvo E, Castaneda S, Largo R, Fernandez-Valle ME, Rodriguez-Salvanes F, Herrero-Beaumont G. Osteoporosis increases the severity of cartilage damage in an experimental model of osteoarthritis in rabbits. Osteoarthr Cartil. 2007;15:69–77.
41. Wang CJ, Huang CY, Hsu SL, Chen JH, Cheng JH. Extracorporeal shockwave therapy in osteoporotic osteoarthritis of the knee in rats: an experiment in animals. Arthritis Res Ther. 2014;16:R139.
42. Reginster JY, Kvasz A, Bruyere O, Henrotin Y. Is there any rationale for prescribing hormone replacement therapy (HRT) to prevent or to treat osteoarthritis? Osteoarthr Cartil. 2003;11:87–91.
43. Kwan Tat S, Lajeunesse D, Pelletier JP, Martel-Pelletier J. Targeting subchondral bone for treating osteoarthritis: what is the evidence? Best Pract Res Clin Rheumatol. 2010;24:51–70.
44. European Medicines Agency (EMA). Recommendation to restrict the use of Protelos/Osseor (strontium ranelate). EMA/258269/2013. 2013. URL: http://www.ema.europa.eu/docs/en_GB/document_library/Press_release/2013/04/WC500142507.pdf. Accessed 25 Apr 2013.
45. European Food Safety Authority (EFSA). Scientific opinion of the panel on food additives and nutrient sources added to food on choline-stabilised orthosilicic acid added for nutritional purposes to food supplements following a request from the European Commission. EFSA J. 2009;948:1–23.
46. Reginster JY, Badurski J, Bellamy N, Bensen W, Chapurlat R, Chevalier X, et al. Efficacy and safety of strontium ranelate in the treatment of knee osteoarthritis: results of a double-blind, randomised placebo-controlled trial. Ann Rheum Dis. 2013;72:179–86.
47. Herrero-Beaumont G, Ivorra JA, Del Carmen Trabado M, Blanco FJ, Benito P, Martin-Mola E, et al. Glucosamine sulfate in the treatment of knee osteoarthritis symptoms: a randomized, double-blind, placebo-controlled study using acetaminophen as a side comparator. Arthritis Rheum. 2007;56:555–67.
48. Geusens P, Chapurlat R, Schett G, Ghasem-Zadeh A, Seeman E, de Jong J, et al. High-resolution in vivo imaging of bone and joints: a window to microarchitecture. Nat Rev Rheumatol. 2014;10:304–13.

Permissions

All chapters in this book were first published in MD, by BioMed Central; hereby published with permission under the Creative Commons Attribution License or equivalent. Every chapter published in this book has been scrutinized by our experts. Their significance has been extensively debated. The topics covered herein carry significant findings which will fuel the growth of the discipline. They may even be implemented as practical applications or may be referred to as a beginning point for another development.

The contributors of this book come from diverse backgrounds, making this book a truly international effort. This book will bring forth new frontiers with its revolutionizing research information and detailed analysis of the nascent developments around the world.

We would like to thank all the contributing authors for lending their expertise to make the book truly unique. They have played a crucial role in the development of this book. Without their invaluable contributions this book wouldn't have been possible. They have made vital efforts to compile up to date information on the varied aspects of this subject to make this book a valuable addition to the collection of many professionals and students.

This book was conceptualized with the vision of imparting up-to-date information and advanced data in this field. To ensure the same, a matchless editorial board was set up. Every individual on the board went through rigorous rounds of assessment to prove their worth. After which they invested a large part of their time researching and compiling the most relevant data for our readers.

The editorial board has been involved in producing this book since its inception. They have spent rigorous hours researching and exploring the diverse topics which have resulted in the successful publishing of this book. They have passed on their knowledge of decades through this book. To expedite this challenging task, the publisher supported the team at every step. A small team of assistant editors was also appointed to further simplify the editing procedure and attain best results for the readers.

Apart from the editorial board, the designing team has also invested a significant amount of their time in understanding the subject and creating the most relevant covers. They scrutinized every image to scout for the most suitable representation of the subject and create an appropriate cover for the book.

The publishing team has been an ardent support to the editorial, designing and production team. Their endless efforts to recruit the best for this project, has resulted in the accomplishment of this book. They are a veteran in the field of academics and their pool of knowledge is as vast as their experience in printing. Their expertise and guidance has proved useful at every step. Their uncompromising quality standards have made this book an exceptional effort. Their encouragement from time to time has been an inspiration for everyone.

The publisher and the editorial board hope that this book will prove to be a valuable piece of knowledge for researchers, students, practitioners and scholars across the globe.

List of Contributors

Junfeng Zhang
Department of Health Statistics / the Publishing house, Public Health of Shanxi Medical University / Chinese Journal of Rheumatology, Taiyuan, Shanxi 030001, China

Tomoko Fujii, Hiroyuki Oka and Ko Matsudaira
Department of Medical Research and Management for Musculoskeletal Pain, 22nd Century Medical & Research Center, Faculty of Medicine, The University of Tokyo, 7-3-1 Hongo, Bunkyo-ku, Tokyo 113-8655, Japan

Junji Katsuhira
Department of Prosthetics & Orthotics and Assistive Technology, Faculty of Medical Technology, Niigata University of Health and Welfare, 1398 Shimami-cho, Kita-ku, Niigata-shi, Niigata 950-3198, Japan

Juichi Tonosu
Department of Orthopaedic Surgery, Kanto Rosai Hospital, 1-1 Kizukisumiyoshi-cho, Nakahara-ku, Kawasaki City, Kanagawa 211-8510, Japan

Satoshi Kasahara
Department of Pain and Palliative Medicine, Faculty of Medicine, The University of Tokyo, 7-3-1 Hongo, Bunkyo-ku, Tokyo 113-8655, Japan

Bo Han
Departments of Surgery and Biomedical Engineering, Keck School of Medicine of USC, 1333 San Pablo St. BMT-302, Los Angeles, CA 90033, USA

Austin K. Mircheff
Department of Physiology & Neuroscience, Keck School of Medicine of USC, 1333 San Pablo St. BMT B-11A, Los Angeles, CA 90033, USA

Shotaro Takano, Kentaro Uchida, Gen Inoue, Jun Aikawa, Dai Iwase, Manabu Mukai, Masayuki Miyagi and Masashi Takaso
Department of Orthopedic Surgery, Kitasato University School of Medicine, 1-15-1 Minami-ku Kitasato, Sagamihara City 252-0374, Japan

Sakae Tanaka
Department of Orthopaedic Surgery, Faculty of Medicine, The University of Tokyo, 7-3-1 Hongo, Bunkyo-ku, Tokyo 113-8655, Japan

Hiroshi Ohi, Eishi Kaneda and Kazuko Ohi
Graduate School of Health and Welfare, Niigata University of Health and Welfare, Niigata, Japan
Ohi Manufacturing Co., Ltd., Kyoto, Japan

Hirotaka Iijima
Department of Physical Therapy, Human Health Sciences, Graduate School of Medicine, Kyoto University, Kyoto, Japan
Department of System Design Engineering, Keio University, Yokohama, Japan
Japan Society for the Promotion of Science, Tokyo, Japan
Nozomi Orthopaedic Clinic, Hiroshima, Japan

Tomoki Aoyama
Department of Physical Therapy, Human Health Sciences, Graduate School of Medicine, Kyoto University, Kyoto, Japan

Kaoru Abe
Graduate School of Health and Welfare, Niigata University of Health and Welfare, Niigata, Japan

Xinxin Wang and Peng Shen
Department of Surgery, Huadong Hospital Affiliated to Fudan University, Shanghai 200040, China
Spine Research Institute, Shanghai University of Traditional Chinese Medicine, Shanghai 200032, China

Dezhi Tang and Hao Xu
Spine Research Institute, Shanghai University of Traditional Chinese Medicine, Shanghai 200032, China

Hongfu Qiu, Tao Wu and Xiang Gao
Department of Surgery, Huadong Hospital Affiliated to Fudan University, Shanghai 200040, China

Toshihide Matsumoto
Department of Pathology, Kitasato University School of Medicine, 1-15-1 Minami-ku Kitasato, Sagamihara City 252-0374, Japan

Emma Parry
NIHR In-Practice Fellow, Arthritis Research UK Primary Care Centre, Research Institute for Primary Care & Health Sciences, Keele University, Keele, Staffordshire ST5 5BG, UK

Reuben Ogollah
Research Fellow in Biostatistics, Arthritis Research UK Primary Care Centre, Research Institute for Primary Care & Health Sciences, Keele University, Keele ST5 5BG, Staffordshire, UK

George Peat
Clinical Epidemiology, Arthritis Research UK Primary Care Centre, Research Institute for Primary Care & Health Sciences, Keele University, Keele ST5 5BG, Staffordshire, UK

Feng-Hang Chang
Graduate Institute of Injury Prevention and Control, College of Public Health, Taipei Medical University, 250 Wu-Hsing Street, Taipei City 11031, Taiwan

Alan M. Jette
MGH Institute of Health Professions, 36 1st Avenue, Charlestown Navy Yard, Boston, MA 02129-4557, USA

Mary D. Slavin
Health Law, Policy and Management, Boston University School of Public Health, 715 Albany St., 5th floor West, Boston, MA 02118, USA

Kristin Baker
Boston University College of Health and Rehabilitation Sciences: Sargent College, Boston, USA

Pengsheng Ni
Health Law, Policy and Management, Boston University School of Public Health, 715 Albany St., 5th floor West, Boston, MA 02118, USA

Julie J. Keysor
MGH Institute of Health Professions, Department of Physical Therapy, 36 1st Avenue, Boston, MA 02129, USA

Masayuki Miyagi, Gen Inoue, Kentaro Uchida and Masashi Takaso
Department of Orthopaedic Surgery, Kitasato University, School of Medicine, 1-15-1, Kitasato, Minami-ku, Sagamihara city, Kanagawa 252-0374, Japan

Tetsuhiro Ishikawa, Hiroto Kamoda, Miyako Suzuki, Yoshihiro Sakuma, Yasuhiro Oikawa, Sumihisa Orita, Kazuhisa Takahashi and Seiji Ohtori
Department of Orthopaedic Surgery, Graduate School of Medicine, Chiba University, Chiba, Japan

Guomin Ren
McCaig Institute for Bone and Joint Health, Faculty of Medicine, University of Calgary, 3330 Hospital Drive NW, Calgary, Alberta T2N 4N1, Canada

Ian Lutz
Department of Surgery, University of Calgary, Calgary, Alberta, Canada

Pamela Railton
Charles Sturt University, Sydney, Australia

J. Preston Wiley
Sports Medicine Centre, Faculty of Kinesiology, University of Calgary, Calgary, Alberta, Canada
McCaig Institute for Bone and Joint Health, Faculty of Medicine, University of Calgary, 3330 Hospital Drive NW, Calgary, Alberta T2N 4N1, Canada

Jenelle McAllister
Sports Medicine Centre, Faculty of Kinesiology, University of Calgary, Calgary, Alberta, Canada

James Powell
McCaig Institute for Bone and Joint Health, Faculty of Medicine, University of Calgary, 3330 Hospital Drive NW, Calgary, Alberta T2N 4N1, Canada
Department of Surgery, University of Calgary, Calgary, Alberta, Canada

Roman J. Krawetz
McCaig Institute for Bone and Joint Health, Faculty of Medicine, University of Calgary, 3330 Hospital Drive NW, Calgary, Alberta T2N 4N1, Canada
Department of Surgery, University of Calgary, Calgary, Alberta, Canada
Department of Anatomy and Cell Biology, University of Calgary, Calgary, Alberta, Canada

Saran Tantavisut, Aree Tanavalee and Srihatach Ngarmukos
Department of Orthopaedics, Faculty of Medicine, Chulalongkorn University, 1873 Rama 4 road, Pathumwan, Bangkok 10330, Thailand

Sittisak Honsawek and Tanyawan Suantawee
Department of Biochemistry, Faculty of Medicine, Chulalongkorn University, Bangkok, Thailand

Sirichai Adisakwatana
Faculty of Allied Health Sciences, Chulalongkorn University, Bangkok, Thailand

John J. Callaghan
Department of Orthopaedics, Faculty of Medicine, University of Iowa Hospitals and Clinics, Iowa City, IA, USA

G. Hirsch and G. Kitas
Department of Rheumatology, Dudley Group for Health (DGH) NHS Foundation Trust, Russells Hall Hospital, Dudley, West Midlands DY1 2HQ, UK

T. W. O'Neill
Faculty of Medical and Human Sciences, Arthritis Research UK Centre for Epidemiology, Institute of Inflammation and Repair, Manchester Academic Health Science Centre, University of Manchester, Manchester, UK
NIHR Manchester Musculoskeletal Biomedical Research Unit, Central Manchester NHS Foundation Trust, Manchester Academic Health Science Centre, Manchester, UK

A. Sinha
Department of Radiology, DGH NHS Foundation Trust, Russells Hall Hospital, Dudley, West Midlands, UK

R. Klocke
Department of Rheumatology, Dudley Group for Health (DGH) NHS Foundation Trust, Russells Hall Hospital, Dudley, West Midlands DY1 2HQ, UK
NIHR Manchester Musculoskeletal Biomedical Research Unit, Central Manchester NHS Foundation Trust, Manchester Academic Health Science Centre, Manchester, UK

Jonathan G. Quicke, Nadine E. Foster, Peter R. Croft, Reuben O. Ogollah and Melanie A. Holden
Arthritis Research UK Primary Care Centre, Research Institute for Primary Care and Health Sciences, Keele University, Keele, Staffordshire ST5 5BG, UK

Vikram Swaminathan and Matthew J Parkes
Arthritis Research UK Centre for Epidemiology, Institute of Inflammation and Repair, Faculty of Medical and Human Sciences, Manchester Academic Health Science Centre, University of Manchester, Stopford Building, Oxford Road, Manchester M13 9PT, UK
NIHR Manchester Musculoskeletal Biomedical Research Unit, Central Manchester NHS Foundation Trust, Manchester Academic Health Sciences Centre, Manchester, UK

Michael J Callaghan
Arthritis Research UK Centre for Epidemiology, Institute of Inflammation and Repair, Faculty of Medical and Human Sciences, Manchester Academic Health Science Centre, University of Manchester, Stopford Building, Oxford Road, Manchester M13 9PT, UK
NIHR Manchester Musculoskeletal Biomedical Research Unit, Central Manchester NHS Foundation Trust, Manchester Academic Health Sciences Centre, Manchester, UK
Faculty of Health, Psychology and Social Care, Department of Health Professions, Manchester Metropolitan University, Manchester, UK
Central Manchester University Hospitals NHS Foundation Trust, Manchester, UK

Terence W O'Neill
Arthritis Research UK Centre for Epidemiology, Institute of Inflammation and Repair, Faculty of Medical and Human Sciences, Manchester Academic Health Science Centre, University of Manchester, Stopford Building, Oxford Road, Manchester M13 9PT, UK
NIHR Manchester Musculoskeletal Biomedical Research Unit, Central Manchester NHS Foundation Trust, Manchester Academic Health Sciences Centre, Manchester, UK
Department of Rheumatology, Salford Royal NHS Foundation Trust, Salford, UK

Richard Hodgson and Andrew D Gait
Centre of Imaging Sciences, Institute of Population Health, University of Manchester, Manchester, UK

David T Felson
Arthritis Research UK Centre for Epidemiology, Institute of Inflammation and Repair, Faculty of Medical and Human Sciences, Manchester Academic Health Science Centre, University of Manchester, Stopford Building, Oxford Road, Manchester M13 9PT, UK
NIHR Manchester Musculoskeletal Biomedical Research Unit, Central Manchester NHS Foundation Trust, Manchester Academic Health Sciences Centre, Manchester, UK
Clinical Epidemiology Unit, Boston University School of Medicine, Boston, MA, USA

Ahmad H. Alghadir and Einas S. Al-Eisa
Rehabilitation Research Chair, College of Applied Medical Sciences, King Saud University, Riyadh 11433, Saudi Arabia

Shahnawaz Anwer
Rehabilitation Research Chair, College of Applied Medical Sciences, King Saud University, Riyadh 11433, Saudi Arabia
Dr. D. Y. Patil College of Physiotherapy, Dr. D. Y. Patil Vidyapeeth, Pune, India

Ivo Valter
Bioclinica, Tallinn, Estonia

Marc C. Hochberg
University of Maryland School of Medicine, Baltimore, USA

Victoria Carmona-Terés and Jenny Moix-Queraltó
Department of Basic, Evolutionary and Educational Psychology, Universitat Autònoma de Barcelona; Psychology Faculty, Building B. UAB Campus, Bellaterra, Barcelona 08193, Spain

Enriqueta Pujol-Ribera and Anna Berenguera
Primary Care University Research Institute (IDIAP Jordi Gol), Gran Via Corts Catalanes, 587, àtic, Barcelona 08007, Spain
Universitat Autònoma de Barcelona, Bellaterra, Cerdanyola del Vallès, Spain

Iris Lumillo-Gutiérrez
Primary Care Centre Can Bou, Ciutat de Màlaga, 18-20, Castelldefels, Barcelona 08860, Spain

Xavier Mas
Primary Care Centre Amadeu Torner, Amadeu Torner, 63, l'Hospitalet de Llobregat, Barcelona 08902, Spain

Enrique Batlle-Gualda
San Juan de Alicante University Hospital; Rheumatology Unit, Ctra N-332, Sant Joan d'Alacant, Alicante-Valencia 03550, Spain

Milena Gobbo-Montoya
Psychology of pain and rheumatological diseases, Av. Presidente Carmona, 10 bis 1°A, Madrid 28020, Spain

Lina Jodar-Fernández
Primary Care Centre Sant Ildefons, Avda República Argentiana s/n, Cornellà de Llobregat, Barcelona 08940, Spain

Vala Flosadottir and Eva Ageberg
Department of Health Sciences, Lund University, 221 00 Lund, Sweden

Richard Frobell
Department of Clinical Sciences, Lund University, Lund, Sweden

Ewa M. Roos
Department of Sports Science and Clinical Biomechanics, Musculoskeletal Function and Physiotherapy, University of Southern Denmark, Odense, Denmark

Joyce A. C. van Tunen and Jonas B. Thorlund
Research Unit for Musculoskeletal Function and Physiotherapy, Department of Sports Science and Clinical Biomechanics, Faculty of Health Sciences, University of Southern Denmark, Campusvej 55, 5230 Odense, Denmark

Andrea Dell'Isola and Martijn Steultjens
School of Health and Life Sciences, Glasgow Caledonian University, Glasgow, Scotland

Carsten Juhl
Department of Rehabilitation, Copenhagen University Hospital, Herlev and Gentofte, Denmark
Research Unit for Musculoskeletal Function and Physiotherapy, Department of Sports Science and Clinical Biomechanics, Faculty of Health Sciences, University of Southern Denmark, Campusvej 55, 5230 Odense, Denmark

Joost Dekker
Department of Rehabilitation Medicine and Department of Psychiatry, EMGO Insitute for Health and Care Research, VU University Medical Center, Amsterdam, the Netherlands

Hans Lund
Centre for Evidence Based Practice, Western Norway University of Applied Sciences, Bergen, Norway

Juhani Multanen
Department of Physical Medicine and Rehabilitation, Central Finland Central Hospital, Keskussairaalantie 19, FI-40620 Jyväskylä, Finland

Mikko Honkanen
Department of Surgery, Mikkeli Central Hospital, Mikkeli, Finland

Arja Häkkinen
Department of Physical Medicine and Rehabilitation, Central Finland Central Hospital, Keskussairaalantie 19, FI-40620 Jyväskylä, Finland
Faculty of Sport and Health Sciences, University of Jyväskylä, Jyväskylä, Finland

Ilkka Kiviranta
Department of Orthopaedics and Traumatology, University of Helsinki and Helsinki University Hospital, Helsinki, Finland

G. Cattaneo, A. De Caro, F. Napoli and A. Camera
Spotorno Foundation c/o San Michele Clinics, Viale Pontelungo, 79, 17031 Albenga, SV, Italy

D. Chiapale and P. Trada
Orthopaedic Department, San Paolo Hospital, Savona, SV, Italy

Kade L. Paterson, Kim L. Bennell, Tim V. Wrigley, Ben R. Metcalf, Penny K. Campbell and Rana S. Hinman
Centre for Health, Exercise and Sports Medicine, Department of Physiotherapy, School of Health Sciences, Faculty of Medicine Dentistry & Health Sciences, The University of Melbourne, Melbourne, VIC, Australia

Jessica Kazsa
Department of Epidemiology and Preventive Medicine, Monash University, Melbourne, Australia

Maik Sliepen and Elsa Mauricio
Institut für Experimentelle Muskuloskelettale Medizin (IEMM), Universitätsklinikum Münster (UKM), Westfälische Wilhelms-Universität Münster (WWU), Albert-Schweitzer Campus 1, Gebäude D3, 48129 Münster, Germany

Matthijs Lipperts and Bernd Grimm
AHORSE, Department of Orthopaedics, Zuyderland Medical Centre, Henri Dunantstraat 5, 6419, PC, Heerlen, the Netherlands

Dieter Rosenbaum
Institut für Experimentelle Muskuloskelettale Medizin (IEMM), Universitätsklinikum Münster (UKM), Westfälische Wilhelms-Universität Münster (WWU), Albert-Schweitzer Campus 1, Gebäude D3, 48129 Münster, Germany
Otto Bock Healthcare GmbH, Hermann-Rein-Str. 2a, 37075 Göttingen, Germany

Ian A. Jones, Ryan Togashi and C. Thomas Vangsness JR
Department of Orthopaedic Surgery, Keck School of Medicine of USC, HCT 1520 San Pablo Street, suite 2000, Los Angeles, CA 90033, USA

Melissa Wilson
Department of Preventive Medicine, Keck School of Medicine of USC, 2001 Soto Street, SSB1 318A, Los Angeles, CA 90033, USA

Piet Geusens
Biomedical Research Institute (BIOMED), Hasselt University, Diepenbeek, Belgium
Rheumatology, Maastricht UMC, Maastricht, The Netherlands
ReumaClinic, Bretheistraat 149, Genk 3600, Belgium

Karel Pavelka
Institute of Rheumatology, Prague, Czech Republic

Jozef Rovensky
Nábrežie I. Krasku 4782/4, Piešťany, Slovakia

Johan Vanhoof
ReumaClinic, Bretheistraat 149, Genk 3600, Belgium

Nathalie Demeester and Mario Calomme
Research & Development, Bio Minerals NV, Destelbergen, Belgium

Dirk Vanden Berghe
Department of Pharmaceutical Sciences, University of Antwerp, Antwerp-Wilrijk, Belgium

Index

CPSIA information can be obtained
at www.ICGtesting.com
Printed in the USA
LVHW062015100122
708212LV00002B/243

9 781639 273973